Bioactive Coatings for Implantable Devices

Bioactive Coatings for Implantable Devices

Editor

Toshiyuki Kawai

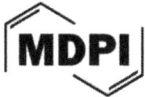 Basel • Beijing • Wuhan • Barcelona • Belgrade • Novi Sad • Cluj • Manchester

Editor
Toshiyuki Kawai
Kyoto University
Kyoto
Japan

Editorial Office
MDPI
St. Alban-Anlage 66
4052 Basel, Switzerland

This is a reprint of articles from the Special Issue published online in the open access journal *Coatings* (ISSN 2079-6412) (available at: https://www.mdpi.com/journal/coatings/special_issues/bio-active_implantable).

For citation purposes, cite each article independently as indicated on the article page online and as indicated below:

Lastname, A.A.; Lastname, B.B. Article Title. *Journal Name* **Year**, *Volume Number*, Page Range.

ISBN 978-3-7258-0597-6 (Hbk)
ISBN 978-3-7258-0598-3 (PDF)
doi.org/10.3390/books978-3-7258-0598-3

© 2024 by the authors. Articles in this book are Open Access and distributed under the Creative Commons Attribution (CC BY) license. The book as a whole is distributed by MDPI under the terms and conditions of the Creative Commons Attribution-NonCommercial-NoDerivs (CC BY-NC-ND) license.

Contents

Seiji Yamaguchi, Koji Akeda, Seine A. Shintani, Akihiro Sudo and Tomiharu Matsushita
Drug-Releasing Gelatin Coating Reinforced with Calcium Titanate Formed on Ti–6Al–4V Alloy Designed for Osteoporosis Bone Repair
Reprinted from: *Coatings* 2022, 12, 139, doi:10.3390/coatings12020139 1

Rubaiya Anjum, Kei Nishida, Haruka Matsumoto, Daiki Murakami, Shingo Kobayashi, Takahisa Anada and Masaru Tanaka
Attachment and Growth of Fibroblast Cells on Poly (2-Methoxyethyl Acrylate) Analog Polymers as Coating Materials
Reprinted from: *Coatings* 2021, 11, 461, doi:10.3390/coatings11040461 14

Jing Yue, Zhichun Jin, Hin Lok Enoch Poon, Guangwei Shang, Haixia Liu, Dan Wang, et al.
Osteogenic and Antibacterial Activity of a Plasma-Sprayed CeO_2 Coating on a Titanium (Ti)-Based Dental Implant
Reprinted from: *Coatings* 2020, 10, 1007, doi:10.3390/coatings10101007 30

Shusen Hou, Weixin Yu, Zhijun Yang, Yue Li, Lin Yang and Shaoting Lang
Properties of Titanium Oxide Coating on MgZn Alloy by Magnetron Sputtering for Stent Application
Reprinted from: *Coatings* 2020, 10, 999, doi:10.3390/coatings10100999 42

Maria Antonia Llopis-Grimalt, Maria Antònia Forteza-Genestra, Víctor Alcolea-Rodriguez, Joana Maria Ramis and Marta Monjo
Nanostructured Titanium for Improved Endothelial Biocompatibility and Reduced Platelet Adhesion in Stent Applications
Reprinted from: *Coatings* 2020, 10, 907, doi:10.3390/coatings10090907 52

Nansi López-Valverde, Beatriz Pardal-Peláez, Antonio López-Valverde and Juan Manuel Ramírez
Role of Melatonin in Bone Remodeling around Titanium Dental Implants: Meta-Analysis
Reprinted from: *Coatings* 2021, 11, 271, doi:10.3390/coatings11030271 66

Catrin Bannewitz, Tim Lenz-Habijan, Jonathan Lentz, Marcus Peters, Volker Trösken, Sabine Siebert, et al.
Evaluation of Antithrombogenic pHPC on CoCr Substrates for Biomedical Applications
Reprinted from: *Coatings* 2021, 11, 93, doi:10.3390/coatings11010093 80

Nansi López-Valverde, Antonio López-Valverde, Juan Manuel Aragoneses, Francisco Martínez-Martínez, María C. González-Escudero and Juan Manuel Ramírez
Bone Density around Titanium Dental Implants Coating Tested/Coated with Chitosan or Melatonin: An Evaluation via Microtomography in Jaws of Beagle Dogs
Reprinted from: *Coatings* 2021, 11, 777, doi:10.3390/coatings11070777 92

Ekaterina S. Marchenko, Kirill M. Dubovikov, Gulsharat A. Baigonakova, Ivan I. Gordienko and Alex A. Volinsky
Surface Structure and Properties of Hydroxyapatite Coatings on NiTi Substrates
Reprinted from: *Coatings* 2023, 13, 722, doi:10.3390/coatings13040722 104

Md Azizul Haque, Daiki Murakami, Takahisa Anada and Masaru Tanaka
Poly(2-Methoxyethyl Acrylate) (PMEA)-Coated Anti-Platelet Adhesive Surfaces to Mimic Native Blood Vessels through HUVECs Attachment, Migration, and Monolayer Formation
Reprinted from: *Coatings* 2022, 12, 869, doi:10.3390/coatings12060869 113

Lavinia Luminita Voina Cosma, Marioara Moldovan, Alexandrina Muntean, Cristian Doru Olteanu, Radu Chifor and Mindra Eugenia Badea
Novel Technology for Enamel Remineralization in Artificially Induced White Spot Lesions: In Vitro Study
Reprinted from: *Coatings* **2022**, *12*, 1285, doi:10.3390/coatings12091285 . . . . **129**

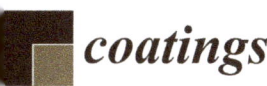

Article

Drug-Releasing Gelatin Coating Reinforced with Calcium Titanate Formed on Ti–6Al–4V Alloy Designed for Osteoporosis Bone Repair

Seiji Yamaguchi [1,*], Koji Akeda [2,*], Seine A. Shintani [1], Akihiro Sudo [2] and Tomiharu Matsushita [1]

[1] Department of Biomedical Sciences, College of Life and Health Sciences, Chubu University, 1200 Matsumoto, Kasugai 487-8501, Aichi, Japan; shintani@isc.chubu.ac.jp (S.A.S.); ma-tommy@isis.ocn.ne.jp (T.M.)
[2] Department of Orthopaedic Surgery, Mie University Graduate School of Medicine, Tsu 514-8507, Mie, Japan; a-sudou@clin.medic.mie-u.ac.jp
* Correspondence: sy-esi@isc.chubu.ac.jp (S.Y.); k_akeda@clin.medic.mie-u.ac.jp (K.A.); Tel.: +81-568-51-6420 (S.Y.); +81-59-231-5022 (K.A.)

Abstract: Ti–6Al–4V alloy has been widely used in the orthopedic and dental fields owing to its high mechanical strength and biocompatibility. However, this alloy has a poor bone-bonding capacity, and its implantation often causes loosening. Osteoporosis increases with the aging of the population, and bisphosphonate drugs such as alendronate and minodronate (MA) are used for the medical treatment. Reliable and multifunctional implants showing both bone bonding and drug releasing functions are desired. In this study, we developed a novel organic-inorganic composite layer consisting of MA-containing gelatin and calcium-deficient calcium titanate (cd–CT) with high bone-bonding and scratch resistance on Ti–6Al–4V alloy. The alloy with the composite layer formed apatite within 7 days in a simulated body fluid and exhibited high scratch resistance of an approximately 50 mN, attributable to interlocking with cd $\pm$ CT. Although the gelatin layer almost completely dissolved in phosphate-buffered saline within 6 h, its dissolution rate was significantly suppressed by a subsequent thermal crosslinking treatment. The released MA was estimated at more than 0.10 μmol/L after 7 days. It is expected that the Ti alloy with the MA-containing gelatin and cd–CT composite layer will be useful for the treatment of osteoporosis bone.

Keywords: bisphosphonate; calcium titanate; titanium alloy; apatite formation; gelatin

1. Introduction

Ti–6Al–4V alloy is widely used for load bearing implants, since it is biocompatible comparatively to pure Ti metal, while it shows superior mechanical strength and corrosion resistance [1]. However, this alloy is poor in its bone bonding ability, and often results in the loosening of the implants [2,3]. This event becomes more serious in osteoporosis bone. Conferring both bone-bonding capabilities on the implant and stimulating surrounding new bone formation is a great challenge in the development of novel implants for osteoporosis bone.

In order to confer bone-bonding on Ti and its alloys, various types of inorganic coatings including a plasma spray apatite coating [4,5], titanate or titania coating by solution and heat [6,7], hydrothermal [8] and anodic oxidation [9] as well as surface roughening by blasting and acid etching [10] have been developed. Direct bone bonding of the metals was observed when coated with apatite or when apatite-formation capability, owing to the titanate or titania coatings, was conferred onto the metal surfaces [11–13]. The titanate coating showed greater adhesion than the plasma-sprayed apatite coating when the chemically graded intermediate layer with a nano-porous structure was produced by means of a solution and heat treatment [13]. Activation of preosteoblast cells was reported on the roughened surfaces with a micro-meter and nano-meter scale and their hierarchical structure [14–16]. Among the inorganic surface coatings, the calcium-deficient calcium titanate (cd–CT) formed by the Ca-heat treatment developed by the present authors has unique surface characteristics of nano-scaled 3D network morphology, high scratch resistance, chemical durability, and abundant Ti–OH groups [17–19]. Thus, the treated metals tightly bind to both cortical and cancerous bone attributed to their high apatite formation capability [7,17–19]. We have also shown that the Ti–6Al–4V pedicle screw treated with cd–CT had a remarkably increased extraction torque compared with the untreated screw [7].

On the other hand, coatings of organic materials including biologically functional molecules composed of peptide, polysaccharide and growth factors and drugs were adhered to metal surfaces to enhance the regeneration of bone at the implant interface [20–22]. However, this type of surface modification does not permanently provide a favorable influence on osteointegration [20,21]. The metrics supporting these biomolecules and drugs are biodegradable, and the bare surface of the metal substrate is exposed after implantation for a certain period of time. Additionally, it is still challenging to achieve high adhesion between the metal substrate and polymer coatings due to large differences in surface energy between the metal and polymer. Gelatin, a biopolymer obtained from the hydrolysis of collagen, is commonly used in tissue engineering for the regeneration of skin [23], cartilage [24] and bone [25,26]. In addition to its availability and biocompatibility, gelatin offers the possibility of modulating its chemical and mechanical properties using its crosslinking capability.

Bisphosphonates (BPs), representative osteoclast inhibitors, are also shown to have a significant capacity for osteogenic induction [27–29]. BPs have been applied to bone tissue engineering technologies to develop functionalized bone tissue scaffolds with controlled release [30]. Previous studies have also shown that BP-coated titanium [31] or calcium phosphate ceramics [32] increased new bone formation around the implant and mechanical fixation. Minodronate monohydrate (MA) is one of the BPs with high potency in inhibiting bone resorption and is developed and approved for clinical use in Japan [33].

In the present study, we propose a novel coating composed of drug-releasing gelatin reinforced with the bioactive cd–CT that exhibits controlled drug release, apatite formation and high scratch resistance. The BP (minodronate) is used as a drug, and its release behavior from the coating was estimated from the degradation rate of the gelatin layer.

2. Materials and Methods

2.1. Sample Preparation

Ti–6Al–4V alloy (Ti = balance, Al = 6.18, V = 4.27 mass%, supplied by Kobelco Research Institute, Inc., Hyogo, Japan) plates with the dimensions of 10 mm × 10 mm × 1 mm were ground with a #400 diamond pad, and cleaned with acetone, 2-propanol and ultrapure water in an ultrasonic bath for 30 min each, then dried at 40 °C in an incubator overnight.

The alloy plates were subjected to NaOH–$CaCl_2$–heat–water treatment according to our previous report to form a cd–CT surface layer with high bone-bonding capability [7,17–19]. In this treatment, the samples were initially soaked in 5 mol/L NaOH (Kanto Chemical Co., Inc., Tokyo, Japan) aqueous solution at 95 °C for 24 h, and subsequently in 100 mmol/L $CaCl_2$ (Kanto Chemical Co., Inc., Tokyo, Japan) at 40 °C for 24 h with shaking in an oil bath. They were subsequently heated to 600 °C at a rate of 5 °C/min and maintained at 600 °C for 1 h, followed by natural cooling in a Fe–Cr electrical furnace. They were soaked in hot water at 80 °C for 24 h. This sequence of treatment is denoted as "Ca–heat" treatment in this study. All the reagents used in this study were of reagent grade.

After the Ca–heat treatment, the samples were dipped in 10 mL of 5–20% gelatin solution (medical grade with 316 g bloom, beMatrix LS–H, Nitta Gelatin, Osaka, Japan) pre-warmed at 60 °C in which 50 µmol/L minodronate monohydrate (minodronate; Tokyo Chemical Industry Co., Ltd., Tokyo, Japan) was dissolved in 20 mmol/L NaOH without or with the additive of 100 mmol/L $CaCl_2$ (Kanto Chemical Co., Inc., Tokyo, Japan) and/or 100 mmol/L $(NH_4)_2HPO_4$ (Kanto Chemical Co., Inc., Tokyo, Japan). The samples were pulled up at a constant speed of 1 cm/min by an electric motor, and then dried in an incubator at 40 °C overnight (This dip coating is denoted as "DC treatment").

Some of the samples with the gelatin coating were subjected to thermal cross-link (TCL) treatment [34] at 140 °C using vacuum oven (VOS-301SD, Tokyo Rikakikai Co., Ltd, Tokyo, Japan) for the desired periods from 3 to 72 h.

The treatments for each sample are summarized in Table 1.

Table 1. Notations of Ti–6Al–4V alloy samples used in this study.

Sample	Treatment		
	Ca-Heat	Dip Coating	Thermal Crosslink
Untreated	Not treated	Not treated	Not treated
CT	Treated	Not treated	Not treated
CT(X)G	Treated	X% gelatin (X = 5–20)	Not treated
CT(X)G + MA	Treated	X% gelatin + 50 μmol/L minodronate	Not treated
CT(X)G + MA + Ca and/or P	Treated	X% gelatin + 50 μmol/L minodronate + 100 mmol/L CaCl$_2$ and/or 100 mmol/L (NH$_4$)$_2$HPO$_4$	Not treated
CT(X)G + MA + Ca and/or P + (Y)TCL	Treated	X% gelatin + 50 μmol/L minodronate + 100 mmol/L CaCl$_2$ and/or 100 mmol/L (NH$_4$)$_2$HPO$_4$	Y hours at 140 °C in vacuum (Y = 6–144)

2.2. Viscosity of Gelatin Solution

The viscosity of the gelatin solution (5–20%) with or without additives as a function of gelatin concentration was measured by Brookfield viscometer (LVDVNextCP; Brookfield Engineering Laboratories, Inc., Middleboro, MA, USA) according to JIS8803 (Japanese Industrial Standards Z8803:2011, Methods for viscosity measurement of liquid). The spindle speeds (and corresponding shear rates) were optimized for each sample between 11.52 and 576 1/s (shear rates were 3 to 150 rpm), and four different spindle speeds were examined for each sample instead of increasing the number of replicates. The measurements were performed using 2 mL samples at 60 °C, and the viscosity (mPa·s) of the sample obtained for each run after a 30 s holding time was used for analysis.

2.3. Surface Characteristics

2.3.1. Scanning Electron Microscopy and Energy Dispersive X-ray Analysis

The surface and cross-sectional area of the prepared samples were coated with a Pt/Pd thin film and observed under a field-emission scanning electron microscope (FE-SEM, S-4300, Hitachi Co., Tokyo, Japan) equipped with energy dispersive X-ray analysis (EDX, EMAX-7000, Horiba Ltd., Kyoto, Japan) at an accelerated voltage of 15 kV and an electric current of 9–11 μA. In EDX analysis, C, O, Ti, Al, V, Ca, P, Na and Cl of the sample surfaces were examined using an accelerated voltage of 9 kV with a electric current of 10 μA. Five locations were measured, and their averaged values (a.v.) and standard deviations (s.d.) were used (described as a.v. ± s.d.).

2.3.2. Thin-Film X-ray Diffraction

Surface crystalline structures of the samples were analyzed using TF-XRD (Model RNT-2500, Rigaku Co., Akishima, Tokyo, Japan), employing a CuKα X-ray source operating at 50 kV and 200 mA. The glancing angle of the incident beam was set to an angle of 1° against the sample surface.

2.3.3. Scratch Resistance Measurements

The scratch resistance of the surface layer formed on the Ca–heat-treated samples with or without gelatin layer was measured using a thin film scratch tester (Model CSR-2000, Rhesca Co., Hino, Tokyo, Japan). A stylus with a diameter of 5 μm with a spring constant of 200 g/mm was employed and pressed onto the samples with a loading rate of 100 mN/min, an amplitude of 100 μm and a scratch speed of 10 μm/s, based on the data in the JIS R-3255 standard (Japanese Industrial Standard R-3255, Test methods for adhesion of thin films on glass substrate). Five areas were measured for each sample, and their averaged values and standard deviations were used.

2.3.4. Dissolution of Gelatin

The samples with the gelatin layer with $CaCl_2$ and MA additives subjected to TCL treatment were immersed in 2 mL of phosphate buffered saline (PBS) and gently shaken at a speed of 50 strokes/min at 36.5 °C. The Ca^{2+} ion concentrations released in PBS as a result of gelatin dissolution (the solvent/sample ratio was 2 mL/2.4 cm^2) were measured by inductively coupled plasma emission spectroscopy (ICP, SPS3100, Seiko Instruments Inc., Chiba, Japan) after the determined periods of soaking up to 7 days. The PBS solution was refreshed at each determined period, and the measurement was repeated 3 times for independently prepared samples. Their averaged values and standard deviations were calculated. The released MA concentration was estimated from the Ca^{2+} ion concentrations under the assumption of homogeneous Ca^{2+} ion distribution in a gelatin layer.

2.4. Apatite Formation

The samples with the gelatin layer with or without additives of $CaCl_2$ and/or $(NH_4)_2HPO_4$ were immersed in 24 mL of a pre-warmed simulated body fluid (SBF, 36.5 °C) with ion concentrations nearly equal to those of human blood plasma for 7 days at 36.5 °C [35]. After removal from the SBF, apatite formation on the sample surface was observed by FE-SEM and TF-XRD.

2.5. Statistical Analysis

Statistical tests were performed with a library of statistical software tools (R language; version 3.6.1, The R Foundation, Vienna, Austria). The normality of the scratch resistance measurement results was tested by the Shapiro–Wilk test. As a result, normality was not rejected for all data. The comparison between the control group and the other groups was tested by the multi-group test (Dunnett's test). The significance level for all statistical analyses was $p < 0.05$.

3. Results

3.1. Viscosity of Gelatin

The viscosity of the 5% gelatin solution was 3.5 mPa·s, and this increased to 15.1 and 184.2 mPa·s with increasing gelatin concentration to 10 and 20%, respectively, as shown in Figure 1. The addition of 100 mmol/L $CaCl_2$ and 50 µmol/L MA into 10% gelatin slightly increased the viscosity to 16.6 mPa·s.

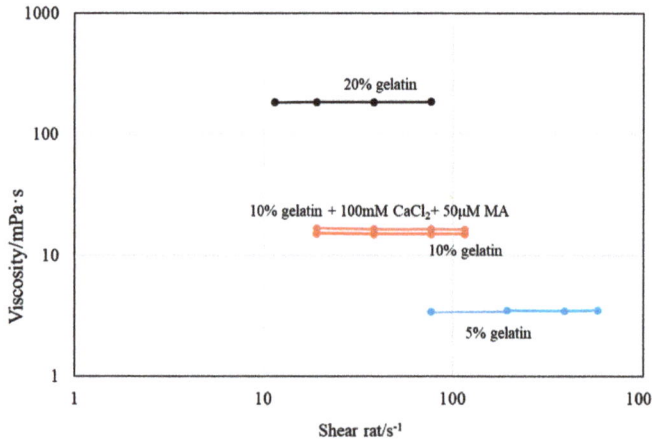

Figure 1. The viscosity of the gelatin solution as a function of gelatin concentration.

3.2. The Surface Characteristics

Figure 2 shows the surface and cross-sectional SEM images of Ti–6Al–4V samples subjected to Ca–heat, and subsequent DC treatment without and with the additives. After the Ca–heat treatment, a nano-structured three-dimensional network surface layer with 1.7 µm thickness was produced on the alloy substrate. This layer was composed of cd–CT, rutile and anatase as reported in our previous study [17].

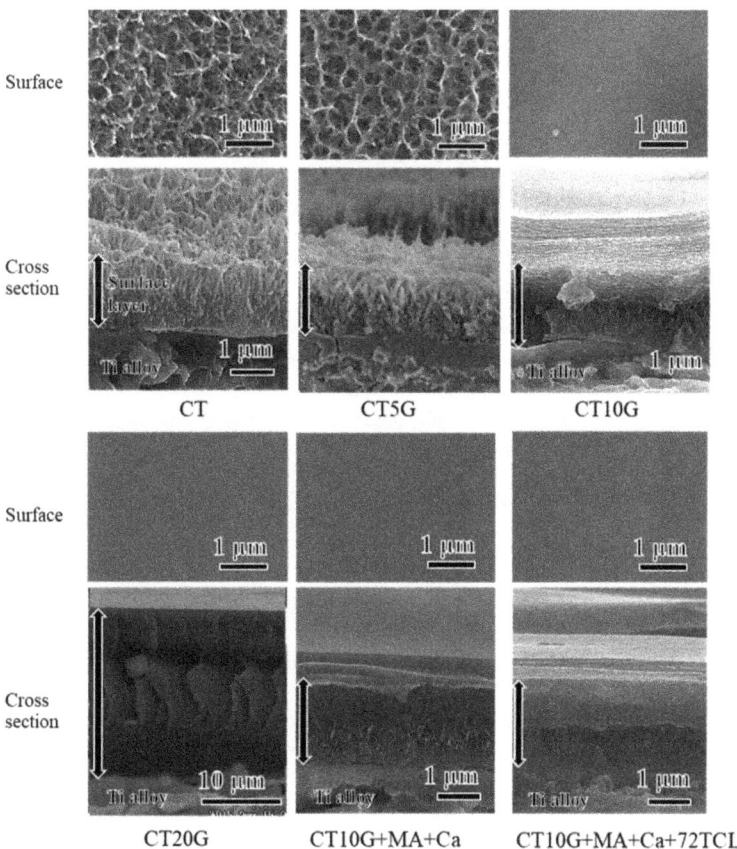

Figure 2. Surface and cross-sectional SEM images of Ca-heat treated Ti–6Al–4V alloy subjected to dip coating with various additives and subsequent thermal cross-link treatment.

When the treated sample was dipped in 5% gelatin solution, only slight modification with the gelatin was observed. In contrast, the surface morphology became smooth due to the complete surface coverage by the gelatin when the metal sample was dipped in 10% gelatin (see CT10G). Cross-sectional observation of CT10G revealed that the gelatin permeated through the nano-structured network to form an inorganic–organic composite layer approximately 2 µm in thickness. The thickness of the gelatin layer increased to about 25 µm by increasing the gelatin concentration to 20%, accompanied by a deposition of a single and thick gelatin layer on the inorganic–organic composite. The additives of 100 mmol/L $CaCl_2$ and 50 µmol/L MA did not apparently affect the thickness of the 10% gelatin coating. The surface and cross-sectional morphologies were maintained even after the TCL treatment.

Table 2 shows the chemical composition of the sample surfaces. The amounts of 2.9% Ca and 23.9% Ti were detected on the sample CT, and these values decreased with the DC treatment using 5–20% gelatin solution: the higher the gelatin concentrations, the lower the Ca and Ti amounts. In contrast, the amount of carbon increased with increasing gelatin concentration. These results are consistent with the SEM results, in which a thicker gelation layer was observed on the DC sample using higher concentration of gelatin. Some amounts of Ca and/or P attributed to the additives were detected on the DC samples when the $CaCl_2$ and/or $(NH_4)_2HPO_4$ were added in the gelatin solution (see the samples of "CT10G + MA + Ca", "CT10G + MA + P" and "CT10G + MA + Ca and P"). The surface chemical composition of CT10G + MA + Ca was maintained even after TCL treatment for 72 h.

Table 2. EDX results on the Ti–6Al–4V alloy surfaces treated with Ca–heat followed by gelatin coating and thermal crosslinking.

Sample	Element/at.%								
	C	O	Ti	Al	V	Ca	P	Na	Cl
Untreated	5.4 ± 1.2	0.0 ± 0.0	80.9 ± 0.9	9.4 ± 0.1	4.3 ± 0.2	0.0 ± 0.0	0.0 ± 0.0	0.0 ± 0.0	0.0 ± 0.0
CT	7.4 ± 0.5	64.4 ± 0.4	23.9 ± 2.9	0.6 ± 0.1	0.8 ± 0.1	2.9 ± 0.2	0.0 ± 0.0	0.0 ± 0.0	0.0 ± 0.0
CT5G	27.9 ± 1.7	53.5 ± 0.9	15.7 ± 0.6	0.4 ± 0.0	0.4 ± 0.1	2.0 ± 0.1	0.0 ± 0.0	0.2 ± 0.0	0.0 ± 0.0
CT10G	61.3 ± 2.9	35.4 ± 1.6	2.3 ± 1.1	0.0 ± 0.0	0.1 ± 0.0	0.5 ± 0.2	0.0 ± 0.0	0.3 ± 0.0	0.2 ± 0.0
CT20G	63.9 ± 1.0	35.6 ± 1.1	0.0 ± 0.0	0.0 ± 0.0	0.0 ± 0.0	0.0 ± 0.0	0.0 ± 0.0	0.3 ± 0.1	0.1 ± 0.0
CT10G + MA + Ca	64.6 ± 0.3	32.1 ± 0.4	0.1 ± 0.0	0.0 ± 0.0	0.0 ± 0.0	0.8 ± 0.1	0.0 ± 0.0	0.3 ± 0.0	2.0 ± 0.1
CT10G + MA + P	66.7 ± 0.2	32.3 ± 0.3	0.2 ± 0.1	0.0 ± 0.0	0.0 ± 0.0	0.0 ± 0.0	0.4 ± 0.0	0.1 ± 0.0	0.2 ± 0.0
CT10G + MA + Ca and P	63.1 ± 3.8	32.6 ± 1.7	0.4 ± 0.8	0.0 ± 0.0	0.0 ± 0.0	0.4 ± 0.6	0.4 ± 0.5	0.4 ± 0.1	2.5 ± 0.6
CT10G + MA + Ca + 72TCL	65.4 ± 0.1	30.8 ± 0.2	0.2 ± 0.0	0.0 ± 0.0	0.0 ± 0.0	1.0 ± 0.0	0.0 ± 0.0	0.3 ± 0.0	2.4 ± 0.1

The TF-XRD profiles in Figure 3 show that the peaks of cd–CT and rutile were detected on the sample CT, and these remained after DC treatment using 5% gelatin solution. In contrast, their intensities decreased with increasing gelatin concentration due to the development of the gelatin layer. Although the sole addition of $CaCl_2$ or $(NH_4)_2HPO_4$ into the MA-containing gelatin solution did not apparently change the profiles of CT10G, the addition of both $CaCl_2$ and $(NH_4)_2HPO_4$ generated large peaks attributed to brushite, indicating precipitation of brushite particles in the gelatin solution. The profile of the sample CT10G + MA + Ca was not apparently changed even after the TCL treatment for 72 h.

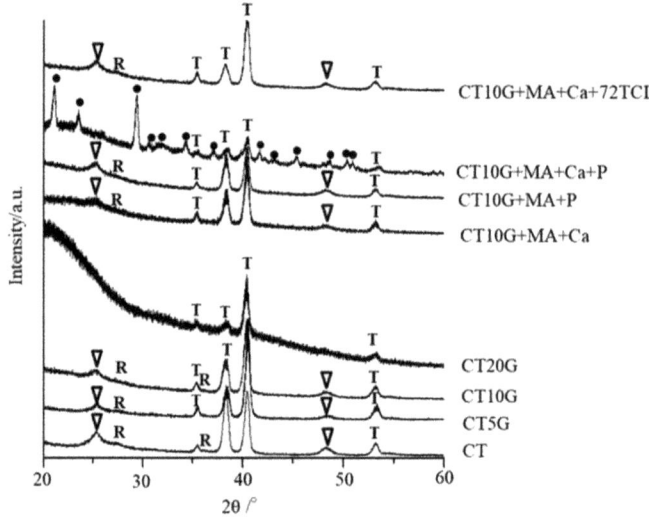

T: α-Ti R: Rutile ●: Brushite $(CaPO_3(OH)\cdot 2H_2O)$
▼: Calcium deficient calcium titanate ($Ca_{1-0.5x}H_xTi_4O_9$, $Ca_{1-0.5x}H_xTi_2O_4$, $Ca_{1-0.5x}H_xTi_4O_5$)

Figure 3. XRD profiles of Ca–heat-treated Ti–6Al–4V alloy subjected to dip coating with various additives and subsequent thermal cross–link treatment.

Critical scratch loads of the samples measured by scratch tester are summarized in Table 3. The critical scratch load was 42.6 mN for the CT sample, and this value increased to 47.2 and 54.0 mN for the CT5G and CT10G samples, respectively. Statistically significant differences were observed between CT and CT10G ($p < 0.001$). Similar values were observed on the 10% DC-treated samples with the additives and subsequent TCL treatment, in which statistically significant differences ($p < 0.001$) were detected on all the samples except CT10G + MA + Ca ($p = 0.092$). For the comparison, the critical scratch load on the 10% DC-treated alloy without cd–CT layer was measured, which was as low as 4.1 mN ($p < 0.001$).

Table 3. Critical scratch loads of the Ti–6Al–4V treated with Ca–heat followed by gelatin coating and thermal crosslinking.

Sample.	Critical Scratch Load/mN	Statistically Significant Difference
CT	42.6 ± 3.3	-
CT5G	47.2 ± 6.6	($p = 0.3428$)
CT10G	54.0 ± 4.6	† ($p < 0.001$)
CT10G + MA + Ca	49.0 ± 2.5	($p = 0.092$)
CT10G + MA + P	59.4 ± 4.4	† ($p < 0.001$)
CT10G + MA + Ca + P	54.6 ± 4.0	† ($p < 0.001$)
CT10G + MA + Ca + 72TCL	55.0 ± 3.7	† ($p < 0.001$)
10G *	4.1 ± 0.3	† ($p < 0.001$)

* 10% gelatin was dip-coated without Ca–heat treatment. † Statistical significant difference toward CT ($p < 0.05$).

3.3. Apatite Formation

Figure 4 shows the SEM images of the treated samples after being soaked in SBF for 7 days. Apatite particles fully deposited on the CT and CT5G samples, while they partially deposited on the CT10G and CT20G samples. When the $CaCl_2$ or $(NH_4)_2HPO_4$ was solely added into the 10% gelatin solution, apatite formation increased to be fully deposited on the sample surfaces (CT10G + MA + Ca, CT10G + MA + P). In contrast, scarce and inhomogeneous apatite formation was observed when both $CaCl_2$ and $(NH_4)_2HPO_4$ were added into the gelatin solution (CT10G + MA + Ca and P).

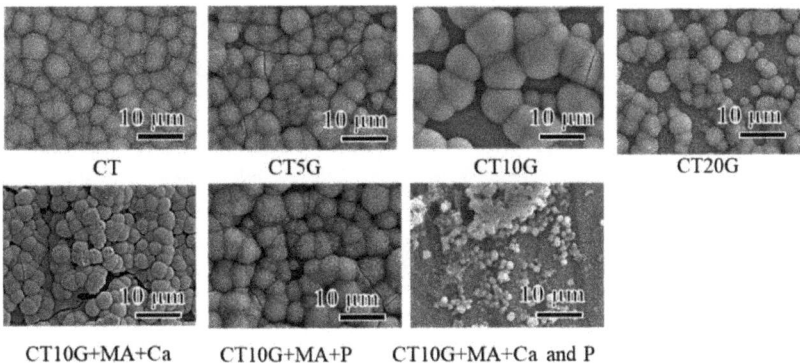

Figure 4. SEM images of surfaces of Ca–heat-treated Ti–6Al–4V alloy soaked in SBF for 7 days following dip coat treatment with various additives.

Figure 5 shows XRD profiles of these samples. The peaks at around 26 and 32 degrees in 2θ that are attributed to hydroxyapatite were observed on all the samples, while CT10G + MA + Ca + P showed the smallest peak intensity.

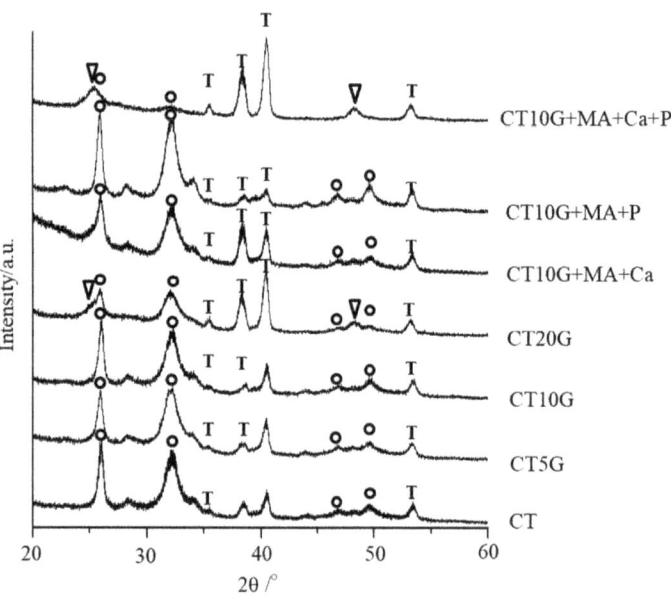

T: α-Ti   R: Rutile   ○: Hydroxyapatite
▽: Calcium deficient calcium titanate ($Ca_{1-0.5x}H_xTi_4O_9$, $Ca_{1-0.5x}H_xTi_2O_4$, $Ca_{1-0.5x}H_xTi_4O_5$)

Figure 5. XRD profiles of surfaces of Ca–heat-treated Ti–6Al–4V alloy soaked in SBF for 7 days following dip coat treatment with various additives.

When the 10%-DC samples with the additives of Ca or P were subjected to TCL treatment, the former maintained its apatite formation even after 72 h of TCL treatment (Figure 6). On the contrary, the latter lost its apatite formation within 3 h of TCL treatment.

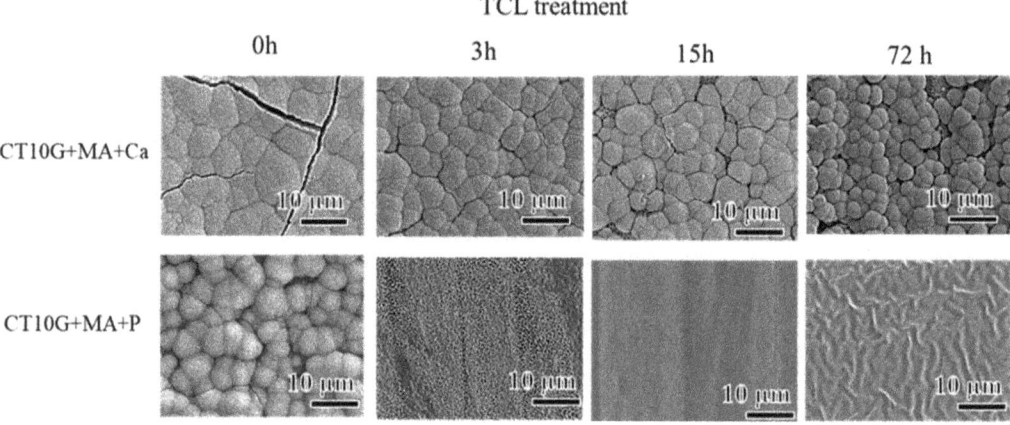

Figure 6. SEM images of surfaces of Ca–heat-treated Ti–6Al–4V alloy soaked in SBF for 7 days following dip coat and subsequent thermal cross-link treatment.

3.4. Gelatin Dissolution

Gelatin dissolution of the sample CT10G + MA + Ca with or without TCL treatment for the periods of 3–72 h was examined by measuring the Ca amount in PBS after the determined soaking period. The released MA concentration was calculated from the dissolution rate under the assumption that Ca is homogeneously distributed in gelatin. It can be seen in Figure 7 that Ca ions were rapidly released within 6 h and reached a stable value after 6 h for CT10G + MA + Ca, suggesting that the gelatin almost completely dissolved within 6 h. The initial gelatin dissolution rate decreased with increasing the periods of TCL treatment up to 72 h, indicating that the TCL treatment effectively suppressed gelatin dissolution. The total amount of MA released into PBS after 7 days was calculated to be 0.13 and 0.10 µmol/L for CT10G + MA + Ca and CT10G + MA + Ca + 72TCL, respectively. When the sample surfaces after being soaked in PBS for 7 days were observed under SEM, it was found that some amount of gelatin remained on the sample treated with TCL for 72 h, while almost complete dissolution of gelatin was observed on other samples (Figure 8). The cd–CT layer with nano-scaled network morphology remained even after the dissolution of gelatin for all of the samples.

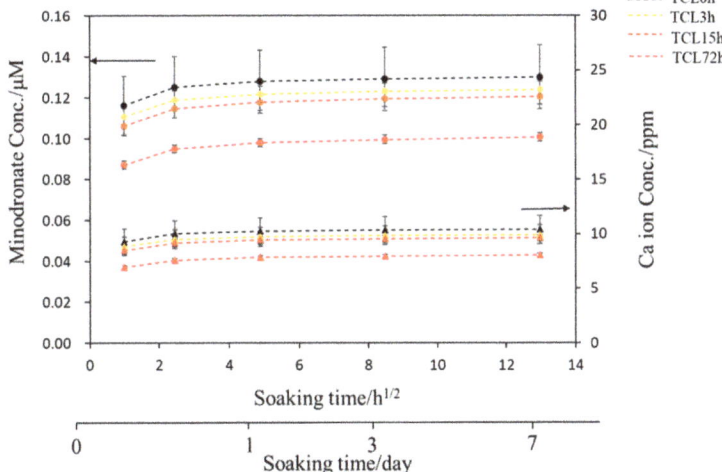

Figure 7. Calcium ion release into PBS from the sample CT10G + MA + Ca without or with thermal cross-link treatment for periods of 3–72 h. The released minodonate was estimated from the Ca ion concentration in PBS for each soaking period.

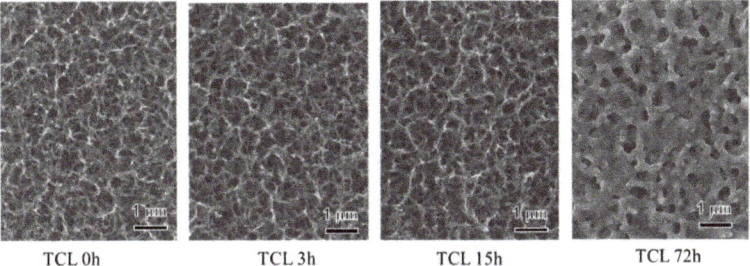

Figure 8. SEM images of the surfaces of the sample CT10G + MA + Ca without or with thermal cross-link treatment for periods of 3–72 h that were soaked in PBS for 7 days.

4. Discussion

A three-dimensional network structure composed of the bioactive cd–CT was initially produced on Ti–6Al–4V alloy by the Ca–heat treatment. It was shown that the cd–CT layer is hydrophilic and has superior scratch resistance, chemical durability, abundant Ti–OH groups, and reliable apatite-formation capability for inducing bone-bonding [7,17–19]. The remarkable bone-bonding capacity of the cd–CT was reported in our previous reports, in which Ti and Ti–Zr–Nb–Ta system alloys such as Ti-15Zr–4Nb–4Ta exhibited significantly higher critical detaching failure load and bone contact area than untreated Ti even in an early period of 4 weeks after implantation [19]. When the cd–CT was formed on the Ti–6Al–4V pedicle screw by the Ca–heat treatment, it exhibited higher extraction torque compared with the untreated screw [7]. It was also demonstrated that many bone fragments remained on the treated metals in both cases [18], indicating that fracture occurred not at the bone–implant interface but in the bone itself. Nevertheless, osteoinductivity and osteogenesis, in addition to osteoconductivity, are also desired in order to achieve further reliable bone regeneration, which are usually induced by functional organic materials such as cytokines, proteins and drugs [36]. In this study, the bioactive cd–CT layer was dipped into the medical-grade gelatin solution including MA to form an inorganic–organic composite releasing a bisphosphonate drug for the treatment of osteoporosis bone.

Generally, it is challenging to achieve high adhesion between the metal substrate and polymer coatings due to large differences in surface energy between the metal and polymer [37]. In the present study, the gelatin easily penetrated into the 3D network structure due to the hydrophilic nature of the cd–CT. Its coating thickness increased with the increase in gelatin concentration as a result of the increased viscosity of the gelatin solution (Figure 1). When the 10% gelatin was used, the thickness of the gelatin coating became comparative to that of the cd–CT layer (Figure 2), which seems to be suitable for practical use. Therefore, we determined the 10% gelatin, and thus the corresponding viscosity of 15.1 mPa·s, as an optimized condition. It was also confirmed that the thickness of the coated gelatin as well as the viscosity of the gelatin solution was almost not affected by the additives such as MA, $CaCl_2$ and $(NH_4)_2HPO_4$ (Figures 1 and 2). Thus, the produced inorganic–organic composite layer exhibits a high scratch resistance of about 50 mN owing to an interlocking effect between the 3D network frames of cd–CT and gelatin matrix.

When the gelatin-coated alloy with the cd–CT layer was soaked in SBF, its apatite formation decreased with an increasing gelatin concentration (Figure 4). Since the apatite formation on the Ti and its alloys with cd–CT was attributed to the release of Ca^{2+} ions from the cd–CT and abundant Ti–OH groups [17,38,39], the decrease in apatite formation on the gelatin-coated alloys was probably due to the suppression of Ca^{2+} ion release and the hiding of Ti–OH groups by the coated gelatin. When the $CaCl_2$ or $(NH_4)_2HPO_4$ as well as MA were solely added to the gelatin, the coated alloys formed apatite fully on their surfaces. The increased apatite formation might be due to the Ca^{2+} or HPO_4^{2-} ions that were released from the dissolved gelatin in SBF. Interestingly, scarce and inhomogeneous precipitation of apatite was observed on the DC-treated alloy with the additives of both $CaCl_2$ and $(NH_4)_2HPO_4$. This may be caused by rapid calcium phosphate precipitation in the gelation solution before the soaking in SBF. Indeed, brushite peaks were detected on the sample surface by XRD (Figure 3). It is seen in Figure 6 that the additives of $CaCl_2$ were also effective in inducing apatite formation even for the TCL-treated alloys while $(NH_4)_2HPO_4$ was not. This might be because the rate of gelatin dissolution was suppressed by the TCL treatment, suggesting that calcium ions are more effective for apatite formation than phosphate ions by effectively increasing the ionic activity product of apatite, $Ca_{10}(PO)_4(OH)_2$, than phosphate ions.

When the gelatin-coated alloy without TCL treatment was soaked in PBS, its gelatin layer rapidly dissolved within 6 h. It has been reported that thermal and chemical crosslinking can enhance the physical durability of gelatin [34,40]. In the present study, the thermal crosslinking method developed by Tsujimoto et al. was adopted to achieve slow dissolution of gelatin. It can be seen in Figure 7 that the dissolution rate was significantly suppressed by TCL treatment for 72 h. The estimated amount of MA released into PBS during the 7 days from the treated alloy was 0.10 μmol/L, which is effective for suppressing the activity of osteoclast cells [41]. Although the gelatin dissolved in a relatively short period of time in the aqueous solution, the cd–CT layer is chemically stable, as shown in Figure 8. It is expected that the treated layer with the composite of MA-containing gelatin and the cd–CT layer slowly releases MA to improve the bone mass of surrounding tissue and bonds to bone because of its apatite formation. Thus, the obtained bone-bonding is expected to be stable even after the dissolution of the gelatin layer, since the cd–CT layer is stable even under a simulated body environment. Further in vivo studies using animal model of osteoporosis are needed to prove the usefulness of the developed material for therapeutic treatment for osteoporosis bone.

5. Conclusions

The novel composite layer of minodronate-containing gelatin and calcium-deficient calcium titanate was produced on Ti–6Al–4V alloy. The treated alloy exhibited high scratch resistance, apatite formation capacity and slow release of minodronate, effective for medical treatment in osteoporosis bone, and thus should be useful for orthopedic implants.

Author Contributions: Conceptualization, S.Y. and K.A. methodology, S.Y.; software, S.A.S.; validation, K.A., A.S., and T.M.; formal analysis, S.Y.; investigation, S.Y.; resources, S.Y.; data curation, K.A., S.A.S., and A.S. and T.M.; writing—original draft preparation, S.Y. and K.A.; writing—review and editing, T.M. and S.A.S.; visualization, S.Y.; supervision, A.S. and T.M.; project administration, S.Y.; funding acquisition, K.A. All authors have read and agreed to the published version of the manuscript.

Funding: This study was supported by Grant-in-Aid for Scientific Research (KAKENHI) (C) (Grant Number 15K10402) and Japan Agency for Medical Research and Development (AMED) seeds A (Grant Number: A78).

Institutional Review Board Statement: Not applicable.

Informed Consent Statement: Not applicable.

Data Availability Statement: The data presented in this study are available on request from the corresponding author.

Conflicts of Interest: The authors declare no conflict of interest and the funders had no role in the design of the study; in the collection, analyses, or interpretation of data; in the writing of the manuscript, or in the decision to publish the results.

References

1. Hanawa, T. Overview of metals and applications. In *Metals for Biomedical Devices*; Niinomi, M., Ed.; Woodhead Publishing: Cambridge, UK, 2019; pp. 3–30.
2. Wu, J.C.; Huang, W.C.; Tsai, H.W.; Ko, C.C.; Wu, C.L.; Tu, T.H.; Cheng, H. Pedicle screw loosening in dynamic stabilization: Incidence, risk, and outcome in 126 patients. *Neurosurg. Focus* **2011**, *31*, E9. [CrossRef] [PubMed]
3. Tokuhashi, Y.; Matsuzaki, H.; Oda, H.; Uei, H. Clinical course and significance of the clear zone around the pedicle screws in the lumbar degenerative disease. *Spine* **2008**, *33*, 903–908. [CrossRef] [PubMed]
4. Wang, H.; Eliaz, N.; Xiang, Z.; Hsu, H.-P.; Spector, M.; Hobbs, L.W. Early bone apposition in vivo on plasma-sprayed and electrochemically deposited hydroxyapatite coatings on titanium alloy. *Biomaterials* **2006**, *23*, 4192–4203. [CrossRef] [PubMed]
5. Su, Y.; Cockerill, I.; Zheng, Y.; Tang, L.; Qin, Y.-X.; Zhu, D. Biofunctionalization of metallic implants by calcium phosphate coatings. *Bioact. Mater.* **2019**, *4*, 196–206. [CrossRef] [PubMed]
6. Kokubo, T.; Yamaguchi, S. Simulated body fluid and the novel bioactive materials derived from it. *J. Biomed. Mater. Res. Part A* **2019**, *107*, 968–977. [CrossRef]
7. Akeda, K.; Yamaguchi, S.; Matsushita, T.; Kokubo, T.; Murata, K.; Takegami, N.; Matsumine, A.; Sudo, A. Bioactive pedicle screws prepared by chemical and heat treatments improved biocompatibility and bone-bonding ability in canine lumbar spines. *PLoS ONE* **2018**, *13*, e196766. [CrossRef]
8. Park, J.-W.; Park, K.-B.; Suh, J.-Y. Effects of calcium ion incorporation on bone healing of Ti6Al4V alloy implants in rabbit tibiae. *Biomaterials* **2007**, *28*, 3306–3313. [CrossRef] [PubMed]
9. Huang, Y.; Wang, W.; Zhang, X.; Liu, X.; Xu, Z.; Han, S.; Su, Z.; Liu, H.; Gao, Y.; Yang, H. A prospective material for orthopedic applications: Ti substrates coated with a composite coating of titania-nanotubes layer and a silver-manganese-doped hydroxyapatite layer. *Ceram. Int.* **2018**, *44*, 5528–5542. [CrossRef]
10. Yang, G.L.; He, F.M.; Yang, X.F.; Wang, X.X.; Zhao, S.F. Bone responses to titanium implants surface-roughened by sandblasted and double etched treatments in a rabbit model. *Oral Surg. Oral Med. Oral Pathol. Oral Radiol. Endod.* **2008**, *106*, 516–524. [CrossRef]
11. Harun, W.S.W.; Harun, W.S.W.; Alias, J.; Zulkifli, F.H.; Kadirgama, K.; Ghani, S.A.C.; Shariffuddin, J.H.M. A comprehensive review of hydroxyapatite-based coatings adhesion on metallic biomaterials. *Ceram. Int.* **2018**, *44*, 1250–1268. [CrossRef]

12. Spriano, S.; Yamaguchi, S.; Baino, F.; Ferraris, S. A critical review of multifunctional titanium surfaces: New frontiers or improving osseointegration and host response, avoiding bacteria contamination. *Acta Biomater.* **2018**, *79*, 1–22. [CrossRef] [PubMed]
13. Kawai, T.; Takemoto, M.; Fujibayashi, S.; Tanaka, M.; Akiyama, H.; Nakamura, T.; Matsuda, S. Comparison between alkali heat treatment and sprayed hydroxyapatite coating on thermally-sprayed rough Ti surface in rabbit model: Effects on bone-bonding ability and osteoconductivity. *J. Biomed. Mater. Res. B Appl. Biomater.* **2015**, *103*, 1069–1081. [CrossRef] [PubMed]
14. Zhang, Z.; Xu, R.; Yang, Y.; Liang, C.; Yu, X.; Liu, Y.; Wang, T.; Yu, Y.; Deng, F. Micro/nano-textured hierarchical titanium topography promotes exosome biogenesis and secretion to improve osseointegration. *J. Nanobiotechnol.* **2021**, *19*, 78. [CrossRef] [PubMed]
15. Le, P.T.M.; Shintani, S.A.; Takadama, H.; Ito, M.; Kakutani, T.; Kitagaki, H.; Terauchi, S.; Ueno, T.; Nakano, H.; Nakajima, Y.; et al. Bioactivation Treatment with Mixed Acid and Heat on Titanium Implants Fabricated by Selective Laser Melting Enhances Preosteoblast Cell Differentiation. *Nanomaterials* **2021**, *11*, 987. [CrossRef] [PubMed]
16. Isaac, J.; Galtayries, A.; Kizuki, T.; Kokubo, T.; Berdal, A.; Sautier, J.M. Bioengineered titanium surfaces affect the gene-expression and phenotypic response of osteoprogenitor cells derived from mouse calvarial bones. *ECM* **2010**, *20*, 178–196. [CrossRef] [PubMed]
17. Yamaguchi, S.; Takadama, H.; Matsushita, T.; Nakamura, T.; Kokubo, T. Apatite-forming ability of Ti-15Zr-4Nb-4Ta alloy induced by calcium solution treatment. *J. Mater. Sci. Mater. Med.* **2010**, *21*, 439–444. [CrossRef]
18. Tanaka, M.; Takemoto, M.; Fujibayashi, S.; Kawai, T.; Yamaguchi, S.; Kizuki, T.; Kokubo, T.; Nakamura, T.; Matsuda, S. Bone bonding ability of a chemically and thermally treated low elastic modulus Ti alloy: Gum metal. *J. Mater. Sci. Mater. Med.* **2014**, *25*, 635–643. [CrossRef]
19. Fukuda, A.; Takemoto, M.; Saito, T.; Fujibayashi, S.; Neo, M.; Yamaguchi, S.; Kizuki, T.; Matsushita, T.; Niinomi, M.; Kokubo, T.; et al. Bone bonding bioactivity of Ti metal and Ti–Zr–Nb–Ta alloys with Ca ions incorporated on their surfaces by simple chemical and heat treatments. *Acta Biomater.* **2011**, *7*, 1379–1386. [CrossRef]
20. Al-Zubaidi, S.M.; Madfa, A.A.; Mufadhal, A.A.; Aldawla, M.A.; Hameed, O.S.; Yue, X.-G. Improvements in clinical durability from functional biomimetic metallic dental implants. *Front. Mater.* **2020**, *7*, 106. [CrossRef]
21. Meng, H.W.; Chien, E.Y.; Chien, H.H. Dental implant bioactive surface modifications and their effects on osseointegration: A review. *Biomark. Res.* **2016**, *4*, 24. [CrossRef]
22. Torres, Y.; Begines, B.; Beltr'an, A.M.; Boccaccini, A.R. Deposition of bioactive gelatin coatings on porous titanium: Influence of processing parameters, size and pore morphology. *Surf. Coat. Technol.* **2021**, *421*, 127366. [CrossRef]
23. Smandri, A.; Nordin, A.; Hwei, N.M.; Chin, K.Y.; Abd Aziz, I.; Fauzi, M.B. Natural 3Dprinted bioinks for skin regeneration and wound healing: A systematic review. *Polymers* **2020**, *12*, 1782. [CrossRef] [PubMed]
24. Ngadimin, K.; Stokes, A.; Gentile, P.; Ferreira-Duarte, A.M. Biomimetic hydrogels designed for cartilage tissue engineering. *Biomater. Sci.* **2021**, *9*, 4246–4259. [CrossRef] [PubMed]
25. Dong, Z.; Yuan, Q.; Huang, K.; Xu, W.; Liu, G.; Gu, Z. Gelatin methacryloyl (GelMA)-based biomaterials for bone regeneration. *RSC Adv.* **2019**, *9*, 17737–17744. [CrossRef]
26. Ranganathan, S.; Balagangadharan, K.; Selvamurugan, N. Chitosan and gelatinbasedelectrospun fibers for bone tissue engineering. *Int. J. Biol. Macromol.* **2019**, *133*, 354–364. [CrossRef] [PubMed]
27. Fleisch, H. Bisphosphonates: Mechanisms of action. *Endocr. Rev.* **1998**, *19*, 80–100. [CrossRef]
28. Garcia-Moreno, C.; Serrano, S.; Nacher, M.; Farre, M.; Diez, A.; Marinoso, M.L.; Carbonell, J.; Mellibovsky, L.; Nogués, X.; Ballester, J.; et al. Effect of alendronate on cultured normal human osteoblasts. *Bone* **1998**, *22*, 233–239. [CrossRef]
29. Wang, C.Z.; Chen, S.M.; Chen, C.H.; Wang, C.K.; Wang, G.J.; Chang, J.K.; Ho, M.L. The effect of the local delivery of alendronate on human adipose-derived stem cell-based bone regeneration. *Biomaterials* **2010**, *31*, 8674–8683. [CrossRef]
30. Cui, Y.; Zhu, T.; Li, D.; Li, Z.; Leng, Y.; Ji, X.; Liu, H.; Wu, W.; Ding, J. Bisphosphonate-Functionalized Scaffolds for Enhanced Bone Regeneration. *Adv. Healthc. Mater.* **2019**, *8*, e1901073. [CrossRef]
31. Kajiwara, H.; Yamaza, T.; Yoshinari, M.; Goto, T.; Iyama, S.; Atsuta, I.; Kido, M.A.; Tanaka, T. The bisphosphonate pamidronate on the surface of titanium stimulates bone formation around tibial implants in rats. *Biomaterials* **2005**, *26*, 581–587. [CrossRef]
32. Peter, B.; Gauthier, O.; Laib, S.; Bujoli, B.; Guicheux, J.; Janvier, P.; van Lenthe, G.H.; Müller, R.; Zambelli, P.-Y.; Bouler, J.-M.; et al. Local delivery of bisphosphonate from coated orthopedic implants increases implants mechanical stability in osteoporotic rats. *J. Biomed. Mater. Res. Part A* **2006**, *76*, 133–143. [CrossRef]
33. Matsumoto, T.; Endo, I. Minodronate. *Bone* **2020**, *137*, 115432. [CrossRef] [PubMed]
34. Tsujimoto, H.; Tanzawa, A.; Miyamoto, H.; Horii, T.; Tsuji, M.; Kawasumi, A.; Tamura, A.; Wang, Z.; Abe, R.; Tanaka, S.; et al. Biological properties of a thermally crosslinked gelatin film as a novel anti-adhesive material: Relationship between the biological properties and the extent of thermal crosslinking. *J. Biomed. Mater. Res. Part B Appl. Biomater.* **2015**, *103*, 1511–1518. [CrossRef]
35. Kokubo, T.; Takadama, H. How useful is SBF in predicting in vivo bone bioactivity? *Biomaterials* **2006**, *27*, 2907–2915. [CrossRef] [PubMed]
36. Botor, M.; Fus-Kujawa, A.; Uroczynska, M.; Stepien, K.L.; Galicka, A.; Gawron, K.; Sieron, A.L. Osteogenesis Imperfecta: Current and Prospective Therapies. *Biomolecules* **2021**, *11*, 1493. [CrossRef] [PubMed]
37. van Tijum, R.; Vellinga, W.P.; De Hosso, J.; Th, M. Adhesion along metal–polymer interfaces during plastic deformation. *J. Mater. Sci.* **2007**, *42*, 3529–3536. [CrossRef] [PubMed]

8. Yamaguchi, S.; Le, P.T.M.; Shintani, S.A.; Takadama, H.; Ito, M.; Ferraris, S.; Spriano, S. Iodine-Loaded Calcium Titanate for Bone Repair with Sustainable Antibacterial Activity Prepared by Solution and Heat Treatment. *Nanomaterials* **2021**, *1*, 2199. [CrossRef] [PubMed]
9. Ferraris, S.; Yamaguchi, S.; Barbani, N.; Cazzola, M.; Cristallini, C.; Miola, M.; Vernè, E.; Spriano, S. Bioactive materials: In vitro investigation of different mechanisms of hydroxyapatite precipitation. *Acta Biomater.* **2019**, *102*, 468–480. [CrossRef]
10. Furuno, K.; Wang, J.; Suzuki, K.; Nakahata, M.; Sakai, S. Gelatin-Based Electrospun Fibers Insolubilized by Horseradish Peroxidase-Catalyzed Cross-Linking for Biomedical Applications. *ACS Omega* **2020**, *5*, 21254–21259. [CrossRef]
11. Dunford, J.E.; Thompson, K.; Coxon, F.P.; Luckman, S.P.; Hahn, F.M.; Poulter, C.D.; Ebetino, F.H.; Rogers, M.J. Structure-activity relationships for inhibition of farnesyl diphosphate synthase in vitro and inhibition of bone resorption in vivo by nitrogen-containing bisphosphonates. *J. Pharmacol. Exp. Ther.* **2001**, *296*, 235–242.

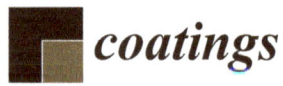

Article

Attachment and Growth of Fibroblast Cells on Poly (2-Methoxyethyl Acrylate) Analog Polymers as Coating Materials

Rubaiya Anjum [1,†], Kei Nishida [2,†], Haruka Matsumoto [1], Daiki Murakami [1,2], Shingo Kobayashi [2], Takahisa Anada [1,2,*] and Masaru Tanaka [1,2,*]

[1] Department of Chemistry and Biochemistry, Graduate School of Engineering, 744 Motooka, Nishi-ku, Fukuoka 819-0395, Japan; anjum.rubaiya.867@s.kyushu-u.ac.jp (R.A.); matsumoto.haruka.093@s.kyushu-u.ac.jp (H.M.); daiki_murakami@ms.ifoc.kyushu-u.ac.jp (D.M.)
[2] Institute for Materials Chemistry and Engineering, Kyushu University, 744 Motooka, Nishi-ku, Fukuoka 819-0395, Japan; kei_nishida@ms.ifoc.kyushu-u.ac.jp (K.N.); shingo_kobayashi@ms.ifoc.kyushu-u.ac.jp (S.K.)
* Correspondence: takahisa_anada@ms.ifoc.kyushu-u.ac.jp (T.A.); masaru_tanaka@ms.ifoc.kyushu-u.ac.jp (M.T.); Tel./Fax: +81-92-802-6238 (T.A. & M.T.)
† These authors contributed equally to this work.

Abstract: The regulation of adhesion and the subsequent behavior of fibroblast cells on the surface of biomaterials is important for successful tissue regeneration and wound healing by implanted biomaterials. We have synthesized poly(ω-methoxyalkyl acrylate)s (PMCxAs; x indicates the number of methylene carbons between the ester and ethyl oxygen), with a carbon chain length of x = 2–6, to investigate the regulation of fibroblast cell behavior including adhesion, proliferation, migration, differentiation and collagen production. We found that PMC2A suppressed the cell spreading, protein adsorption, formation of focal adhesion, and differentiation of normal human dermal fibroblasts, while PMC4A surfaces enhanced them compared to other PMCxAs. Our findings suggest that fibroblast activities attached to the PMCxA substrates can be modified by changing the number of methylene carbons in the side chains of the polymers. These results indicate that PMCxAs could be useful coating materials for use in skin regeneration and wound dressing applications.

Keywords: PMEA analog polymers; coating materials; fibroblasts; cell behavior; wound dressing

1. Introduction

Coatings on implanted biomaterials play a pivotal role in regulating biological reactions after implantation [1,2]. Various coating approaches such as covalent and physically adsorbed coating have been developed to reduce biological reaction and improve biocompatibility [3,4]. To ensure biocompatibility, it is critical to control the contact between the biomaterial surface and biological components, including proteins and cells [5]. Cell adhesion and growth on biomaterials are indicators of biocompatibility, as these behaviors are involved in the adsorbed biological components and biological response on the surface of the biomaterial [6,7]. Therefore, in order to develop better biomaterials, it is necessary to understand the regulation of cell adhesion and its subsequent behavior on the implant surface. The selection of a suitable surface for the implanted biomaterials is also an important issue from the perspective of cell–material interactions. The interactions between the surface of biomaterials and cells are responsible for regulating cell fate and tissue regeneration.

Fibroblasts play an important role in tissue remodeling and wound healing [8,9]. Because their functions are related to the epidermal proliferation, differentiation, and formation of extracellular matrix (ECM), fibroblast regulation is linked to the integration or disintegration of biomaterials in tissue engineering and wound healing [8]. In the regeneration of functional tissues, extracellular signals occasionally convert a quiescent state of fibroblasts into an active phenotype known as myofibroblasts, which are required for inducing tissue connection and contraction [10,11]. Myofibroblasts create a type of environment/network during tissue regeneration that results in cell differentiation, proliferation, quiescence, and apoptosis. In the case of natural healing processes, they release an excess amount of matrix proteins to promote faster healing. However, the over and prolonged activation of myofibroblasts induces the formation of fibrotic tissues [12–14]. This promotes the development of numerous diseases and plays a major role in most organ failure cases. Therefore, it is important to regulate the balance between fibroblast recruitment and differentiation on the surface of implanted biomaterials.

Several groups have demonstrated that fibroblast behavior is controlled by modulating surface properties, including wettability, roughness, elasticity, micro and nanostructure, polarity, and hydrophobicity [6,15–17]. These properties contribute to altering the signal transduction via focal adhesion signaling, which is responsible for the dynamic relationship between the integrins of cells adhered on surfaces and adhesive proteins, including fibronectin (FN) and vitronectin [7,18,19]. In this regard, the surface properties, including cell adhesiveness on the biomaterials, can be modified by a polymer coating on the surface [20–22]. Therefore, the use of synthetic polymeric coatings on implanted biomaterials can be a suitable approach for controlling cellular behavior. Our group has developed a biocompatible poly(2-methoxyethyl acrylate) (PMEA) and its analogs as coating materials that exhibit excellent non-thrombogenicity and selective cell adhesivity [23–25]. In addition, the mechanism underlying these properties is related to the hydrated water on the PMEA analogs. Hydrated water can be classified into three types: non-freezing water (NFW), intermediate water (IW), and free water, based on the mode of binding defined by time-resolved infrared spectroscopy, nuclear magnetic resonance correction time, and differential scanning calorimetry (DSC) [26–28]. In particular, PMEA analogs modulate protein adsorption and conformational changes on the surface according to the IW content [29–31]. Furthermore, PMEA analogs promote the adipogenesis of mouse adipocyte precursor cells by suppressing the conformational change of adsorbed proteins and subsequent integrin signaling [32]. These results indicate that PMEA analogs can modulate the amount and conformation of the adsorbed protein, thereby regulating cellular behavior. Thus, we hypothesized that PMEA analogs could be used as coating materials on biomaterials to regulate fibroblast behavior, including adhesion, recruitment, and differentiation. However, the relationship between fibroblast behavior and PMEA analogs with varying hydration water contents has yet to be clarified.

Poly(ω-methoxyalkyl acrylate) (PMCxAs; where x indicates the number of methylene carbons between the ester and ethyl oxygen) has been reported to be a PMEA analog polymer that can systemically modulate hydrophobicity, hydration water content, and protein adsorption [33]. Thus, we anticipated that PMCxAs with changes in carbon chain length would modulate fibroblast behavior. Here, we evaluated fibroblast behavior, including adhesion, migration, differentiation, and collagen secretion, on PMCxAs. PMCxAs were developed as coating materials to regulate fibroblast behavior. Therefore, we examined the attachment and growth of normal human dermal fibroblasts (NHDFs) on PMCxA-coated substrates. To estimate the focal adhesion signaling activity, the formation of focal adhesions and the amount of adsorbed FN were evaluated. Moreover, the expression of specific proteins, cell migration, and collagen production were assessed to determine the activation of NHDFs in response to the PMCxA properties.

2. Materials and Methods

2.1. Preparation of Polymer-Coated Substrates

Poly(2-methoxyethyl acrylate) (PMC2A), poly(3-methoxypropyl acrylate) (PMC3A), poly(4-methoxybutyl acrylate) (PMC4A), poly(5-methoxypentyl acrylate) (PMC5A), and poly(6-methoxyhexyl acrylate) (PMC6A) were synthesized as described previously [33], and their chemical structures are represented in Figure 1. The toluene solutions (0.5 wt.%/vol.%) of each polymer were used to prepare the polymer substrates. Each polymer was spin-coated on a polyethylene terephthalate (PET) disc (thickness = 125 μm) (Mitsubishi Plastics, Tokyo, Japan) of 14 and 30 mm in diameter at 3000 rpm for 40 s. Then, the polymer-coated substrates were dried and stored in a desiccator. Prior to each experiment, the prepared substrate was sterilized by exposure to UV for 1 h.

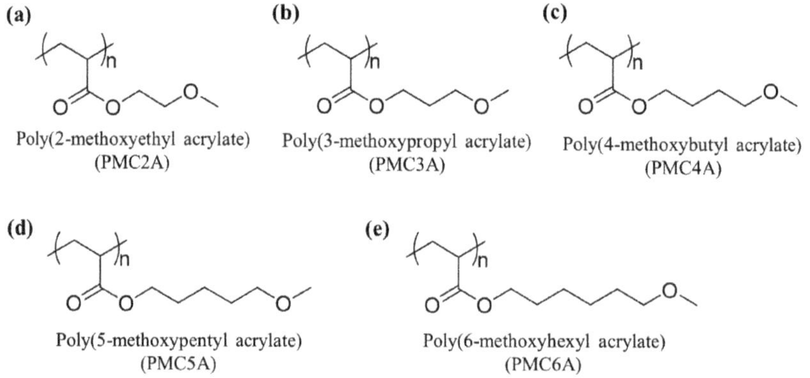

Figure 1. Chemical structures of poly(ω-methoxyalkyl acrylates) (PMCxAs): (**a**) poly(2-methoxyethyl acrylate) (PMC2A); (**b**) poly(3-methoxypropyl acrylate) (PMC3A); (**c**) poly(4-methoxybutyl acrylate) (PMC4A); (**d**) poly(5-methoxypentyl acrylate) (PMC5A); (**e**) poly(6-methoxyhexyl acrylate) (PMC6A).

2.2. Contact Angle Measurement

The contact angles of each prepared polymer substrate were measured using two techniques: sessile water droplet and captive air bubble. The droplet method was executed by placing 2 μL of water droplets on the five positions of the substrate. For captive bubble measurement, the prepared polymer substrates were immersed in water for 24 h. Then, 2 μL of air bubbles were injected at the three positions beneath the substrate.

2.3. Cell Culture

NHDFs (Lonza, Warsaw, Poland) were cultured in a media consisting of Dulbecco's modified Eagle's medium/nutrient mixture (DMEM/F12) (1:1), 10% (v/v) fetal bovine serum, and 1% (v/v) penicillin-streptomycin (all from Thermo Fisher Scientific, Waltham, MA, USA). Prior to the experiment, cells were isolated from the culture dish using 0.25% trypsin/EDTA solution (Thermo Fisher Scientific, Rockford, IL, USA).

2.4. Cell Attachment and Proliferation Assays

Cell proliferation assays were performed using 24-well plates. For the proliferation assay, NHDFs were cultured on each PMCxA-coated PET substrate (φ = 14 mm) at a density of 5×10^3 cells/cm^2 for 24, 96, and 168 h. All substrates were pre-soaked in phosphate-buffered saline (PBS) (−) and incubated for 1 h at 37 °C prior to cell seeding. After the specified incubation time, the number of cells was determined from a standard curve prepared using the colorimetric WST-8 assay (Dojindo Laboratories, Kumamoto, Japan). The calcein reagent (Thermo Fisher Scientific, Rockford, IL, USA) was used to stain living cells after 24 h of cultivation. Fluorescence images were captured to observe living cells.

2.5. Quantification of Adsorbed Protein on Polymer Substrates

The amount of total adhered proteins was measured by performing a bicinchoninic acid assay with the micro-BCA protein assay kit (Thermo Fisher Scientific, Rockford, IL, USA) according to the manufacturer's instructions. All polymer substrates with a diameter of 30 mm were used in this experiment. First, the substrates were pre-soaked in PBS (−) for 1 h at room temperature. Then, protein solution (10 μg/mL in PBS (−)) was added to each well and incubated for 1 h at 37 °C. After protein adsorption, the substrates were rinsed three times with PBS. Next, 5% (w/v) sodium dodecyl sulfate (SDS) (Bio-Rad Laboratories, Tokyo, Japan) and 0.1 M NaOH solutions were added to 6-well plates and incubated at 37 °C for 2 h. The surface of the substrate was scratched using a cell scraper to peel off the adsorbed protein from the substrate. Finally, the extracted protein solution was mixed with BCA solution to measure the absorbance at a wavelength of 562 nm. The amount of adsorbed protein was calculated using the standard curve.

2.6. Immunocytochemical Analysis

Before starting the experiment, the prepared substrates were pretreated with PBS, following cell attachment and proliferation assays. NHDFs (1×10^4 cells/cm^2) were seeded on each PMCxA-coated substrate (φ = 14 mm) and incubated for 24 h. After culturing, the cells were fixed using 4% (w/v) paraformaldehyde (Fujifilm Wako Pure Chemical Corporation, Osaka, Japan) and incubated at 37 °C for 10 min. Then, 0.5% (v/v) Triton X-100 (Fujifilm Wako Pure Chemicals Co., Ltd., Osaka, Japan) in PBS (−) was added to permeabilize the cell membranes. The substrates were then treated with mouse monoclonal anti-human vinculin antibody (VIN-11-5; Sigma-Aldrich, St. Louis, MO, USA) (1:400) diluted in 1% (w/v) BSA dissolved in PBS (−) for 90 min at room temperature, and subsequently treated with Alexa Fluor 488-conjugated anti-mouse IgG (H + L) antibody (1:1000 dilution), Alexa Fluor 568-conjugated phalloidin (1:100 diluted), and 4′,6-diamidino-2-phenylindole (1:1000 diluted) (all from Thermo Fisher Scientific, Waltham, MA, USA) for 1 h at room temperature. After performing these steps, the fluorescence images were captured using a confocal laser-scanning microscope (CLSM) (FV-1000; Olympus, Tokyo, Japan). Cell area and circularity were evaluated quantitatively using ImageJ software (version 1.53C, Bethesda, MD, USA).

2.7. Western Blotting

NHDFs (1×10^4 cells/cm^2) were cultured on PMCxA substrates (φ = 30 mm) for 24 h. The cells were washed twice with PBS and lysed with RIPA buffer (Fujifilm Wako Pure Chemical Corporation, Osaka, Japan) containing phosphatase (Nacalai Tesque, Kyoto, Japan) and protease inhibitors (Nacalai Tesque, Kyoto, Japan). The collected cell lysate was centrifuged at 12,000 rpm for 10 min at 4 °C. The supernatant was mixed with Laemmli buffer (Bio-Rad) containing 10% 2-mercaptoethanol and incubated at 95 °C for 3 min. For the collected solution, SDS-polyacrylamide gel electrophoresis (SDS-PAGE) was performed on a 4–20% gradient polyacrylamide gel (Bio-Rad, Hercules, CA, USA) for 50 min at 150 V. The separated proteins on the gels were transferred onto a polyvinylidene fluoride membrane (Bio-Rad, Hercules, CA, USA) using a Trans-Blot turbo transfer system (Bio-Rad, Hercules, CA, USA). The protein-transferred membrane was blocked with 5% skim milk or 5% BSA dissolved in TBS-T (20 mM Tris-HCl, 500 mM NaCl, 0.1% Tween-20, pH 7.5) for 60 min at room temperature. The primary antibodies were diluted with 5% skim milk or 3% BSA dissolved in TBS-T, added to the membrane, and incubated at 4 °C overnight. Rabbit monoclonal anti-Snail antibody (C15D3; Cell Signaling Technology, Tokyo, Japan) (1:1000 dilution), rabbit monoclonal anti-α-SMA antibody (E184; Abcam, Cambridge, UK) (1:1000 dilution), mouse monoclonal anti-vimentin antibody (10366-1-AP; Proteintech, Rosemont, IL, USA) (1:2000 dilution), and mouse monoclonal anti-β-actin antibody (6D1; MBL, Tokyo, Japan) (1:1000 dilution) were used as primary antibodies. Next, the membrane was washed with TBS-T and treated with horseradish peroxidase (HRP)-conjugated goat anti-mouse IgG (MBL, Tokyo, Japan) (1:10,000 dilution) or HRP-conjugated goat anti-rabbit IgG (MBL, Tokyo, Japan) (1:10,000 dilution) for 60 min at room temperature. The membrane was then washed with TBS-T and treated with ImmunoStar Zeta (Wako, Tokyo, Japan). Chemiluminescence images of the membrane were acquired using LuminoGraphI (WSE-6100; ATTO, Amherst, NY, USA). The band intensity of the captured images was measured using ImageJ software (version 1.53C, Bethesda, MD, USA).

2.8. Cell Migration Test

Cell migration experiments were performed in 6-well plates. First, NHDFs were cultured on PMCxA-coated substrates (φ = 30 mm) at 1×10^4 cells/cm² in 6-well plates and incubated at 37 °C. Then, the cell monolayer surface was scratched using a rubber cell scraper. Finally, cell migration was observed at 0, 24, and 48 h after the scratch and the images were captured using a phase-contrast microscope. The migration area was determined using Image J software and estimated as ($A_0 - A_t$), where A_0 is the initial wound area and A_t is the wound area at the desired time (t). Then, the migration area was plotted against migration time, and finally, the rate of migration was calculated from the slope of this curve as slope/2l, where l is the length of the wounded region [34].

2.9. Collagen Production Measurement

NHDFs-secreted collagen was quantified using a collagen assay kit. For this experiment, the cells were seeded at a density of 2×10^4 cells/cm². L (+)-ascorbic acid sodium salt (1 mM) (Fujifilm Wako Pure Chemical Corporation, Osaka, Japan) was added as a supplement after 24 h of incubation at 37 °C to increase collagen production [35,36]. The media were collected after 7 days of cell culturing with supplements. The amount of collagen was normalized to the DNA concentration, as determined by the Picogreen assay (Thermo Fisher Scientific, Rockford, IL, USA).

2.10. Statistical Analysis

Data from at least three separate tests are presented as the mean ± standard deviation (SD). Significance tests were performed using one-way analysis of variance (ANOVA) followed by Tukey's post hoc test for multiple comparisons. Statistical significance was set at $p < 0.05$.

3. Results and Discussion

3.1. Physicochemical Properties of PMCxA-Coated Substrates

Poly(ω-methoxyalkyl acrylate)s (PMCxAs; where x indicates the number of methylene carbons between the ester and ether oxygen) was synthesized following a previously reported method [33]. PMCxAs with a carbon chain length of x = 2–6 were used. PMC2A has the same chemical structure as PMEA. As per the previous report, the physicochemical properties, including molecular weight (M_n), glass transition temperature (T_g), IW content, and NFW content, were determined (Table 1). T_g, the transition temperature of the polymer from the glassy state to the rubbery state, is ascribed to the mobility of the polymer chain [37]. T_g decreased with an increasing length of the alkyl side chain under both dry and wet conditions, suggesting that the mobility of the polymer chains increased with the length of the alkyl side chain. Under wet conditions, the T_g values of PMCxAs were lower than those under dry conditions. The values of T_g decreased in the following order: PMC2A > PMC3A > PMC4A > PMC5A > PMC6A. Because the hydration of the polymer influences T_g, we calculated the hydration water content, such as IW and NFW, in PMCxAs [33]. The hydration water content of PMCxAs showed a steady decrease in the amount of IW along with the amount of NFW upon the introduction of the hydrophobic methylene carbon in the side chain.

To evaluate the cell adhesion behavior on PMCxAs, PMCxA-coated PET substrates were fabricated using spin-coating methods. Because the hydrophilicity on the surface is one of the parameters to modulate cell behavior, PMCxA-coated substrates were characterized by evaluating the contact angle to determine the hydrophilicity on the surface (Table 2). The contact angle values derived from each polymer-coated substrate were distinct from those of the uncoated PET substrate (86.4° in air and 129.2° in water), indicating that every polymer was coated properly. In the case of the sessile drop technique, the water contact angle increased with an increasing side chain alkyl length, suggesting that the hydrophilicity of polymers decreased with increasing side chain alkyl length. The contact angle values obtained with the captive air bubble method showed similar tendencies as the sessile water drop, indicating that the hydrophilicity of the hydrated PMCxAs was similar before hydration. Therefore, the physicochemical properties of the PMCxAs showed that the side chain length affected the properties of the polymers.

Table 1. Physicochemical and thermal properties of PMCxAs [33] Copyright © 2017, American Chemical Society.

Scheme	M_n (kg/mol)	M_w/M_n	$T_{g\,dry}$ [a] (°C)	$T_{g\,wet}$ [a] (°C)	IW [b] (wt.%)	NFW [c] (wt.%)
PMC2A	32	1.3	−35	−51	3.7	2.5
PMC3A	33	2.7	−48	−58	2.8	3.1
PMC4A	24	2.4	−65	−67	1.7	1.3
PMC5A	31	2.8	−74	−78	1.0	1.5
PMC6A	42	2.7	−77	−78	0.8	1.3

[a] Measured by DSC performed at a rate of 5 °C/min, [b] intermediate water (IW), and [c] non-freezing water (NFW).

Table 2. Contact angle of PET substrate coated with PMCxAs. The data represent the mean ± SD (n = 5).

Samples	Contact Angle (°)	
	Sessile Water Drops [a]	Captive Air Bubble [a]
PET	86.4 (± 1.1)	129.2 (± 1.0)
PMC2A	44.2 (± 0.6)	133.6 (± 1.0)
PMC3A	51.1 (± 0.4)	129.5 (± 1.7)
PMC4A	54.4 (± 0.7)	125.7 (± 1.7)
PMC5A	57.3 (± 0.2)	120.3 (± 0.6)
PMC6A	61.0 (± 0.6)	119.4 (± 3.7)

[a] Sessile water drops method by placing a 2 μL water droplet for 30 s and a captive air bubble method by placing 2 μL air bubble on the substrates immersed in water for 24 h.

3.2. Cell Attachment and Proliferation Assay

In the field of designing and improving biomaterials, the capacity for cell attachment is considered an important factor. The physicochemical properties of the surface affect the behavior of adhered cells on the substrates, including proliferation, cell signaling pathways, and cell differentiation [38]. Initially, we examined NHDFs' morphology on each PMCxA substrate at 24 h. To visualize adhered NHDFs, they were stained using a calcein reagent, as shown in Figure 2a. Most of the adhered NHDFs on every substrate showed green fluorescence signals attributed to living cells. The cells were found to spread on uncoated PET substrate as well as on PMC4A, PMC5A, and PMC6A-coated substrates after 24 h of culture. In contrast, on the PMC2A- and PMC3A-coated substrates, cells retained their circular shape. In addition, the number of adhered cells on PMCxA substrates at a predetermined time was measured using the colorimetric WST-8 assay, as shown in Figure 2b. Over 60% of the initially seeded cells adhered to the uncoated PET, PMC4A, PMC5A, and PMC6A-coated substrates within 24 h. The number of adhered cells on the PMC4A was approximately 76% of initially seeded cells and the highest among all substrates. The PMC2A and PMC3A significantly reduced the number of attached cells compared to other substrates. After 96 h and 168 h of incubation, the number of cells on the substrates decreased in the following order: PMC4A > PMC6A > PMC5A > PET > PMC3A > PMC2A. Although there was an almost two-fold increase in the number of adhered cells on all substrates at 96 h, it showed a five-fold and a seven-fold increase on PMC2A and PMC4A at 196 h, respectively. Therefore, the proliferation of cells on PMC2A was significantly lower than that on PET and other substrates at all time intervals, while the proliferation of cells on PMC4A was significantly higher than that of other substrates.

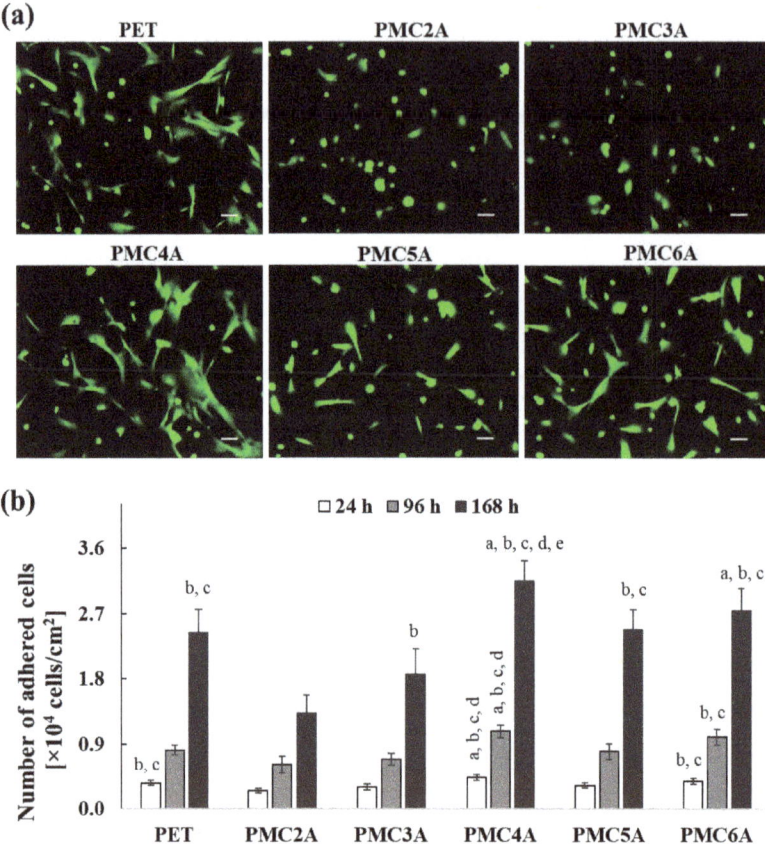

Figure 2. (a) Calcein staining images for NHDFs adhered on PET, PMC2A, PMC3A, PMC4A, PMC5A, and PMC6A after 24 h of incubation (scale bars = 100 μm). (b) The number of adhered NHDF on PMCxA-coated substrates at 24, 96, and 168 h. The data represent the mean ± SD (n = 3, [a] $p < 0.05$ compared with PET, [b] $p < 0.05$ compared with PMC2A, [c] $p < 0.05$ compared with PMC3A, [d] $p < 0.05$ compared with PMC5A, [e] $p < 0.05$ compared with PMC6A; Tukey's multiple comparisons test).

Guerra et al. reported that the stiffness of the substrate has an impact on cellular behavior [39]. In their study, MC3T3-E1 cells were cultured on substrates coated with poly(n-alkyl acrylate)s with various lengths of side-chain alkyl groups with different mechanical stiffnesses. The substrate stiffness declined linearly with an increasing side chain alkyl length, leading to better cellular interactions on the stiffer substrate compared to the flexible substrate. In our results, we found that the cell adhesion and proliferation of NHDFs were modulated on the substrates coated with PMCxAs, of which the chemical structures were similar to the methoxy groups at the side chains. This suggests that the mechanical stiffness of substrates based on the side chain of PMCxAs might be one of the factors affecting cell adhesion and proliferation, although the stiffness of the surface of PMCxA coatings has not been measured in the present study. However, PMC4A exhibited excellent cell adhesion behavior and proliferation (Figure 2a). The physicochemical properties, such as wettability, surface energy, the balance of hydrophilicity and hydrophobicity, roughness, polymer chain mobility, chemical functionalities, and hydration water content, are known to affect cell behavior [16,40]. Since PMCxA altered these properties, the cells adhered to the PMCxAs would be influenced by the balance of the hydrophilicity and hydrophobicity of polymers, and the hydration water content of polymers.

3.3. Quantification of Adsorbed Protein on Polymer Substrates

The amount and conformational changes of adsorbed proteins, such as FN and vitronectin, are another important factor that may be involved in the cell attachment process [41,42]. The amount of adsorbed FN on the substrates is likely to affect NHDFs' adhesion. Therefore, the amount of adsorbed FN on the PMCxA-coated substrate was analyzed, as shown in Figure 3. The amount of adsorbed FN on the substrates increased with an increase in the carbon length up to PMC4A but decreased for PMC5A and PMC6A compared to PMC4A. The amount of adsorbed FN on PMC2A was significantly lower, while that on PMC4A was significantly higher than that on PET and other substrates, except for PMC6A. Considering the number of adhered NHDFs on the PMCxA substrates, the adsorbed FN on PMC4A enhanced the adhesion and proliferation of NHDFs, whereas PMC2A suppressed NHDFs' adhesion. Our group has previously clarified that the presence of IW within or on the hydrated polymer surface acts as a repulsive barrier between the proteins and the substrate, leading to poor interactions between them [9,10]. A previous study on a PMEA analog PMCxA-coated substrate demonstrated that the amount of adsorbed fibrinogen increased as the side chain increased, implying that hydrophobicity was an essential factor [33]. Moreover, another study indicated that the enhancement of the adsorbed protein layer was correlated with the mobility of the polymer surface [37]. Therefore, the FN adsorption was also modulated by hydration water, the balance of hydrophilicity and hydrophobicity, and polymer mobility.

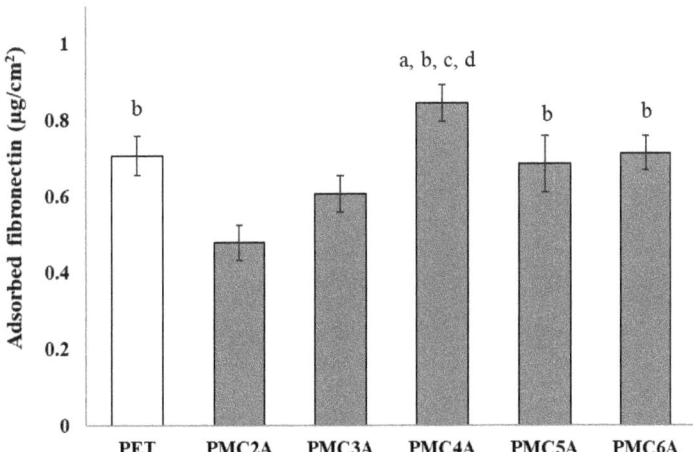

Figure 3. Evaluation of adsorbed fibronectin on substrates coated with PMCxAs. The data represent the mean ± SD (n = 15, [a] $p < 0.05$ compared with PET, [b] $p < 0.05$ compared with PMC2A, [c] $p < 0.05$ compared with PMC3A, [d] $p < 0.05$ compared with PMC5A; Tukey's multiple comparisons test).

3.4. Immunocytochemical Assay

The physicochemical properties and adsorbed proteins on the biomaterial surface affect cell adhesion behavior, cell signaling pathways, and cell differentiation. Focal adhesion plays a crucial role in transmitting mechanochemical signals, together with integrin clusters, providing strength between integrin and actin connections, and is a crucial factor in tissue regeneration, maintenance, and repair via cell signaling for direct cell migration, proliferation, and differentiation [43]. Therefore, cell morphology and the formation of focal adhesions in cells are initial indicators of cell signaling pathways with cell adhesion on biomaterial surfaces. Immunocytochemical assays for F-actin and vinculin were conducted to evaluate the cellular functions of adhered NHDFs on the substrates (Figure 4a). Focal adhesions were identified via the localization of actin filaments and vinculin [44]. NHDFs were found to be entirely spread on PET, and several focal adhesions in the cells were observed on the PET through the thicker extension of actin filaments and the observation of vinculin localization at the tip of actin filaments as a dot. However, on the PMC2A- and PMC3A-coated substrates, actin, and vinculin were not fully developed, suggesting that very few focal adhesions were observed on PMC2A and PMC3A. Although the shape of the NHDFs showed spreading on PMC4A, PMC5A, and PMC6A, focal adhesion with denser actin filament extension and vinculin localization was significant on the NHDFs adhered to PMC4A compared to those on PMC5A and PMC6A. In addition, the cells adhered to a coated substrate of PMCxAs were calculated using confocal images for various parameters, including area, circularity, and aspect ratio (Figure 4b–d). The round shape of the cells was observed on PMC2A- and PMC3A-coated substrates because of the limited spreading area, high circularity, and low aspect ratio. Contrasting results, such as a larger spreading area, a low circularity, and a higher aspect ratio, were observed on the PMC4A-coated substrate. Typically, focal adhesions are known to occur through interactions between integrin and ECM proteins [45,46]. In our previous reports, protein adsorption has already been shown to be suppressed on PMEA analog-coated surfaces compared with tissue culture polystyrene (TCPS) [25,32]. Hence, because of the adsorption of a limited amount of ECM proteins, focal adhesion formation was suppressed on PMC2A- and PMC3A-coated substrates. In contrast, the strong focal adhesion of cells on the PMC4A-coated substrate was attributed to the higher amount of adsorbed FN (Figure 3).

3.5. Immunoblotting Studies

The adhesion of fibroblasts onto biomaterial surfaces is generally carried out through the interaction between $\alpha 5\beta 1$ or $\alpha v\beta 3$ integrins and the cell-binding motif of adhesive proteins [9,19]. Integrin signaling in fibroblasts is related not only to cell adhesion and proliferation but also to fibroblast differentiation. Fibroblasts differentiate into α-SMA-expressing myofibroblasts [47]. As a marker of fibroblast-to-myofibroblast differentiation, the expression of α-SMA has already been recognized, the differentiation of which plays a vital role in accelerating wound repair [21,48]. Snail and vimentin expression is also associated with fibroblast differentiation and proliferation [49,50]. To further clarify the cell behavior on the PMCxAs, we measured the differential expression of cytoskeletal proteins, which could be a phenotypic marker of myofibroblasts, such as Snail, α-SMA, and vimentin, by immunoblotting (Figure 5). The ratio of band strength was calculated to assess the expression levels of proteins in cells (Figure 5b–d). Snail, α-SMA, and vimentin were more highly expressed in cells cultured on the PMC4A-coated substrate than in those cultured on other substrates. These results indicate that a robust integrin-dependent interaction between PMC4A and NHDF may induce myofibroblast differentiation. The function of FN in controlling cellular adhesion, migration, and differentiation has already been reported [42].

3.6. Cell Migration Test

The modulation of fibroblast-to-myofibroblast differentiation and fibroblast migration is essential for the development of wound dressing materials [51]. Cell migration is the directionality of cells migrating toward the wounded area. To evaluate whether PMCxA substrates could be utilized in wound healing, a migration test was performed using the scratch procedure. The migration of NHDFs, migration area, and healing rate in the wound region are shown in Figure 6a–c, respectively. Figure 6a shows that the area of the scratch was significant at 0 h, while the region decreased from 0 to 24 and 48 h. The migration area was found to increase over time (Figure 6b), which implies the migration of cells towards the wound via autocrine or paracrine mechanisms [51]. Figure 6c also shows that the migration rate of cells on the substrate coated with PMC2A (4.81 µm/h; slope from Figure 6b and PMC3A (5.72 µm/h) was lower than that on the other substrates. It is crucial that the cells on PMC4A substrates migrate rapidly to the scratched area, resulting in a rapid decline in the area (12.47 µm/h). For PMC5A- and PMC6A-coated substrates, cells also migrated to the scratched area. Although the migration rate was lower than that on PMC4A, the differences were not significant compared with those on PET and other substrates. The fibroblast-to-myofibroblast differentiation is attributed to the expression of a phenotypic marker of myofibroblasts and the increase in the migration of cells [49,50]. Therefore, it suggested that the increase in the migration of NHDFs on PMC4A was accompanied by the fibroblast-to-myofibroblast differentiation, whereas PMC2A suppressed the migration of NHDFs and the differentiation.

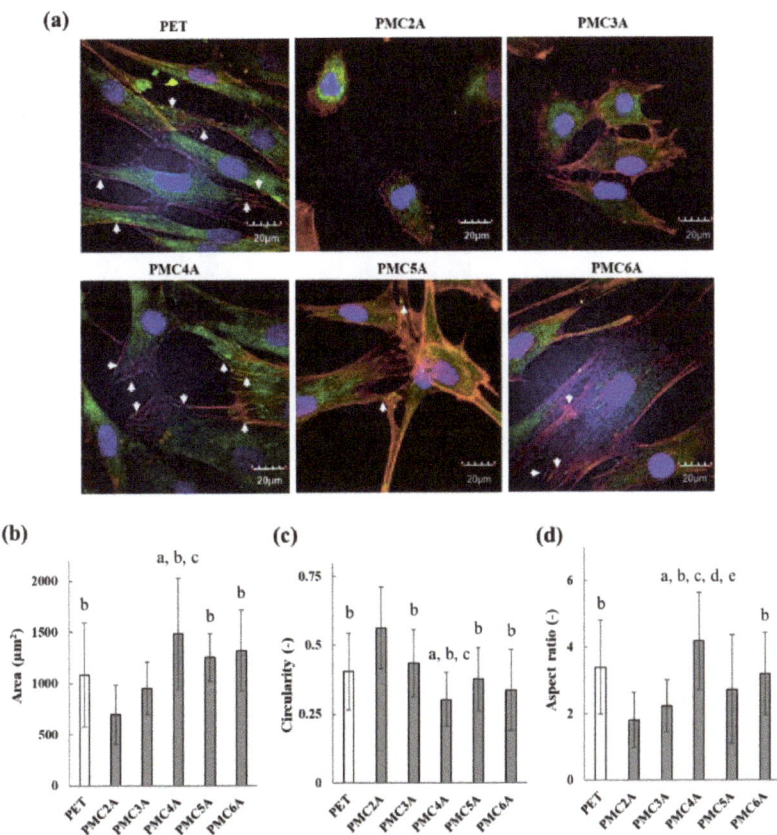

Figure 4. (a) CLSM photos of PMC*x*A-coated substrates for focal adhesion formation. Blue: cell nuclei; green: vinculin; red: actin fibers. Arrows indicate focal adhesion. Cell morphologies were determined by (b) spreading area, (c) circularity, and (d) aspect ratios of NHDFs on PMC*x*A-coated substrates calculated from CLSM images. The data represent the mean ± SD (n = 15, [a] $p < 0.05$ compared with PET, [b] $p < 0.05$ compared with PMC2A, [c] $p < 0.05$ compared with PMC3A, [d] $p < 0.05$ compared with PMC5A, [e] $p < 0.05$ compared with PMC6A; Tukey's multiple comparisons test). Each experiment was carried out at least three times.

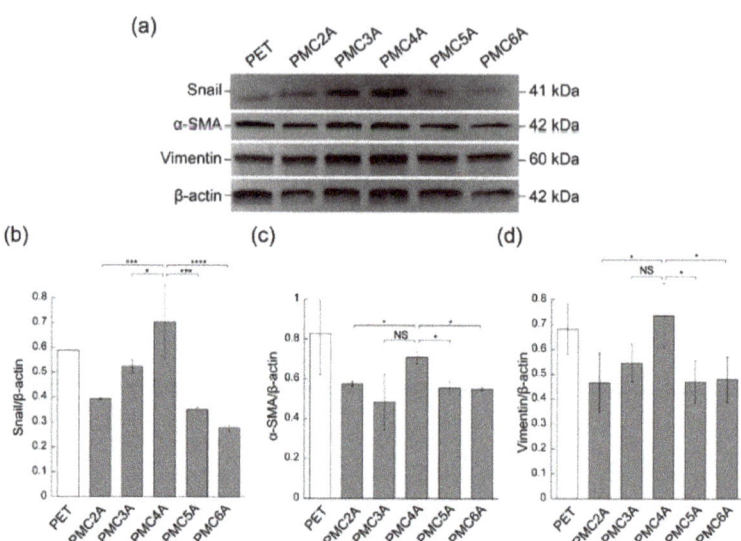

Figure 5. (**a**) Immunoblotting analysis for Snail, α-SMA, vimentin, and β-actin in NHDF cultured on PET, PMC2A, PMC3A, PMC4A, PMC5A, and PMC6A. (**b–d**) The band intensity for (**b**) Snail/β-actin, (**c**) α-SMA/β-actin, and (**d**) vimentin/β-actin ($n = 3$, * $p < 0.05$, *** $p < 0.001$, **** $p < 0.0001$; Tukey's multiple comparisons test).

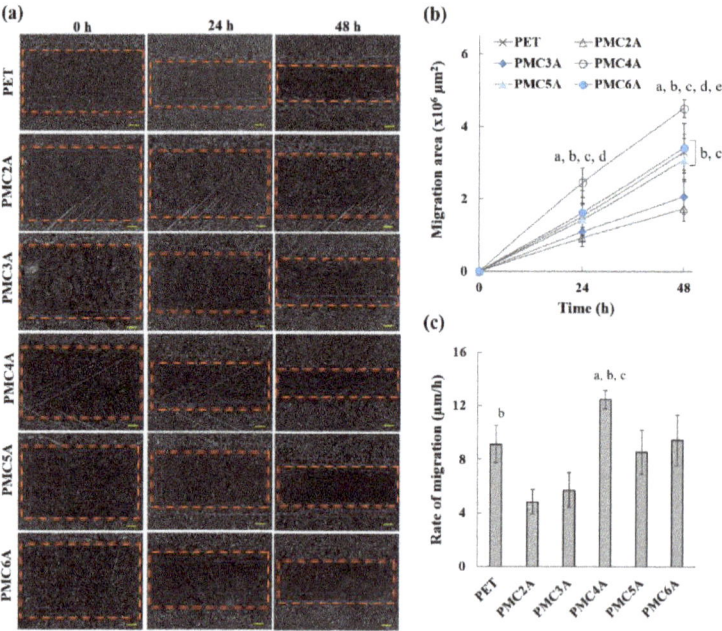

Figure 6. (**a**) Microscopic images of cell migration of NHDFs, (**b**) migration area, and (**c**) rate of migration on PMCxA-coated substrates (scale bar = 300 μm). The data represent the mean ± SD ($n = 5$, [a] $p < 0.05$ compared with PET, [b] $p < 0.05$ compared with PMC2A, [c] $p < 0.05$ compared with PMC3A, [d] $p < 0.05$ compared with PMC5A, [e] $p < 0.05$ compared with PMC6A; Tukey's multiple comparisons test).

3.7. Total Collagen Measurement

In wound healing, the function of collagen is associated with the attraction of fibroblasts and the secretion of new collagen at the injured location [52]. To verify the possibility of wound healing, it is important to determine whether the secretion of collagen from NHDFs is promoted on PMCxA-coated substrates. In this experiment, a comparatively higher density of NHDFs was plated on PMCxA-coated substrates to prevent proliferation and accelerate collagen growth. The concentration of secreted collagen from the cells was measured (Figure 7). Collagen secretion was significantly higher for substrates coated with PMC4A than for other substrates. Collagen secretion for PMC5A- and PMC6A-coated substrates was similar to that for PET. For PMC2A, however, a significantly lower collagen output was observed in NHDFs. Hence, it suggested PMC4A could recruit the fibroblast which secreted a large amount of collagen while the secretion of collagen from fibroblast was reduced by PMC2A. The regulation of the amount of collagen plays an important role in restoring the strength and function of wound tissue [52]. PMCxA may be utilized in the wound healing process to adjust the amount of collagen to be suitable for the tissue.

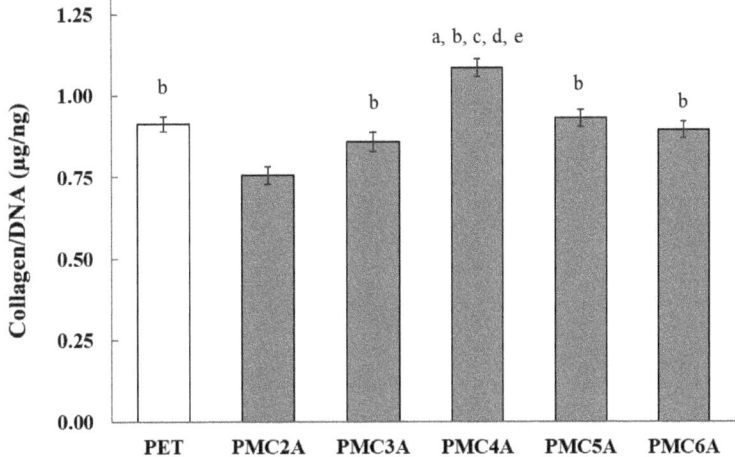

Figure 7. Total soluble collagen production by NHDFs on PMCxA substrates. The data represent the mean ± SD (n = 5, [a] p < 0.05 compared with PET, [b] p < 0.05 compared with PMC2A, [c] p < 0.05 compared with PMC3A, [d] p < 0.05 compared with PMC5A, [e] p < 0.05 compared with PMC6A; Tukey's multiple comparisons test).

In the present study, we revealed that PMC4A enhanced fibroblast-to-myofibroblast differentiation, cell migration, and collagen synthesis and secretion in adhered NHDFs, while PMC2A suppressed these functions in the cells. PMCxAs were polymers whose properties, such as hydrophobicity, T_g, and hydration water content, were modulated systematically with the change in the number of methylene carbons on the side chain. Several studies have reported that cell migration, proliferation, and differentiation are influenced by physicochemical properties such as stiffness and hydration water content on the substrates. Engler et al. demonstrated that mesenchymal stem cells migrated to stiffer regions on hydrogels with different degrees of stiffness, known as durotaxis [53,54]. Han et al. reported that vascular smooth muscle cells were perceived to migrate towards the low hydration side of poly(sodium 4-styrenesulfonate)/poly(diallyl dimethylammonium) chloride multilayers with swelling differences [55]. Evans et al. reported that cells can sense underlying stiff material through a soft layer at low (<10 µm) thickness [56]. Because the thickness of the PMEA derivative polymer-coated layer, which was coated by almost the same procedure as used in the present study on the PET substrates and was determined to be around 80 nm, the effect of stiffness attributed to the PMCxA layer would not be predominant, but that of PET was [57]. Therefore, hydration water content, hydrophobicity, and mobility of PMCxAs might affect the NHDFs' behavior. We summarized the behavior of NHDFs adhered to the PMCxAs as shown in Figure 8. By changing the number of methylene carbons, PMCxAs-coating modulated the amount of adsorbed fibronectin, hydrophobicity, and hydration water content on the substrates, leading to the change in NHDFs' behavior. However, the cell behavior did not change with the increasing number of methylene carbons of PMCxAs, resulting in PMC4A bearing the intermediate properties among PMCxAs' significantly activated fibroblast behavior. Therefore, it suggested that there was an optimal value of parameters of polymer to activate the cells. The detailed mechanism of activation of cells by PMCxAs requires further investigation.

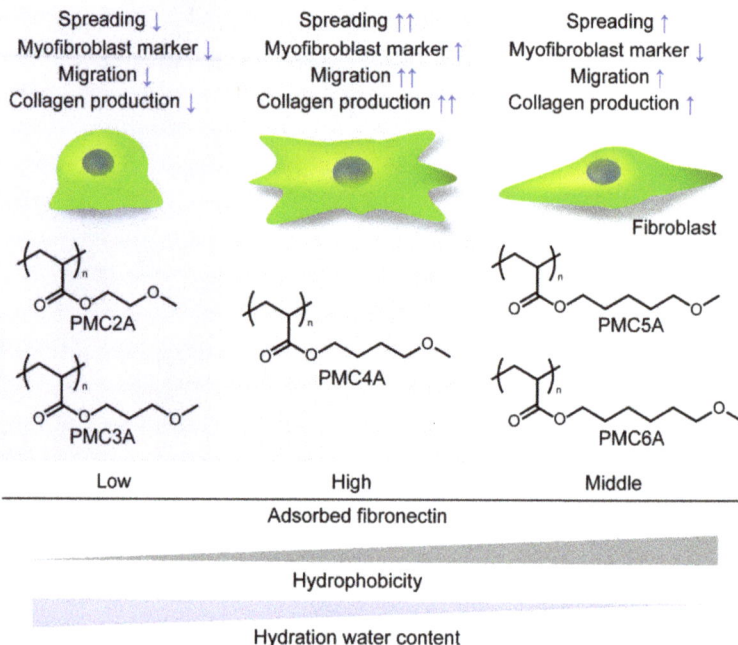

Figure 8. Schematic drawing of cellular behavior on PMCxA-coated substrates.

The required function of wound healing materials is different for wound type, phase, and size [58]. In this regard, PMCxAs could tune the fibroblast behavior such as fibroblast-to-myofibroblast differentiation, cell migration, and collagen synthesis and secretion with the number of methylene carbon on the side chain. Hence, PMCxAs are anticipated to be successful materials for use in wound healing, with the ability to modulate cellular function.

4. Conclusions

One aspect of modern medical treatment is the control of cellular behavior, including adhesion, recruitment, and differentiation on the implant surface to avoid biological rejection and accelerate tissue repair. Fibroblast cells have a variety of functions that are mainly involved in the secretion of several cytokines and matrix proteins in the regulation of the immune response and tissue regeneration [10]. Differentiated myofibroblasts from fibroblasts induce the production of matrix proteins that allow dermal regeneration [11]. In the present study, PMEA analog polymers (PMCxAs) were chosen as coating materials to control the cell adhesion and growth behavior of fibroblasts, as the series of polymers modulate hydrophobicity, hydration water content, and protein adsorption by increasing the number of methylene groups in the side chain. As a result, PMC4A coating was found to induce a greater spreading of cells, protein adsorption, focal adhesion formation, migration, expression of α-SMA on NHDFs, and collagen production. By contrast, the activation of NHDF adhered to PMC2A was lower than that adhered to other PMCxAs. According to the analysis of fibroblast behavior regulation, PMCxAs show promise as coating materials for biomaterials, such as biodegradable mesh-like materials for applications in wound healing.

Author Contributions: Conceptualization: T.A. and K.N.; methodology: R.A., K.N., H.M., S.K., T.A. and M.T.; formal analysis: R.A., K.N. and T.A.; investigation: R.A., K.N., H.M., S.K. and T.A.; data curation: R.A., K.N., T.A. and M.T.; writing—original draft preparation: R.A., K.N., T.A. and M.T.; writing—review and editing: R.A., K.N., D.M., S.K., T.A. and M.T.; visualization: R.A., K.N. and T.A.; supervision: T.A. and M.T.; project administration: M.T.; funding acquisition: M.T. All authors have read and agreed to the published version of the manuscript.

Funding: This study was funded by the Japan Society for the Promotion of Science (JSPS) (19H05720) from the Ministry of Education, Culture, Sports, Science, and Technology of Japan.

Institutional Review Board Statement: Not applicable.

Informed Consent Statement: Not applicable.

Data Availability Statement: The data presented in this study are available on request from the corresponding author.

Acknowledgments: We thank the Government of Japan (MEXT) for providing the scholarship for conducting a higher study and research at Kyushu University. We also thank the Cooperative Research Program "Dynamic Alliance for Open Innovation Bridging Human, Environment and Materials".

Conflicts of Interest: The authors declare no conflict of interest.

References

1. Schindhelm, K.; Milthorpe, B.K. Overview of biomaterials. *Australas. Phys. Eng. Sci. Med.* **1986**, *9*, 29–32. [CrossRef] [PubMed]
2. Teo, A.J.; Mishra, A.; Park, I.; Kim, Y.J.; Park, W.T.; Yoon, Y.J. Polymeric biomaterials for medical implants and devices. *ACS Biomater. Sci. Eng.* **2016**, *2*, 454–472. [CrossRef]
3. Saini, M. Implant biomaterials: A comprehensive review. *World J. Clin. Cases* **2015**, *3*, 52–57. [CrossRef]
4. Ou, S.F.; Chen, C.S.; Hosseinkhani, H.; Yu, C.H.; Shen, Y.D.; Ou, K.L. Surface properties of nano-structural silicon-doped carbon films for biomedical applications. *Int. J. Nanotechnol.* **2013**, *10*, 945–958. [CrossRef]
5. Chen, H.; Yuan, L.; Song, W.; Wu, Z.; Li, D. Biocompatible polymer materials: Role of protein-surface interactions. *Prog. Polym. Sci.* **2008**, *33*, 1059–1087. [CrossRef]
6. Rahmati, M.; Silva, E.A.; Reseland, J.E.; Heyward, C.A.; Haugen, H.J. Biological responses to physicochemical properties of biomaterial surface. *Chem. Soc. Rev.* **2020**, *49*, 5178–5224. [CrossRef]
7. Cai, S.; Wu, C.; Yang, W.; Liang, W.; Yu, H.; Liu, L. Recent advance in surface modification for regulating cell adhesion and behaviors. *Nanotechnol. Rev.* **2020**, *9*, 971–989. [CrossRef]
8. Wong, T.; McGrath, J.A.; Navsaria, H. The role of fibroblasts in tissue engineering and regeneration. *Br. J. Dermatol.* **2007**, *156*, 1149–1155. [CrossRef]
9. Sriram, G.; Bigliardi, P.L.; Bigliardi-Qi, M. Fibroblast heterogeneity and its implications for engineering organotypic skin models in vitro. *Eur. J. Cell Biol.* **2015**, *94*, 483–512. [CrossRef] [PubMed]
10. Ko, U.H.; Choi, J.; Choung, J.; Moon, S.; Shin, J.H. Physicochemically tuned myofibroblasts for wound healing strategy. *Sci. Rep.* **2019**, *9*, 16070. [CrossRef]
11. Mori, L.; Bellini, A.; Stacey, M.A.; Schmidt, M.; Mattoli, S. Fibrocytes contribute to the myofibroblast population in wounded skin and originate from the bone marrow. *Exp. Cell Res.* **2005**, *304*, 81–90. [CrossRef]
12. Bharath Rao, K.; Malathi, N.; Narashiman, S.; Rajan, S.T. Evaluation of myofibroblasts by expression of alpha smooth muscle actin: A marker in fibrosis, dysplasia and carcinoma. *J. Clin. Diagn. Res.* **2014**, *8*, 14–17. [CrossRef]
13. Honda, E.; Park, A.M.; Yoshida, K.; Tabuchi, M.; Munakata, H. Myofibroblasts: Biochemical and proteomic approaches to fibrosis. *Tohoku J. Exp. Med.* **2013**, *230*, 67–73. [CrossRef] [PubMed]
14. Witherel, C.E.; Abebayehu, D.; Barker, T.H.; Spiller, K.L. Macrophage and fibroblast interactions in biomaterial-mediated fibrosis. *Adv. Healthc. Mater.* **2019**, *8*, 1–35. [CrossRef] [PubMed]
15. Kerch, G. Polymer hydration and stiffness at biointerfaces and related cellular processes. *Nanomed. Nanotechnol. Biol. Med.* **2018**, *14*, 13–25. [CrossRef] [PubMed]
16. Chen, L.; Yan, C.; Zheng, Z. Functional polymer surfaces for controlling cell behaviors. *Mater. Today* **2018**, *21*, 38–59. [CrossRef]
17. Bacakova, L.; Filova, E.; Parizek, M.; Ruml, T.; Svorcik, V. Modulation of cell adhesion, proliferation and differentiation on materials designed for body implants. *Biotechnol. Adv.* **2011**, *29*, 739–767. [CrossRef]

18. Wang, X.; Hu, X.; Dulinska-Molak, I.; Kawazoe, N.; Yang, Y.; Chen, G. Discriminating the independent influence of cell adhesion and spreading area on stem cell fate determination using micropatterned surfaces. *Sci. Rep.* **2016**, *6*, 28708. [CrossRef] [PubMed]
19. Wozniak, M.A.; Modzelewska, K.; Kwong, L.; Keely, P.J. Focal adhesion regulation of cell behavior. *Biochim. Biophys. Acta Mol. Cell Res.* **2004**, *1692*, 103–119. [CrossRef]
20. Wysotzki, P.; Gimsa, J. Surface coatings modulate the differences in the adhesion forces of eukaryotic and prokaryotic cells as detected by single cell force microscopy. *Int. J. Biomater.* **2019**, *2019*, 7024259. [CrossRef]
21. Nedela, O.; Slepicka, P.; Švorčík, V. Surface modification of polymer substrates for biomedical applications. *Materials* **2017**, *10*, 1115. [CrossRef]
22. Ye, Z.; Hiroyasu, K.; Yuya, S.; Kano, M.; Tada-Aki, K.; Shimizu, Y. MPC polymer regulates fibrous tissue formation by modulating cell adhesion to the biomaterial surface. *Dent. Mater. J.* **2010**, *29*, 518–528. [CrossRef]
23. Tanaka, M.; Motomura, T.; Kawada, M.; Anzai, T.; Kasori, Y.; Shiroya, T.; Shimura, K.; Onishi, M.; Mochizuki, A. Blood compatible aspects of poly(2-methoxyethylacrylate) (PMEA)-relationship between protein adsorption and platelet adhesion on PMEA surface. *Biomaterials* **2000**, *21*, 1471–1481. [CrossRef]
24. Hoshiba, T.; Nikaido, M.; Tanaka, M. Characterization of the attachment mechanisms of tissue-derived cell lines to blood-compatible polymers. *Adv. Healthc. Mater.* **2014**, *3*, 775–784. [CrossRef]
25. Hoshiba, T.; Nemoto, E.; Sato, K.; Orui, T.; Otaki, T.; Yoshihiro, A.; Tanaka, M. Regulation of the contribution of integrin to Cell attachment on poly(2-methoxyethyl acrylate) (PMEA) analogous polymers for attachment-based cell enrichment. *PLoS ONE* **2015**, *10*, e0136066. [CrossRef] [PubMed]
26. Tanaka, M.; Hayashi, T.; Morita, S. The roles of water molecules at the biointerface of medical polymers. *Polym. J.* **2013**, *45*, 701–710. [CrossRef]
27. Miwa, Y.; Ishida, H.; Saitô, H.; Tanaka, M.; Mochizuki, A. Network structures and dynamics of dry and swollen poly(acrylate)s. Characterization of high- and low-frequency motions as revealed by suppressed or recovered intensities (SRI) analysis of 13C NMR. *Polymer* **2009**, *50*, 6091–6099. [CrossRef]
28. Morita, S.; Tanaka, M.; Ozaki, Y. Time-resolved in situ ATR-IR observations of the process of sorption of water into a poly(2-methoxyethyl acrylate) film. *Langmuir* **2007**, *23*, 3750–3761. [CrossRef] [PubMed]
29. Tanaka, M.; Mochizuki, A. Effect of water structure on blood compatibility—Thermal analysis of water in poly(meth)acrylate. *J. Biomed. Mater. Res. Part A* **2004**, *68*, 684–695. [CrossRef]
30. Tanaka, M.; Sato, K.; Kitakami, E.; Kobayashi, S.; Hoshiba, T.; Fukushima, K. Design of biocompatible and biodegradable polymers based on intermediate water concept. *Polym. J.* **2015**, *47*, 114–121. [CrossRef]
31. Tanaka, M.; Kobayashi, S.; Murakami, D.; Aratsu, F.; Kashiwazaki, A.; Hoshiba, T.; Fukushima, K. Design of polymeric biomaterials: The "Intermediate water concept.". *Bull. Chem. Soc. Jpn.* **2019**, *92*, 2043–2057. [CrossRef]
32. Hoshiba, T.; Nemoto, E.; Sato, K.; Maruyama, H.; Endo, C.; Tanaka, M. Promotion of adipogenesis of 3T3-L1 cells on protein adsorption-suppressing poly(2-methoxyethyl acrylate) analogs. *Biomacromolecules* **2016**, *17*, 3808–3815. [CrossRef]
33. Kobayashi, S.; Wakui, M.; Iwata, Y.; Tanaka, M. Poly(ω-methoxyalkyl acrylate)s: Nonthrombogenic polymer family with tunable protein adsorption. *Biomacromolecules* **2017**, *18*, 4214–4223. [CrossRef] [PubMed]
34. Jonkman, J.E.; Cathcart, J.A.; Xu, F.; Bartolini, M.E.; Amon, J.E.; Stevens, K.M.; Colarusso, P. An introduction to the wound healing assay using live-cell microscopy. *Cell Adhes. Migr.* **2014**, *8*, 440–451. [CrossRef] [PubMed]
35. Kumar, P.; Satyam, A.; Fan, X.; Collin, E.; Rochev, Y.; Rodriguez, B.J.; Gorelov, A.; Dillon, S.; Joshi, L.; Raghunath, M.; et al. Macromolecularly crowded in vitro microenvironments accelerate the production of extracellular matrix-rich supramolecular assemblies. *Sci. Rep.* **2015**, *5*, 8729. [CrossRef] [PubMed]
36. Bachhuka, A.; Hayball, J.; Smith, L.E.; Vasilev, K. Effect of surface chemical functionalities on collagen deposition by primary human dermal fibroblasts. *ACS Appl. Mater. Interfaces* **2015**, *7*, 23767–23775. [CrossRef]
37. Bathawab, F.; Bennett, M.; Cantini, M.; Reboud, J.; Dalby, M.J.; Salmerón-Sánchez, M. Lateral chain length in polyalkyl acrylates determines the mobility of fibronectin at the cell/material interface. *Langmuir* **2016**, *32*, 800–809. [CrossRef]
38. Xing, F.; Li, L.; Zhou, C.; Long, C.; Wu, L.; Lei, H.; Kong, Q.; Fan, Y.; Xiang, Z.; Zhang, X. Regulation and directing stem cell fate by tissue engineering functional microenvironments: Scaffold physical and chemical cues. *Stem Cells Int.* **2019**, *2019*, 2180925. [CrossRef]
39. Guerra, N.B.; González-García, C.; Llopis, V.; Rodríguez-Hernández, J.C.; Moratal, D.; Rico, P.; Salmerón-Sánchez, M. Subtle variations in polymer chemistry modulate substrate stiffness and fibronectin activity. *Soft Matter* **2010**, *6*, 4748–4755. [CrossRef]
40. Wong, J.Y.; Leach, J.B.; Brown, X.Q. Balance of chemistry, topography, and mechanics at the cell-biomaterial interface: Issues and challenges for assessing the role of substrate mechanics on cell response. *Surf. Sci.* **2004**, *570*, 119–133. [CrossRef]
41. Ngandu Mpoyi, E.; Cantini, M.; Reynolds, P.M.; Gadegaard, N.; Dalby, M.J.; Salmerón-Sánchez, M. Protein adsorption as a key mediator in the nanotopographical control of cell behavior. *ACS Nano* **2016**, *10*, 6638–6647. [CrossRef] [PubMed]
42. Parisi, L.; Toffoli, A.; Ghezzi, B.; Mozzoni, B.; Lumetti, S.; Macaluso, G.M. A glance on the role of fibronectin in controlling cell response at biomaterial interface. *Jpn. Dent. Sci. Rev.* **2020**, *56*, 50–55. [CrossRef] [PubMed]
43. Khalili, A.A.; Ahmad, M.R. A Review of cell adhesion studies for biomedical and biological applications. *Int. J. Mol. Sci.* **2015**, *16*, 18149–18184. [CrossRef]
44. Kanchanawong, P.; Shtengel, G.; Pasapera, A.M.; Ramko, E.B.; Davidson, M.W.; Hess, H.F.; Waterman, C.M. Nanoscale architecture of integrin-based cell adhesions. *Nature* **2010**, *468*, 580–584. [CrossRef] [PubMed]

25. Ziegler, W.H.; Liddington, R.C.; Critchley, D.R. The structure and regulation of vinculin. *Trends Cell Biol.* **2006**, *16*, 453–460. [CrossRef] [PubMed]
26. Gu, J.; Sumida, Y.; Sanzen, N.; Sekiguchi, K. Laminin-10/11 and fibronectin differentially regulate integrin-dependent Rho and Rac activation via p130Cas-CrkII-DOCK180 pathway. *J. Biol. Chem.* **2001**, *276*, 27090–27097. [CrossRef]
27. Hinz, B.; Celetta, G.; Tomasek, J.J.; Gabbiani, G.; Chaponnier, C. Alpha-smooth muscle actin expression upregulates fibroblast contractile activity. *Mol. Biol. Cell* **2001**, *12*, 2730–2741. [CrossRef]
28. Shinde, A.V.; Humeres, C.; Frangogiannis, N.G. The role of α-smooth muscle actin in fibroblast-mediated matrix contraction and remodeling. *Biochim. Biophys. Acta Mol. Basis Dis.* **2017**, *1863*, 298–309. [CrossRef]
29. Franz, M.; Spiegel, K.; Umbreit, C.; Richter, P.; Codina-Canet, C.; Berndt, A.; Altendorf-Hofmann, A.; Koscielny, S.; Hyckel, P.; Kosmehl, H.; et al. Expression of Snail is associated with myofibroblast phenotype development in oral squamous cell carcinoma. *Histochem. Cell Biol.* **2009**, *131*, 651–660. [CrossRef]
30. Cheng, F.; Shen, Y.; Mohanasundaram, P.; Lindström, M.; Ivaska, J.; Ny, T.; Erikss, J.E. Vimentin coordinates fibroblast proliferation and keratinocyte differentiation in wound healing via TGF-β-Slug signaling. *Proc. Natl. Acad. Sci. USA* **2016**, *113*, E4320–E4327. [CrossRef]
31. Tottoli, E.M.; Dorati, R.; Genta, I.; Chiesa, E.; Pisani, S.; Conti, B. Skin wound healing process and new emerging technologies for skin wound care and regeneration. *Pharmaceutics* **2020**, *12*, 735. [CrossRef]
32. Rangaraj, A.; Harding, K.; Leaper, D. Role of collagen in wound management. *Drug Invent. Today* **2020**, *13*, 55–57.
33. Kennedy, K.M.; Bhaw-Luximon, A.; Jhurry, D. Cell-matrix mechanical interaction in electrospun polymeric scaffolds for tissue engineering: Implications for scaffold design and performance. *Acta Biomater.* **2017**, *50*, 41–55. [CrossRef]
34. Tse, J.R.; Engler, A.J. Stiffness gradients mimicking in vivo tissue variation regulate mesenchymal stem cell fate. *PLoS ONE* **2011**, *6*, e15978. [CrossRef] [PubMed]
35. Han, L.; Mao, Z.; Wu, J.; Guo, Y.; Ren, T.; Gao, C. Directional cell migration through cell-cell interaction on polyelectrolyte multilayers with swelling gradients. *Biomaterials* **2013**, *34*, 975–984. [CrossRef] [PubMed]
36. Tusan, C.G.; Man, Y.H.; Zarkoob, H.; Johnston, D.A.; Andriotis, O.G.; Thurner, P.J.; Yang, S.; Sander, E.A.; Gentleman, E.; Sengers, B.G.; et al. Collective cell behavior in mechanosensing of substrate thickness. *Biophys. J.* **2018**, *114*, 2743–2755. [CrossRef] [PubMed]
37. Hoshiba, T.; Orui, T.; Endo, C.; Sato, K.; Yoshihiro, A.; Minagawa, Y.; Tanaka, M. Adhesion-based simple capture and recovery of circulating tumor cells using a blood-compatible and thermo-responsive polymer-coated substrate. *RSC Adv.* **2016**, *6*, 89103–89112. [CrossRef]
38. Okur, M.E.; Karantas, I.D.; Şenyiğit, Z.; Üstündağ Okur, N.; Siafaka, P.I. Recent trends on wound management: New therapeutic choices based on polymeric carriers. *Asian J. Pharm. Sci.* **2020**, *15*, 661–684. [CrossRef]

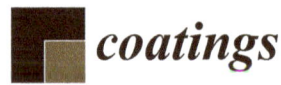

Article

Osteogenic and Antibacterial Activity of a Plasma-Sprayed CeO$_2$ Coating on a Titanium (Ti)-Based Dental Implant

Jing Yue [1,†], Zhichun Jin [2,†], Hin Lok Enoch Poon [3,4], Guangwei Shang [1], Haixia Liu [1], Dan Wang [3,4], Shengcai Qi [1], Fubo Chen [1,*] and Yuanzhi Xu [1,*]

1. Department of Stomatology, Shanghai Tenth People's Hospital, Tongji University School of Medicine, Shanghai 200072, China; jingyue624@163.com (J.Y.); gwshang99@yahoo.com (G.S.); 13673530995@163.com (H.L.); dentistqi@163.com (S.Q.)
2. Jiangsu Key Laboratory of Oral Diseases, Affiliated Hospital of Stomatology, Nanjing Medical University, Nanjing 211166, China; jinzhichun@126.com
3. Institute for Tissue Engineering and Regenerative Medicine, The Chinese University of Hong Kong, Hong Kong 999077, China; enochhlpoon@link.cuhk.edu.hk (H.L.E.P.); wangmd@cuhk.edu.hk (D.W.)
4. School of Biomedical Sciences, Faculty of Medicine, The Chinese University of Hong Kong, Hong Kong 999077, China
* Correspondence: chenfubo@126.com (F.C.); amyxyz01@hotmail.com (Y.X.); Tel.: +86-02166301722 (F.C.)
† Both contributed equally to this work.

Received: 11 September 2020; Accepted: 9 October 2020; Published: 21 October 2020

Abstract: Peri-implantitis, often induced by oral pathogens, is one of the main reasons for the clinical failure of dental implants. The aim of this study was to investigate the biocompatibility, osteogeneic, and antibacterial properties of a cerium oxide (CeO$_2$) coating containing high proportions of Ce^{4+} valences on a titanium-based dental implant biomaterial, Ti-6Al-4V. MC3T3-E1 cells or bone marrow stem cells (BMSCs) were seeded onto Ti-6Al-4V disks with or without CeO$_2$ coating. Compared to the control, the plasma-sprayed CeO$_2$ coating showed enhanced cell viability based on cell counting kit-8 (CCK-8) and flow cytometry assays. CCK-8, colony-forming unit test (CFU), and live-dead staining illustrated the antibacterial activity of CeO$_2$ coating. Additionally, CeO$_2$ coating upregulated the gene expression levels of osteogenic markers *ALP*, *Bsp* and *Ocn*, with a similar increase in protein expression levels of OCN and Smad 1 in both MC3T3-E1 cells and BMSCs. More importantly, the viability and proliferation of *Enterococcus faecalis*, *Prevotella intermedia*, and *Porphyromonas gingivalis* were significantly decreased on the CeO$_2$-coated Ti-6Al-4V surfaces compared to non-treated Ti-6Al-4V. In conclusion, the plasma-sprayed CeO$_2$ coating on the surface of Ti-6Al-4V exhibited strong biocompatibility, antibacterial, and osteogenic characteristics, with potential for usage in coated dental implant biomaterials for prevention of peri-implantitis.

Keywords: CeO$_2$ coating; antibacterial activity; biocompatibility; osteogenic differentiation

1. Introduction

Dental implantation, an indispensable and established dental therapy, is a widely adopted replacement for missing teeth in various clinical situations. Nevertheless, evidence from recent decades has shown an increasing presence of peri-implantitis associated with the use of dental implants [1]. Peri-implant mucositis was detected in approximately 60.2% of implants in 73.1% of patients, while peri-implantitis affected 12% of implants in 15.4% of patients [2]; The resultant inflammatory processes damage both soft and hard tissues surrounding the implants, which were attributed as a major cause of dental implant failures [3]. The occurrence of peri-implantitis is primarily traced to the presence of gram-negative anaerobic microflora [4], of which the species

Porphyromonas gingivalis (*P.g.*) and *Prevotella intermedia* (*P.i.*) are the dominant cause of periodontitis and peri-implantitis [5]. In addition, traces of *Enterococcus faecalis* (*E.f.*) can be found in the osseous environs of infected implants, indicating its involvement in peri-implantitis [6]. *E.f.* has been pervasive in dental infections and was adopted as a test for abutment seals in dental implant designs [7,8]. Furthermore, *E.f.* is known to tolerate physiologically harsh environments such as high-pH alkaline conditions and nutritional deficiency. Thus, it has been a recurrent challenge for dentists to eliminate *E.f. P.g.* and *P.i.* in peri-implantitis.

Titanium (Ti)-based dental implants are widely employed due to their superior osseointegration properties beneficial to the structural integrity and durability of the implants [9,10], with the titanium alloy Ti-6AL-4V frequently adopted due to its intrinsic mechanical strength and resistance as compared to pure titanium [11]. Due to severe consequences of peri-implantitis brought on the integrity of dental implants, strategies for treatment or prevention of peri-implantitis are an important area of discussion [12]. Much of the published strategies for peri-implantitis therapy focus on treatments similar to those adopted for periodontitis [13–17]. Compared to treatment, prevention is the more important strategy along with appropriate treatment planning, continuous check-up intervals, and professional teeth/implant cleaning [1]. Currently, antibacterial surface coatings on dental implants have attracted great attention due to the ease in applying on dental implant surfaces without impacting its physical properties [18]. Various titanium-based dental implant surfaces can be obtained in different ways, such as machining, acid etching, anodization, plasma spraying, grit blasting, or combination techniques yielding materials with smooth or microroughened surfaces [19]. Thus, ideal surface coatings for dental implants should prevent polymicrobial infection while enabling excellent osseointegration [20]. Plasma-sprayed biocoatings on Ti-6Al-4V, which have a significantly greater bonding strength compared with Ti-6Al-4V substrata, are potential biomaterials for implant applications [21,22]. Previous research has elucidated the osteogenic properties of cerium oxide (CeO_2)-incorporated hydroxyapatite coatings on Ti-6Al-4V [23]. Furthermore, previous work has shown that a higher percentage of Ce^{4+} valence states promoted the osteogenic behaviors of bone marrow stem cells (BMSCs), potentially benefitting its inclusion in dental implant applications [24]. However, the antibacterial of the high percentage of Ce^{4+} in CeO_2 coatings on Ti-6Al-4V implants has yet to be reported in literature.

In this study, a CeO_2 coating with high percentage of Ce4+ valences was applied via plasma spraying technique onto Ti-6Al-4V substrates. The antibacterial effects of CeO_2 on *E.f.*, *P.g.*, and *P.i.* were investigated in vitro via CCK-8, CFU, and live-dead cell staining assays, with flow cytometry performed as further validation of the results. The biocompatibility and osteogenic activity of the CeO_2 coating on both MC3T3-E1 cells and human bone marrow stem cells (BMSCs) was evaluated by CCK-8, real-time PCR, and Western blot.

2. Materials and Methods

The entire study was performed according to informed protocols approved by the Ethics Committee of Shanghai Tenth People's Hospital, Tongji University School of Medicine.

2.1. Preparation and Characterization of the CeO_2 Coating

CeO_2 powder was prepared via a high-temperature solid-state reaction using CeO_2 (A.R., SCRC, China) as the raw material. An atmosphere plasma spraying (APS) system (F4-MB, Sulzer Metco, Switzerland) was applied to fabricate the coating on the Ti-6Al-4V substrate with dimensions of ø 34 mm × 1 mm and ø 10 mm × 1 mm. Detailed preparation of the powders and coating was described in a previous study [25]. Briefly, the plasma spray process used a direct current (DC) electric arc to generate a stream of high temperature ionized plasma gas, which acted as the spraying heat source. The CeO_2 powder was carried in an inert gas stream into the plasma jet where it was heated and propelled towards the Ti alloy substrate. The phase chemical composition of the powder-sprayed coating was measured using an X-ray diffractometer (XRD, D/max 2500 V, Rigiku, Tokyo, Japan) with Cu Kα radiation. Surface microstructure of the sprayed coating was observed by field emission scanning electron microscopy (FE-SEM, SU8200, Hitachi, Tokyo, Japan). The test samples were dehydrated using alcohol and sputter-coated with gold before the FE-SEM. Additionally, in order to quantify the ratio of Ce^{3+}/Ce^{4+} valence state in the CeO_2 coating, the coating samples were analyzed by X-ray photoelectron spectroscopy (XPS, MICRO-LAB 310F, Thermo Fisher Scientific, Waltham, MA, USA) Al ka X-ray source.

2.2. Cell Biocompatibility and Osteogenic Behaviors of the CeO_2 Coating

2.2.1. Cell Viability Assay

Primary mouse bone marrow-derived mesenchymal stem cells (BMSCs) were isolated from the bone marrow cavity of the tibias of 3-week-old C57BL/6 mice and cultured in BMSC growth medium (α-MEM medium containing 10% FBS, 100 U/mL penicillin and 100 mg/mL streptomycin). Briefly, aspirates were flushed with growth medium and seeded in 10 cm Petri dishes for 3 days. Adherent BMSCs were further cultured and expanded. Passage 3–6 cells were used in experiments.

Cell counting kit-8 (CCK-8; Dojindo Kagaku Co., Kumamoto, Japan) was used to analyze cell viability according to the manufacturer's protocols. BMSCs and MC3T3-E1 cells were used in this section. A total of 5×10^4 cells/well were seeded on the coating surfaces (φ 10 mm × 1 mm) in 24 well plate and cultured in 1 mL culture medium. After culturing for 3 days, the medium was replaced with 0.9 mL of culture medium and 0.1 mL of CCK-8 working solution for an additional culture duration of 3 h, with 100 μL of the reacted reagent extracted and transferred to a 96-well plate. Wells with identical concentrations CCK-8 working solution without cells were used as blank controls. Absorbance was measured using a microplate reader at 450 nm absorbance to reflect the number of viable cells per well. Cell viability was represented as the mean ± standard deviation (SD) of the absorbance obtained from five wells per group.

2.2.2. Cell Apoptosis Assay

Cellular apoptosis was determined using the Annexin V/FITC apoptosis detection kit (Beyotime, Nantong, China) conducted under flow cytometry. Briefly, MC3T3-E1 cells were seeded in a 6-well plate with a Ti-6Al-4V disk (φ 34 mm × 1 mm) coated with CeO_2 at a density of 2×10^5 cells/well. Cells cultured on 6-well plates with Ti-6Al-4V disks served as the control group. After culturing in 2 mL 10% FBS for 24 h, the cells were harvested by trypsinization and rinsed twice with PBS. The cell suspension was subsequently centrifuged at 1000 rpm for 3 min. Obtained cells were then resuspended in Annexin V and propidium iodide (PI) (BD Pharmingen, Franklin Lakes, NJ, USA) stain according to the manufacturer's instructions. Apoptotic cell fractions were analyzed by FACScan flow cytometry (Becton-Dickinson, San Jose, CA, USA). Early apoptotic cells (Q2: Annexin V+/PI− staining) and late apoptotic cells (Q4: Annexin V+/PI+ staining) were classified as undergoing apoptosis, with the proportion of these cells out of the total cell count was determined and presented.

2.2.3. Osteogenic Differentiation Assay

BMSCs cells with 2 mL culture medium were seeded on Ti-6Al-4V disks (φ 34 mm × 1 mm) with or without CeO_2 coating in 6-well plates at a density of 10^5 cells/well. After 24 h of incubation, the culture medium was replaced with equal volumes of osteoinduction medium. Cells seeded on Ti-6Al-4V disks without CeO_2 coating served as controls. The osteoinduction medium was composed of DMEM supplemented with 10% FBS, 1% antibiotics, 50 μg/mL ascorbic acid (Sigma, St Louis, MO, USA), 10 mmol/L sodium β-glycerophosphate (Sigma, St Louis, MO, USA), and 10 nmol/L dexamethasone (Sigma, St Louis, MO, USA). Quantitative real-time PCR (qPCR) was applied to test the expression of osteogenesis-associated genes including alkaline phosphatase (ALP), bone sialoprotein (BSP) and osteocalcin (OCN), with their respective primer sequences listed below. TRIzol reagent (Invitrogen, Carlsbad, CA, USA) was used to extract RNA at 0, 7, and 14 days. Then, the extracted RNA was translated into cDNA with a PCR kit (Takara, Japan). Finally, qPCR was performed with an ABI 7500

Real-Time PCR system (Applied Biosystems, Waltham, MA, USA) as follows: Hot start at 95 °C for 5 min in the holding stage; 95 °C for 10 s and 60 °C for 30 s for 40 cycles in the cycling stage; and 95 °C for 15 s, 60 °C for 1 min, and 60 °C for 15 s in the melt curve stage. The PCR products were normalized to GAPDH, and relative gene expression was calculated using the $2^{-\Delta\Delta Ct}$ method. Each sample was examined in triplicate. Sequences for the primers used in qPCR are as listed in Table 1.

Table 1. Sequences for the primers used in qPCR.

ALP	forward	5′-GCC CTC TCC AAG ACA TAT A-3′
	reverse	5′-CCA TGA TCA CGA TAT CC-3′
Bsp	forward	5′-AGG ACT GCC GAA AGG AAG GTT A-3′
	reverse	5′-AGT AGC GTG GCC GGT ACT TAA A-3′
Ocn	forward	5′-AGG GAG GAT CAA GTC CCG-3′
	reverse	5′-GAA CAG ACT CCG GCG CTA-3′
GAPDH	forward	5′-GGG AAG CCC ATC ACC ATC TT-3
	reverse	5′-GGG AAG CCC ATC ACC ATC TT-3

Following 14 days of culturing in osteogenic induction, BMSCs in respective groups were lysed using a protein extraction kit (Piece, Rockford, IL, USA). Protein concentrations were determined using a bicinchoninic acid protein assay kit (Piece, Rockford, IL, USA) according to the manufacturer's protocols. Briefly, equal amounts of protein per sample (25 µg) were separated and transferred onto nitrocellulose membranes (Millipore Corporation, Billerica, MA, USA). After blocking with 5% skim milk, the primary antibodies of rabbit anti-mouse Smad 1 (1:1000, Bioworld Technology, Inc., St Louis Park, MN, USA), rabbit anti-mouse OCN (1:500, Abcam, Inc., Cambridge, MA, USA), and rabbit anti-mouse GAPDH (1:5000, Proteintech, Inc., Wuhan, China) were applied to each group. The membranes were subsequently washed three times and incubated with goat anti-rabbit IRDye 680 (1:10,000; Invitrogen, USA). After the final wash, the membranes were visualized using an Odyssey LI-CDR system, with representative images captured.

2.3. Antibacterial Effects of the CeO$_2$ Coating on Ti-6Al-4V Disks

2.3.1. Direct Contact (DCT) and CCK-8 Tests

E.f. ATCC 29,212 (American Type Culture Collection, Manassas, VA, USA), P.g. ATCC 33,277 and P.i. ATCC 25,611 were chosen for this study. The bacteria were grown overnight in 3% tryptic soy broth (TSB) (3 g of TSB powder in 100 g of water), at 37 °C in an anaerobic environment (80% N_2, 10% H_2 and 10% CO_2). The bacteria were subsequently suspended and diluted to 10^6 cells/mL in 3% TSB culture medium.

For antibacterial analysis, direct contact tests were conducted to analyze antimicrobial activity. In brief, diluted cell suspensions (0.5 mL, 1×10^6/mL) of E.f., P.g., and P.i. were seeded onto six Ti-6Al-4V disks (ø 10 mm × 1 mm) coated with CeO2 in 24-well plates. Identical cell suspensions seeded on Ti-6Al-4V disks without coating were used as negative controls; simultaneously, wells with TSB culture medium but without bacteria were used as blank controls. After 24 h incubation, the bacteria on the disks were collected and resuspended in 1 mL of 3% TSB culture medium. Five duplicates per group, each containing 100 uL of the above bacterial suspension, was transferred into in 96-well plates. The absorbance of each well was measured at 630 nm with a microplate reader (Bio-Tek, Winooski, VT, USA).

Bacterial proliferation was evaluated by a CCK-8 assay kit (Dojindo Molecular Technologies, Inc., Kumamoto, Japan) in accordance with the manufacturer's protocols. 200 uL E.f., P.g., and P.i. cell suspension (1×10^6/mL) were seeded onto five CeO$_2$-coated Ti-6Al-4V disks per group (ø 10 mm × 1 mm) placed in 24-well plates. Then, 100 µL of the above surplus diluted bacterial suspensions with 10 µL of CCK-8 was added to a 96-well plate for another 2 h of culture. Wells with CCK-8 solution but without bacteria were used as blank controls. The absorbance of each well was measured by using a microplate reader at 450 nm. Cell viability was represented as the mean ± standard deviation (SD) of the absorbance for five wells from each group.

2.3.2. Colony-Forming Unit Test (CFU)

Two hundred microliters E.f., P.g., and P.i. cell suspension (1×10^6/mL) were seeded onto five CeO_2-coated Ti-6Al-4V disks per group (ø 34 mm × 1 mm). A film over the disk was used to help create contact and in an anaerobic environment. Ti-6Al-4V disks without coating were used as blanks. After 24 h culture, the microorganisms were subsequently removed from the samples and suspended in 1 mL of PBS in a cell culture dish. Twenty microliters of the above bacterial suspensions were then inoculated onto nutrient agar plates and cultured at 37 °C for 24 h. Colonies formed on the agar were viewed under light microscopy, with representative images captured and the number of cell colonies counted.

2.3.3. Live/dead Bacteria Staining

Antibacterial effects of the CeO_2 coating were further evaluated via live/dead staining. One hundred microliters of surplus E.f. bacteria suspended in PBS (from Section 2.3.2) were transferred to a culture plate and stained using a live/dead BacLight bacterial viability kit, in accordance with the manufacturer's instructions, and bacterial suspensions were chosen and imaged using confocal laser scanning microscopy (CLSM) (Carl Zeiss, Oberkochen, German) at excitation wavelengths of 488 nm (Calcein-AM) and 555 nm (propidium iodide). Then, the percent distribution of live and dead bacteria was analyzed according to the green and red fluorescence. Images were obtained with a 20× objective, and at least three images were collected randomly from each sample.

2.4. Statistical Analysis

All experiments were repeated thrice. Statistical analyses were conducted with using GraphPad Prism software, version 5.0 (GraphPad Software, Inc., La Jolla, CA, USA). Obtained results are expressed as the mean ± standard deviation (SD) and analyzed using one-way ANOVA with a post hoc test, with a p-value < 0.05 considered as statistically significant.

3. Results

3.1. Characterization of the CeO_2-Sprayed Coating

X-ray diffraction (XRD) patterns of the CeO_2 sprayed coating is used to infer its phase composition, with the results illustrated in Figure 1A. The coating was composed of the CeO_2 phase (JCPDS no. 34-0394) corresponding to the planes of (111, 200, 220, 311). The X-ray photoelectron spectra (XPS) of the CeO2 coating are shown in Figure 1B. The spectra revealed the presence of a mixed valence state (Ce^{3+} and Ce^{4+}) on the surface of the CeO_2-modified coating. For quantitative estimation of Ce^{3+} concentration in the CeO_2 coating, the ratio of Ce^{3+} in the total Ce content was calculated from the total areas under the Gaussian fitting peaks for each respective Ce^{3+} and Ce^{4+} state, using the equation for the ratio of peak areas reported in literature [26]; the percent of Ce^{4+} in the CeO_2 coating was calculated to be approximately 72.8%, indicating a major composition of Ce^{4+} valences present. SEM results shows the roughness of the CeO_2 coating in Figure 1C. The as-sprayed coating exhibited rough and uneven surfaces in the third electron image.

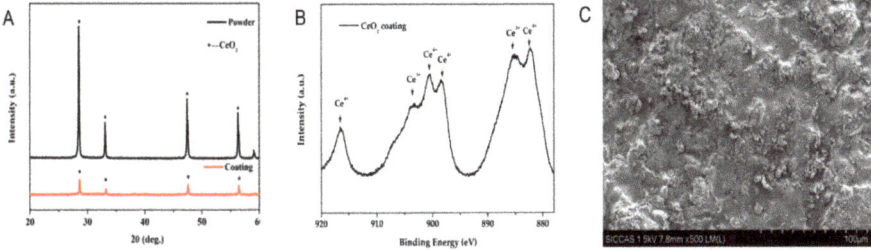

Figure 1. Structural and compositional characterization of the plasma-sprayed CeO_2 coating. (**A**) X-ray diffraction (XRD) patterns of the CeO_2 coating. Distribution of peaks were characteristic of CeO_2. (**B**) X-ray photoelectron spectroscopy spectra of the CeO_2 coating. The spectra revealed the presence of a mixed valence state (Ce^{3+} and Ce^{4+}) on the surface of the CeO_2 modified coatings, with Ce^{4+} accounting for 72.8% as calculated from the distribution ratio of their respective Gaussian fitting peaks. (**C**) SEM result revealed a rough texture present on the surface of the CeO_2 coating.

3.2. Biocompatibility of CeO_2 Coating

The biocompatibility of the CeO_2 coating in BMSCs and MC3T3-E1 cells was assessed by CCK-8 and cell apoptosis assays. CCK-8 results demonstrated no statistically significant difference in viability of BMSCs (Figure 2A) and MC3T3-E1 cells (Figure 2B) seeded on the CeO_2 coating, as compared to equivalent groups seeded on Ti-6Al-4V surface (#: $p > 0.05$). Similar results were observed from the flow cytometry analysis. Additionally, the percentage of apoptotic MC3T3-E1 cells (Q2 + Q4) seeded on the CeO_2 coating was statistically significantly lower than that on the Ti-6Al-4V surface (6.7% compared to 24.0%) as shown in Figure 2C. The above results indicated that the CeO_2 coating on the Ti-6Al-4V disks demonstrated good biocompatibility.

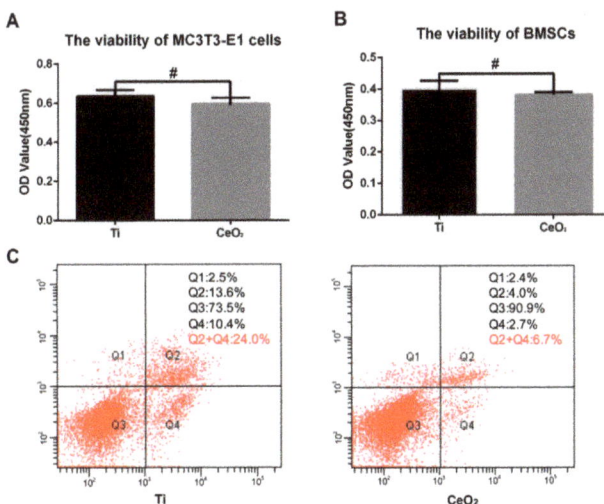

Figure 2. Biocompatibility of CeO_2 coating towards bone marrow stem cells (BMSCs) and MC3T3-E1 cells. (**A**,**B**) CCK-8 results demonstrated improved viability of BMSCs (**A**) and MC3T3-E1 cells (**B**) seeded on CeO2 coating after a 3-day culture period, as compared to uncoated Ti-6Al-4V surfaces (#: $p > 0.05$) ($n = 5$). (**C**) Flow cytometry analysis conducted on MC3T3-E1 cells cultured on CeO_2 coated Ti-6Al-4V surfaces. Percentage of apoptotic cells (Q2 + Q4) on the CeO_2 coating was measured at 6.7%, significantly lower than the percentage of apoptotic cells measured on the Ti-6Al-4V surface at 24.0% ($p < 0.05$) ($n = 3$).

3.3. Osteogenic Ability of the CeO$_2$ Coating

To directly address a functional role for the CeO$_2$ coating in osteogenic ability, the mRNA and protein expression of mineralization-related genes *ALP*, *Ocn*, and *Bsp* were measured after 7-day and 14-day BMSCs cell culture in osteoinduction medium. Compared with the control group, the CeO$_2$ coating significantly increased the mRNA levels of *ALP* (A), *Bsp* (B), and *Ocn* (C) ($p < 0.05$) at 7 and 14 days ($p < 0.01$), as shown in Figure 3A–C. Additionally, compared to groups cultivated on nontreated Ti-6Al-4V surface, the protein levels of OCN and Smad 1 were upregulated in the CeO$_2$ coating group at 14 days as shown in Figure 3D. These combined results indicate the ability of Ce^{4+}-rich CeO$_2$ coating in promoting osteogenesis in BMSCs.

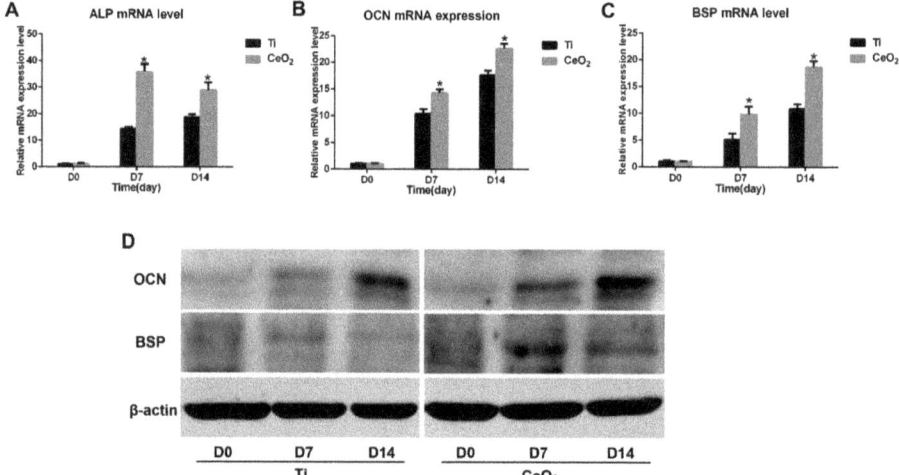

Figure 3. Osteogenic effect of CeO$_2$ coatings induced on BMSCs. (**A–C**) Expression levels of the osteogenic mRNA markers alkaline phosphatase (ALP), osteocalcin (OCN), and bone sialoprotein (BSP) at days 7 and 14 were significantly increased in CeO$_2$ groups as compared with uncoated Ti-6Al-4V control groups (*, $p < 0.05$;) ($n = 3$). (**D**) Western blot analysis of OCN, BSP, and β-actin protein expression levels level. Upregulation of both OCN and BSP of were observed in the CeO$_2$ coating group compared to the Ti-6Al-4V control group ($n = 3$).

3.4. Antibacterial Activity

E.f., P.g., and P.i. viability on the CeO$_2$ coating was assessed by DCT and CCK-8 assays to ascertain the antibacterial effects of the CeO$_2$ coating. DCT (Figure 4A) and CCK-8 (Figure 4B) results indicate a significant decrease in viability of E.f., P.g. and P.i. bacteria seeded on CeO$_2$ coating, as compared with corresponding groups seeded on pure Ti-6Al-4V discs. As shown in Figure 5, CFU results affirm similar findings with significantly lower bacterial viability on the CeO$_2$ coating compared to the respective control groups for E.f., P.g., and P.i. To further elucidate the antibacterial effects of the CeO$_2$ coating, live/dead staining of seeded E.f. bacteria (Figure 6A) show a significantly higher percent of dead bacteria (approximately 74.3%, stained in red) in the CeO$_2$ coating group, compared to the control group (approximately 4.1%) in Figure 6B. The combined results illustrate the antibacterial activity of the CeO$_2$ coating on the Ti-6Al-4V surface against E.f., P.g., and P.i., which are the main pathogens involved in peri-implantitis.

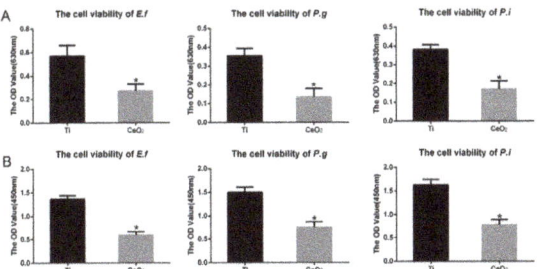

Figure 4. Viability of *E.f.*, *P.g.*, and *P.i.* seeded on CeO_2 coating. (**A**) DCT results indicate a significantly decreased viability of *E.f.*, *P.g.*, and *P.i.* on CeO_2 coatings as compared to the uncoated Ti-6Al-4V control group after 24 h culture. (**B**) CCK-8 results illustrate a similar trend of decreased viability among all CeO_2-coated groups after 24 h culture (*, $p < 0.05$;) ($n = 5$).

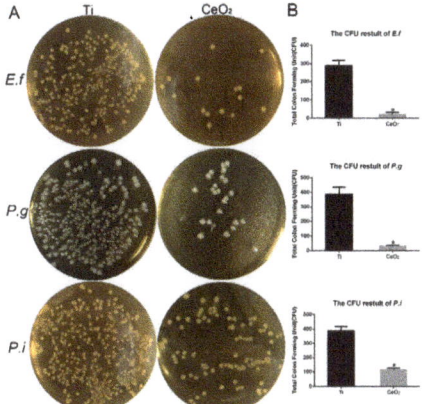

Figure 5. Colony-forming ability of *E.f.*, *P.g.*, and *P.i.* seeded on CeO_2 coating. (**A**) Observed under light microscopy, colony-forming unit (CFU) assays conducted after 24 h culture indicate a significant decrease in the number of *E.f.*, *P.g.*, and *P.i.* colonies on the CeO_2 coating as compared to the control group. (**B**) Statistical analysis indicates significantly reduced CFU numbers among all CeO_2 experimental groups. (*, $p < 0.05$;) ($n = 3$).

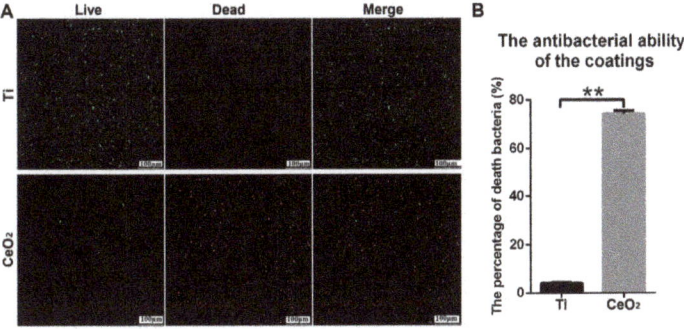

Figure 6. Live/dead staining of *E.f* seeded on CeO_2 coating. (**A**) Staining results of live *E.f* cells (staining with green) and dead *E.f* cells (staining with red) illustrate decreased viability in *E.f* cells seeded on CeO_2-coated Ti-6Al-4V discs. (**B**) Statistical analysis reveals the percentage of dead *E.f* cells was approximately 74.3% in the CeO_2-coated group, significantly higher than the percentage of dead *E.f* cells (4.1%) measured in the control group. (**, $p < 0.01$).

4. Discussion

Titanium and its alloys (most significantly grade 5 titanium alloy, Ti-6Al-4V) have favorable biocompatibility and mechanical properties, contributing to their widespread use as dental implants [2]. Correspondingly, the amount of bacterial colonization and the osteogenic ability of cells around the titanium alloy implants affect the final survival rate of dental implants [27]; prevention is the ideal method for implant-associated infection, with professional implant surface cleaning for bacterial adherence. Therefore, antibacterial surface coatings on dental implants have attracted great attention due to the development of their surface properties [28,29].

Amongst newly developed or adopted biomaterials, some have demonstrated strong antibacterial activity potentially useful for clinical usage or dental implant applications [30]; one of which is ceria (CeO_2). CeO_2 as a rare earth oxide has been gaining wide attention in various biomedical applications, such as anti-inflammatory and tissue regeneration applications, due to its free radical scavenging activity [31]. In our previous study, we found that incorporating CeO_2 into a calcium silicate coating enhances ALP activity and antibacterial activity [26]. The aim of our current study was to determine the osteogenic activity and antibacterial activity of a CeO_2 coating containing high Ce^{4+} valence proportion on a Ti-6Al-4V surface, with the express purpose of evaluating CeO_2-coated Ti-6Al-4V as a potential dental implant biomaterial.

As the use of CeO_2 coatings containing high proportions of Ce^{4+} valences on Ti-6Al-4V metal surfaces has yet to be reported, we first sought to classify and characterize our CeO_2 coating from a structural point of view. Both X-ray diffraction (Figure 1A) and X-ray photoelectron spectroscopy (Figure 1B) results verify the CeO_2 chemical composition and indicate the major contribution of Ce^{4+} over Ce^{3+} valences in the coating. The additional SEM images (Figure 1C) allows visualization of the microtexture present owing to the spray-coating process; the corresponding coarseness may help attachment of BMSCs and prove beneficial to the osteogenesis process critical to the survival rate of dental implants [2–4].

We then tested the osteogenic activity of the CeO_2 coating in vitro to optimize the mechanical performance of dental implants and to improve their survival rate. In our study, the CeO_2 coating demonstrated good biocompatibility on both BMSCs and MC3T3-E1 cells, as shown in Figure 2. Further evidence could be ascertained from the flow cytometry results, in which the percentage of apoptotic MC3T3-E1 cells (Q2 + Q4) seeded on the CeO_2 coating was statistically significantly lower than that on the Ti-6Al-4V surface (6.7% compared to 24.0%) as shown in Figure 2C. Additionally, the CeO_2 coating promoted the osteogenic ability of BMSCs with a corresponding significant increase in expression levels of all three selected osteogenesis gene markers (Figure 3A–C), along with a similar increase in protein expression (Figure 3D). This illustrates a similar trend as discovered in our previous study [24].

From an etiological point of view, an imbalance between the host response and bacteria is a significant contributing factor in inducing peri-implant disease, as observed in susceptible patients [32]. Because of the complex and varied oral consortium, it is extremely difficult to pinpoint a single or a group of microorganisms as the cause of peri-implant disease [33]. We chose E.f., P.g., and P.i. as representative targets in identifying the antibacterial activity of our coating. E.f., P.g., and P.i. are oral pathogens that are difficult to eliminate, and have been implicated to play at least a significant role in developing periodontitis or peri-implantitis [34], with further evidence highlighting their roles in individuals with chronic and refractory periodontitis [35,36]. Correspondingly, our results indicate the antibacterial activity of the CeO_2 coating against E.f., P.g., and P.i. in vitro. The proliferation and viability of E.f., P.g., and P.i. were significantly inhibited after CeO_2 coating compared with the Ti-6Al-4V surface alone by the DCT (Figure 4A) and CCK-8 (Figure 4B) assays. CFU and live/dead bacterial staining were further used to detect bacterial viability. Both results showed that the bacterial viabilities of E.f., P.g., and P.i. on the CeO_2 coating were significantly lower than that of the control groups, demonstrating that the CeO_2 coating has the ability to impact the survivability of E.f., P.g., and P.i., which are major pathogens involved in peri-implantitis. Both the inflammation and source of pathogens (e.g., E.f., P.g., and P.i.) observed in peri-implantitis result in reactive oxygen species (ROS) production; Selvaraj et al. reported that CeO_2 decreased cellular ROS production, which inhibited proinflammatory mediator expression by attenuating the activity of NF-κB [37]. Scavenging of free radicals is a way of eliminating ROS production and reducing the inflammatory response; CeO_2 coating with a high level of Ce^{4+} on the surface was demonstrated to possess catalase mimetic activity, which could breakdown H_2O_2 into molecular oxygen and therefore scavenge free radicals present from ROS production. This may be a major mechanism achieved by the Ce^{4+}-containing CeO_2 coating in our study.

Despite having discovered significant results on the antimicrobial and osteogenic activity of our CeO_2 coating, there are certain limitations of our study that could possibly be further addressed to ascertain the suitability of CeO_2-coated titanium as a dental implant biomaterial. The first of which would direct towards the absence of in vivo biocompatibility results to determine whether CeO_2-coated Ti-6Al-4V elicits significant immune response; despite the novel combination of the two materials in a dental clinical usage setting, both CeO_2 and Ti-6Al-4V have previously been reported in the literature to possess positive biocompatibility in vivo [38–40]. Henceforth, we believe the physical combination of CeO_2 and Ti-6Al-4V as observed in our study to possess a low risk of inciting significant immune response; this could be a possible investigation area for a future study. Additionally, owing to the complex interactions between various cell types in the oral cavity, it would have been a closer reflection of the oral cavity if BMSCs and/or MC3T3-E1 cells were co-cultured with other cell types (such as oral mucosal epithelial cells and oral keratinocytes) in our experiments. However, owing to the focus of our study being the antimicrobial activity of CeO_2 coating towards oral microbiota and its osteogenic activity elicited towards BMSCs/MC3T3-E1 cells, it may have been an unnecessary complication to co-culture with further oral cell types as they are not directly involved in CeO_2 activity and may potentially confound results.

5. Conclusions

In this study, plasma-sprayed CeO_2 coating on Ti-6Al-4V surfaces with high composition of Ce^{4+} valences significantly enhanced antibacterial activity towards oral microbiota, along with increased osteogenic activity in BMSCs and MC3T3-E1 cells. These results illustrate the potential of CeO_2-coated Ti-6Al-4V constructs in dental implant applications, to reduce the occurrence of peri-implantitis and implant failures as induced by oral microbiota.

Author Contributions: J.Y. and Y.X. conceived and designed the experiments, S.Q., Z.J. and H.L. performed the experiments, J.Y., G.S. and F.C. acquired and analysed the data, J.Y.Z.J. and S.Q. wrote the manuscript, D.W. and H.L.E.P. revised the manuscript. All authors have read and agreed to the published version of the manuscript.

Funding: This work was funded by the Natural Science Foundation of Shanghai (grant no. 19ZR1439600).

Conflicts of Interest: The authors claim to have no financial interest, either directly or indirectly, in the products or information listed in the article.

References

1. Smeets, R.; Henningsen, A.; Jung, O.; Heiland, M.; Hammaecher, C.; Stein, J.M. Definition, etiology, prevention and treatment of peri-implantitis—A review. *Head Face Med.* **2014**, *10*, 34. [CrossRef]
2. Tenenbaum, H.; Bogen, O.; Séverac, F.; Elkaim, R.; Davideau, J.L.; Huck, O. Long-term prospective cohort study on dental implants: Clinical and microbiological parameters. *Clin. Oral. Implant. Res.* **2017**, *28*, 86–94. [CrossRef] [PubMed]
3. Norowski, P.A.; Bumgardner, J.D. Biomaterial and antibiotic strategies for peri-implantitis: A review. *J. Biomed. Mater. Res. B Appl. Biomater.* **2009**, *88*, 530–543. [CrossRef] [PubMed]
4. Leonhardt, Å.; Renvert, S.; Dahlén, G. Microbial findings at failing implants. *Clin. Oral. Implant. Res.* **1999**, *10*, 339–345. [CrossRef] [PubMed]
5. Zhuang, L.F.; Watt, R.M.; Mattheos, N.; Si, M.S.; Lai, H.C.; Lang, N.P. Periodontal and peri-implant microbiota in patients with healthy and inflamed periodontal and peri-implant tissues. *Clin. Oral. Implant. Res.* **2016**, *27*, 13–21. [CrossRef] [PubMed]

6. Cardoso, M.; Sangalli, J.; Koga-Ito, C.Y.; Ferreira, L.L.; da Silva Sobrinho, A.S.; Nogueira, L. Abutment Coating with Diamond-Like Carbon Films to Reduce Implant—Abutment Bacterial Leakage. *J. Periodontol.* **2016**, *87*, 168–174. [CrossRef]
7. Chatzistavrou, X.; Fenno, J.C.; Faulk, D.; Badylak, S.; Kasuga, T.; Boccaccini, A.R.; Papagerakis, P. Fabrication and characterization of bioactive and antibacterial composites for dental applications. *Acta Biomater.* **2014**, *10*, 3723–3732. [CrossRef]
8. Razavian, H.; Barekatain, B.; Shadmehr, E.; Khatami, M.; Bagheri, F.; Heidari, F. Bacterial leakage in root canals filled with resin-based and mineral trioxide aggregate-based sealers. *Dent. Res. J. Isfahan* **2014**, *11*, 599–603.
9. Kirmanidou, Y.; Sidira, M.; Drosou, M.-E.; Bennani, V.; Bakopoulou, A.; Tsouknidas, A.; Michailidis, N.; Michalakis, K. New Ti-Alloys and Surface Modifications to Improve the Mechanical Properties and the Biological Response to Orthopedic and Dental Implants: A Review. *Biomed Res. Int.* **2016**, *2016*, 1–21. [CrossRef]
10. Romeo, E.; Ghisolfi, M.; Murgolo, N.; Chiapasco, M.; Lops, D.; Vogel, G. Therapy of peri-implantitis with resective surgery. A 3-year clinical trial on rough screw-shaped oral implants. Part I: Clinical outcome. *Clin. Oral. Implant. Res.* **2005**, *16*, 9–18. [CrossRef]
11. Elias, C.N.; Lima, J.H.C.; Valiev, R.; Meyers, M.A. Biomedical applications of titanium and its alloys. *JOM* **2008**, *60*, 46–49. [CrossRef]
12. Li, K.; Yu, J.; Xie, Y.; Huang, L.; Ye, X.; Zheng, X. Effects of Zn content on crystal structure, cytocompatibility, antibacterial activity, and chemical stability in Zn-modified calcium silicate coatings. *J. Therm. Spray Technol.* **2013**, *22*, 965–973. [CrossRef]
13. Romeo, E.; Lops, D.; Chiapasco, M.; Ghisolfi, M.; Vogel, G. Therapy of peri-implantitis with resective surgery. A 3-year clinical trial on rough screw-shaped oral implants. Part II: Radiographic outcome. *Clin. Oral. Implant. Res.* **2007**, *18*, 179–187. [CrossRef]
14. Serino, G.; Turri, A. Outcome of surgical treatment of peri-implantitis: Results from a 2-year prospective clinical study in humans. *Clin. Oral. Implant. Res.* **2011**, *22*, 1214–1220. [CrossRef] [PubMed]
15. Thierbach, R.; Eger, T. Clinical outcome of a nonsurgical and surgical treatment protocol in different types of peri-implantitis: A case series. *Quintessence Int.* **2013**, *44*, 137–148.
16. Roccuzzo, M.; Bonino, F.; Bonino, L.; Dalmasso, P. Surgical therapy of peri-implantitis lesions by means of a bovine-derived xenograft: Comparative results of a prospective study on two different implant surfaces. *J. Clin. Periodontol.* **2011**, *38*, 738–745. [CrossRef]
17. Kaluđerović, M.R.; Schreckenbach, J.P.; Graf, H.L. Titanium dental implant surfaces obtained by anodic spark deposition—From the past to the future. *Mater. Sci. Eng. C* **2016**, *69*, 1429–1441. [CrossRef]
18. Li, K.; Xie, Y.; Ao, H.; Huang, L.; Ji, H.; Zheng, X. The enhanced bactericidal effect of plasma sprayed zinc-modified calcium silicate coating by the addition of silver. *Ceram. Int.* **2013**, *39*, 7895–7902. [CrossRef]
19. Li, K.; Liu, S.; Hu, T.; Razanau, I.; Wu, X.; Ao, H.; Huang, L.; Xie, Y.; Zheng, X. Optimized Nanointerface Engineering of Micro/Nanostructured Titanium Implants to Enhance Cell–Nanotopography Interactions and Osseointegration. *ACS Biomater. Sci. Eng.* **2020**, *6*, 969–983. [CrossRef]
20. Thill, A.; Zeyons, O.; Spalla, O.; Chauvat, F.; Rose, J.; Auffan, M.; Flank, A.M. Cytotoxicity of CeO_2 Nanoparticles for Escherichia coli. Physico-Chemical Insight of the Cytotoxicity Mechanism. *Environ. Sci. Technol.* **2006**, *40*, 6151–6156. [CrossRef]
21. Li, K.; Hu, D.; Xie, Y.; Huang, L.; Zheng, X. Sr-doped nanowire modification of Ca–Si-based coatings for improved osteogenic activities and reduced inflammatory reactions. *Nanotechnology* **2018**, *29*, 84001. [CrossRef] [PubMed]
22. Hu, D.; Li, K.; Xie, Y.; Pan, H.; Zhao, J.; Huang, L.; Zheng, X. Different response of osteoblastic cells to Mg^{2+}, Zn^{2+} and Sr^{2+} doped calcium silicate coatings. *J. Mater. Sci. Mater. Med.* **2016**, *27*, 56. [CrossRef] [PubMed]
23. Li, K.; Shen, Q.; Xie, Y.; You, M.; Huang, L.; Zheng, X. Incorporation of cerium oxide into hydroxyapatite coating regulates osteogenic activity of mesenchymal stem cell and macrophage polarization. *J. Biomater. Appl.* **2017**, *31*, 1062–1076. [CrossRef]
24. You, M.; Li, K.; Xie, Y.; Huang, L.; Zheng, X. The Effects of Cerium Valence States at Cerium Oxide Coatings on the Responses of Bone Mesenchymal Stem Cells and Macrophages. *Biol. Trace Elem. Res.* **2017**, *179*, 259–270. [CrossRef] [PubMed]

25. Li, K.; Xie, Y.; You, M.; Huang, L.; Zheng, X. Plasma sprayed cerium oxide coating inhibits H_2O_2-induced oxidative stress and supports cell viability. *J. Mater. Sci. Mater. Med.* **2016**, *27*, 100. [CrossRef]
26. Li, K.; Yu, J.; Xie, Y.; You, M.; Huang, L.; Zheng, X. The Effects of Cerium Oxide Incorporation in Calcium Silicate Coating on Bone Mesenchymal Stem Cell and Macrophage Responses. *Biol. Trace Elem. Res.* **2017**, *177*, 148–158. [CrossRef] [PubMed]
27. Zhou, X.; Hu, X.; Lin, Y. Coating of Sandblasted and Acid-Etched Dental Implants With Tantalum Using Vacuum Plasma Spraying. *Implant Dent.* **2018**, *27*, 202–208. [CrossRef]
28. Chouirfa, H.; Bouloussa, H.; Migonney, V.; Falentin-Daudré, C. Review of titanium surface modification techniques and coatings for antibacterial applications. *Acta Biomater.* **2019**, *83*, 37–54. [CrossRef]
29. Mehdikhani-Nahrkhalaji, M.; Fathi, M.H.; Mortazavi, V.; Mousavi, S.B.; Hashemi-Beni, B.; Razavi, S.M. Novel nanocomposite coating for dental implant applications in vitro and in vivo evaluation. *J. Mater. Sci. Mater. Med.* **2012**, *23*, 485–495. [CrossRef]
30. Maria Magdalane, C.; Kaviyarasu, K.; Raja, A.; Arularasu, M.V.; Mola, G.T.; Isaev, A.B.; Al-Dhabi, N.A.; Arasu, M.V.; Jeyaraj, B.; Kennedy, J.; et al. Photocatalytic decomposition effect of erbium doped cerium oxide nanostructures driven by visible light irradiation: Investigation of cytotoxicity, antibacterial growth inhibition using catalyst. *J. Photochem. Photobiol. B Biol.* **2018**, *185*, 275–282. [CrossRef]
31. Estevez, A.Y.; Pritchard, S.; Harper, K.; Aston, J.W.; Lynch, A.; Lucky, J.J.; Ludington, J.S.; Chatani, P.; Mosenthal, W.P.; Leiter, J.C.; et al. Neuroprotective mechanisms of cerium oxide nanoparticles in a mouse hippocampal brain slice model of ischemia. *Free Radic. Biol. Med.* **2011**, *51*, 1155–1163. [CrossRef] [PubMed]
32. Mombelli, A.; Décaillet, F. The characteristics of biofilms in peri-implant disease. *J. Clin. Periodontol.* **2011**, *38*, 203–213. [CrossRef] [PubMed]
33. Belibasakis, G.N. Microbiological and immuno-pathological aspects of peri-implant diseases. *Arch. Oral Biol.* **2014**, *59*, 66–72. [CrossRef] [PubMed]
34. Canullo, L.; Orlato Rossetti, P.H.; Penarrocha, D. Identification of Enterococcus Faecalis and Pseudomonas Aeruginosa on and in Implants in Individuals with Peri-implant Disease: A Cross-Sectional Study. *Int. J. Oral Maxillofac. Implant.* **2015**, *30*, 583–587. [CrossRef]
35. Rams, T.E.; Feik, D.; Mortensen, J.E.; Degener, J.E.; van Winkelhoff, A.J. Antibiotic Susceptibility of Periodontal Enterococcus faecalis. *J. Periodontol.* **2013**, *84*, 1026–1033. [CrossRef]
36. Sun, J.; Sundsfjord, A.; Song, X. Enterococcus faecalis from patients with chronic periodontitis: Virulence and antimicrobial resistance traits and determinants. *Eur. J. Clin. Microbiol. Infect. Dis.* **2012**, *31*, 267–272. [CrossRef]
37. Selvaraj, V.; Manne, N.D.; Arvapalli, R.; Rice, K.M.; Nandyala, G.; Fankhanel, E.; Blough, E.R. Effect of cerium oxide nanoparticles on sepsis induced mortality and NF-κB signaling in cultured macrophages. *Nanomedicine* **2015**, *10*, 1275–1288. [CrossRef]
38. Varini, E.; Sánchez-Salcedo, S.; Malavasi, G.; Lusvardi, G.; Vallet-Regí, M.; Salinas, A.J. Cerium (III) and (IV) containing mesoporous glasses/alginate beads for bone regeneration: Bioactivity, biocompatibility and reactive oxygen species activity. *Mater. Sci. Eng. C* **2019**, *105*, 109971. [CrossRef]
39. Strobel, C.; Förster, M.; Hilger, I. Biocompatibility of cerium dioxide and silicon dioxide nanoparticles with endothelial cells. *Beilstein J. Nanotechnol.* **2014**, *5*, 1795–1807. [CrossRef]
40. Haslauer, C.M.; Springer, J.C.; Harrysson, O.L.A.; Loboa, E.G.; Monteiro-Riviere, N.A.; Marcellin-Little, D.J. In vitro biocompatibility of titanium alloy discs made using direct metal fabrication. *Med. Eng. Phys.* **2010**, *32*, 645–652. [CrossRef]

Publisher's Note: MDPI stays neutral with regard to jurisdictional claims in published maps and institutional affiliations.

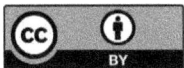

© 2020 by the authors. Licensee MDPI, Basel, Switzerland. This article is an open access article distributed under the terms and conditions of the Creative Commons Attribution (CC BY) license (http://creativecommons.org/licenses/by/4.0/).

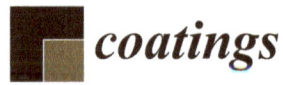

Article

Properties of Titanium Oxide Coating on MgZn Alloy by Magnetron Sputtering for Stent Application

Shusen Hou [1,2], Weixin Yu [2], Zhijun Yang [2], Yue Li [2], Lin Yang [1,*] and Shaoting Lang [2]

1. School of Chemistry and Chemical Engineering, Henan Normal University, Xinxiang 453007, China; shusen.hou@xxu.edu.cn
2. School of Mechanical and Electrical Engineering, Xinxiang University, Xinxiang 453003, China; yuweixin@xxu.edu.cn (W.Y.); yangzhijun@xxu.edu.cn (Z.Y.); liyue@xxu.edu.cn (Y.L.); shaotinglang@xxu.edu.cn (S.L.)
* Correspondence: yanglin1819@xxu.edu.cn; Tel.: +86-373-3328117

Received: 14 September 2020; Accepted: 16 October 2020; Published: 19 October 2020

Abstract: Constructing surface coatings is an effective way to improve the corrosion resistance and biocompatibility of magnesium alloy bioabsorbable implants. In this present work, a titanium oxide coating with a thickness of about 400 nm was successfully prepared on a MgZn alloy surface via a facile magnetron sputtering route. The surface features were characterized using scanning electron microscopy (SEM), atomic force microscopy (AFM), X-ray diffraction (XRD), X-ray photoelectron spectroscopy (XPS), and the contact angle method. The corrosion behavior and biocompatibility were evaluated. The results indicated that the amorphous TiO_2 coating with a flat and dense morphology was obtained by magnetron-sputtering a titanium oxide target. The corrosion current density decreased from 1050 (bare MgZn alloy) to 49 $\mu A/cm^2$ (sample with TiO_2 coating), suggesting a significant increase in corrosion resistance. In addition, the TiO_2 coating showed good biocompatibilities, including significant reduced hemolysis and platelet adhesion, and increased endothelial cell viability and adhesion.

Keywords: titanium oxide; magnetron sputtering; magnesium alloy; corrosion resistance; biocompatibility

---

1. Introduction

Magnesium alloy (Mg alloy) is an excellent biological material for bioabsorbable implant applications, due to its low corrosion resistance, good biocompatibility, and mechanical properties [1,2]. In recent years, cardiovascular stents made from absorbable Mg alloys have been developed to overcome the drawbacks of permanent metallic stents, including late-term restenosis, delayed re-endothelialization, and persistent inflammation [3,4]. However, the main disadvantage of Mg alloys for medical applications is the rapid and inhomogeneous corrosion in the physiological environment; hence, Mg alloy implants may lose their mechanical integrity before the complete healing of the tissue. In order to solve this problem, surface modifications have been widely carried out to prepare suitable coatings onto Mg alloys as corrosion protective layers, and also to improve their biocompatibility and mechanical stability [5–9]. Therefore, modifying the surface with ideal coatings is of high significance for Mg alloy stents.

For Mg alloy cardiovascular stents, some organic-based coatings, such as polylactic acid (PLA) [7], polydopamine (PDA) [10,11], poly (lactic-co-glycolic acid) (PLGA) [12], and polytrimethylene carbonate (PTMC) [13], have been commonly used as corrosion protection layers or drug delivery carriers to prevent the in-stent restenosis (ISR). However, the adhesion of organic coatings still needs to be improved. On the other hand, inorganic coatings can be prepared by various methods, providing a superior adhesion with substrates. More importantly, inorganic coatings are remarkably corrosion-resistant, and thus, they should be suitable for Mg alloy stents to improve the rapid corrosion behavior. Some inorganic coatings including magnesium fluoride (MgF_2) [14] and titanium dioxide (TiO_2) [15,16] have been used to endow the Mg alloy with greater corrosion resistance and improved biocompatibility.

It is well known that titanium oxide is chemically stable, and the biocompatibility of a titanium oxide coating has been demonstrated [17–19]. In a representative literature, Huang et al. [20] synthesized titanium oxide film on a cobalt alloy by ion beam-enhanced deposition at below 180 °C, and proved that titanium oxide was an excellent blood contact material because of the semiconductor nature. In our previous studies, the anatase titanium dioxide coating with sheet-like nanoscale features was fabricated via the solvothermal route at 160 °C, which improved the corrosion resistance of degradable MgZn alloy [21].

In view of the current research status and progress, there is still a lack of comprehensive evaluation on the application prospects of the titanium oxide-coated absorbable Mg alloy stent. In this paper, titanium oxide was prepared on Mg alloy substrates at room temperature by a facile and clean magnetron sputtering. The comprehensive properties including corrosion resistance, blood compatibility, and endothelial cells (ECs) adhesion of the as-prepared coating were discussed.

2. Materials and Methods

2.1. Preparation of the Coating

In the current study, titanium oxide coatings were deposited onto the surface of biomedical MgZn alloy (composition: 2.0 wt.% Zn, 0.46 wt.% Y, 0.5 wt.% Nd, balance Mg), developed by Zhengzhou University, China [12,22]. Firstly, rectangular samples with dimensions of $10 \times 10 \times 1$ mm^3 were cut from the as-cast MgZn ingots by wire-electrode machining, then mechanically polished and sonicated in ethanol for 5 min. Finally, samples were dried before magnetron sputtering. Titanium oxide was deposited on the MgZn samples for 2 h, with a radio-frequency magnetron sputtering system by sputtering a high-purity TiO_2 target under a constant power of 150 W. The working pressure was 0.6 Pa with an argon flow of 30 sccm.

2.2. Characterizations

The characteristics of the as-prepared coatings were analyzed by a scanning electron microscope (SEM, Hitachi SU8000, Tokyo, Japan), energy-dispersive spectrometer (EDS), and atomic force microscope (AFM, Bruker MultiMode8, Billerica, MA, USA). The crystal structure was determined by employing an X-ray diffractometer (XRD, PANalytical X'Pert3 Powder, Malvern Instruments, Malvern, UK) with Cu Kα radiation at 45 kV and 40 mA. The valence states of the elements were detected using an X-ray photoelectron spectrometer (XPS). The water contact angle (CA) of samples ($n = 3$) was measured with 10 μL droplets of deionized water at ambient temperature, using a contact angle meter.

2.3. Corrosion Tests

For corrosion tests, bare and Ti-O-coated MgZn samples ($n = 3$) were immersed in simulated body fluids (SBFs, containing 8.035 g of NaCl, 0.355 g of $NaHCO_3$, 0.225 g of KCl, 0.231 g of $K_2HPO_4 \cdot 3H_2O$, 0.311 g of $MgCl_2 \cdot 6H_2O$, 40 mL of 1.0M-HCl, 0.292 g of $CaCl_2$, 0.072 g of Na_2SO_4, and 6.118 g of Na_2HPO_4, in 1000 mL of deionized water, pH = 7.4, 37 °C) [23]. The solution volume-to-specimen area ratio was 40 mL/cm^2. After a decent interval, samples were rinsed with deionized water and dried. Then, the corrosion products were analyzed by SEM and XRD.

The electrochemical corrosion behavior of samples ($n = 3$) was measured through a three-electrode system (CorrTest CS2350, Corrtest Instruments, Wuhan, China). A saturated calomel electrode, platinum electrode, and the sample were respectively utilized as the reference electrode, counter-electrode, and working electrode. The polarization curve of tested samples (with a 1 cm^2 area exposed in 150 mL of SBF) was measured with a scanning rate of 0.5 mV/s, after a steady open-circuit potential (OCP) value was achieved.

2.4. Biocompatibility Evaluation

Blood compatibility was evaluated including hemolysis and platelet adhesion. The samples ($n = 3$) were put into the test tubes containing 10 mL normal saline at 37 °C for 30 min. Subsequently, 0.2 mL of diluted blood was added into every tube and incubated for 60 min at 37 °C. The solution was centrifuged at 3000 rpm for 5 min and the absorbance (OD_t) of the supernatant at 545 nm was determined by a microplate reader. Normal saline was used as a negative control (OD_{nc}), and deionized water as a positive control (OD_{pc}). The hemolysis ratio was calculated by the following equation:

$$\text{Hemolysis ratio (\%)} = \frac{OD_t - OD_{nc}}{OD_{pc} - OD_{nc}} \times 100\% \quad (1)$$

For the platelet adhesion test, fresh human anticoagulant blood was centrifuged at 1500 rpm for 15 min and the upper yellow liquid was separated to obtain platelet-rich plasma (PRP). Then, 0.5 mL of PRP was taken and dropped onto every sample ($10 \times 10 \times 1$ mm^3, $n = 3$) in 24-well culture plates, incubated at 37 °C for 120 min. After that, samples were taken out, rinsed with normal saline, and fixed with 0.2% glutaraldehyde solution for 6 h. Finally, samples were washed with normal saline and dehydrated with 50%, 75%, 90%, and 100% ethanol for 15 min, respectively, then dried and examined by SEM.

Human umbilical vein endothelial cells (HUVECs, Ea.hy926, Cell Bank of the Chinese Academy of Sciences, Shanghai, China) were selected to evaluate the cytocompatibility. The sterilized samples ($10 \times 10 \times 1$ mm^3) were put into 24-well culture plates ($n = 3$). The cells were cultured in Dulbecco's modified Eagle medium (DMEM), then digested by 0.25% trypsin and seeded on the surface of the samples at a concentration of 2×10^4 cells/mL. After incubating for 1 and 3 d, 20 µL of MTT solution (5 mg/mL in PBS) was added to the wells for 4 h incubation at 37 °C, then 150 µL of DMSO was added and shaken for 10 min. The absorbance (OD_t) of 100 µL of supernatant in 96-well plates was tested by a microplate reader at 490 nm. DMEM solution with 10% serum was used as a negative control. Cell viability was calculated by the following equation:

$$\text{Viability (\%)} = \frac{OD_t}{OD_{nc}} \times 100\% \quad (2)$$

To observe the adhered cells, samples were taken out and washed with PBS buffer several times, then put into PBS buffer containing 2.5% glutaraldehyde for 12 h at 4 °C, and dehydrated in increasing concentrations of ethanol. After drying and spraying with gold, the cell morphology on the surface of samples was observed by SEM.

3. Results and Discussion

3.1. Coating Characteristics

Figure 1a,b present the surface and cross-sectional microstructure of the 400 nm-thick titanium oxide coating deposited on the MgZn substrate after 2 h of magnetron sputtering. The obtained coating was flat macroscopically but slightly rough on the microscopic level. There is a clear boundary visible in the SEM image between the substrate and the coating. This is determined by the sputtering process. Under the action of the electric field, the electrons collide with argon atoms in the process of flying to the substrate, which makes them ionize to produce Ar^+ ions and new electrons. The new electrons fly to the substrate, and Ar^+ ions accelerate to fly to the cathode TiO_2 target and bombard the target surface with high energy to make the target sputtering. The sputtered neutral target molecules, i.e., TiO_2, deposited and gathered more and more on the substrate to form a thin coating in the form of nanoparticles. According to the results of AFM measurement, as shown in Figure 2c, the particle size was ~100 nm and the coating showed a smooth surface with a roughness (R_a) of 51 nm. The micro-characteristic of the coating caused a change in the surface water contact angle (CA), from 8.4° of the polished MgZn substrate to 79.6° after magnetron sputtering, indicating a decreased hydrophilicity, as shown in Figure 2a,b.

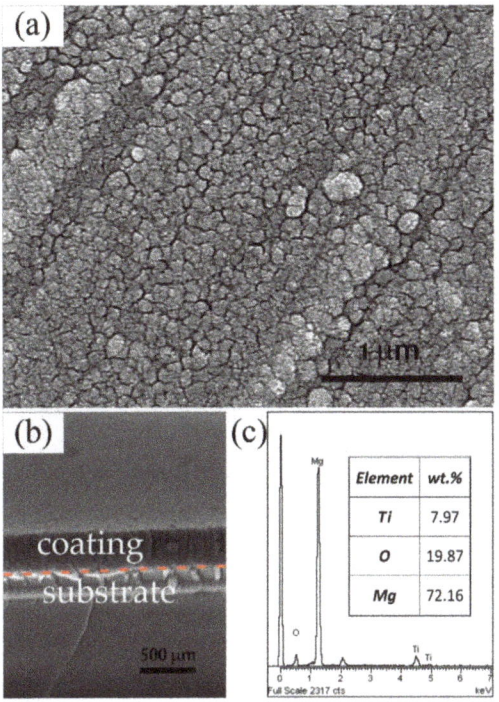

Figure 1. SEM morphologies of (**a**) surface and (**b**) cross-sectional microstructures, and (**c**) the EDS spectra of the titanium oxide-coated MgZn alloy.

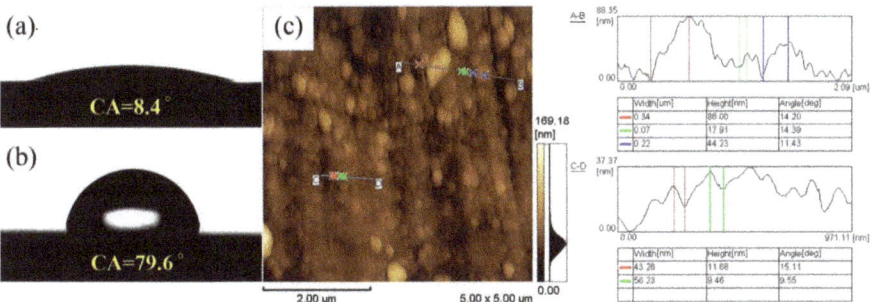

Figure 2. The contact angles of the (**a**) MgZn substrate, (**b**) TiO$_2$ coating, and (**c**) the AFM micrograph of the TiO$_2$ coating.

In Figure 1c, Ti and O were detected in the coating by EDS, which confirmed the existence of the Ti-O compound. Meanwhile, the phase composition of the coating and the chemical state of Ti were investigated by XRD and XPS (see Figure 3). The result of XPS shows that all Ti in the coating exists in the form of TiO$_2$, because the peak positions of Ti 2p$_{3/2}$ and Ti 2p$_{1/2}$ are 458.4 and 464.1 eV, respectively, which are consistent with the electronic binding peak position of Ti^{4+} in TiO$_2$ [17]. Figure 3a shows the XRD pattern of the TiO$_2$ coating deposited on the Mg alloy substrate. Clear peaks are found in the XRD pattern, which are all characteristics of the Mg alloy substrate. In addition, there are no other diffraction peaks corresponding to the titanium dioxide. A noisy pattern proves the amorphous structure of the coating. The result shows that the structure of the TiO$_2$ coating deposited by magnetron sputtering is amorphous at a low temperature [18].

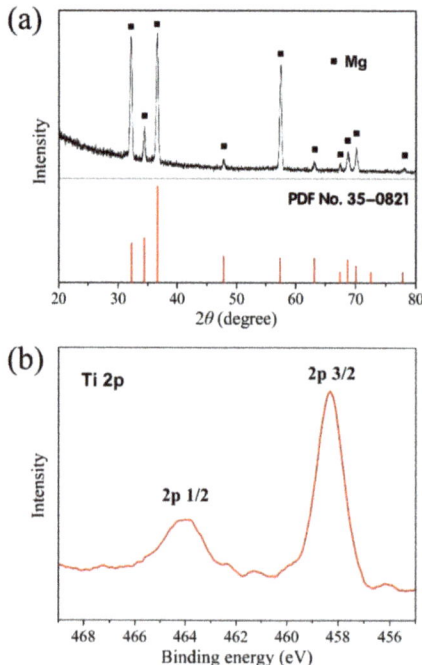

Figure 3. (a) XRD pattern of the titanium oxide coating along with the substrate and (b) XPS pattern of high-resolving Ti 2p on the titanium oxide surface.

3.2. Corrosion Behavior

The corrosion behavior was studied by the immersion test and electrochemical technique. The surface micrographs of the bare and TiO$_2$-coated Mg alloys after 14 d immersion in SBF are shown in Figure 4a,b respectively. The surface of the bare MgZn sample is heavily corroded, with abundant corrosion products deposited. It has been evidenced that during the corrosion process of Mg alloys, insoluble Mg(OH)$_2$ is formed and falls off the surface of the matrix gradually with time, leaving an uneven surface morphology [14]. By contrast, the corrosion extent of the TiO$_2$-coated sample is obviously lesser than that of the substrate. It can be seen that the surface was flat and the corrosion products were smaller and discontinuous. In fact, the better corrosion resistance is mainly conditional on the chemical stability of the TiO$_2$ coating. In Figure 4c, it was observed that the uncorroded area is where the TiO$_2$ coating remains, even if the coating has been broken and incomplete. The results prove that the 400 nm-thick TiO$_2$ coating can provide effective corrosion protection for the Mg alloy. The corrosion products are primarily Mg(OH)$_2$, as shown in Figure 4d.

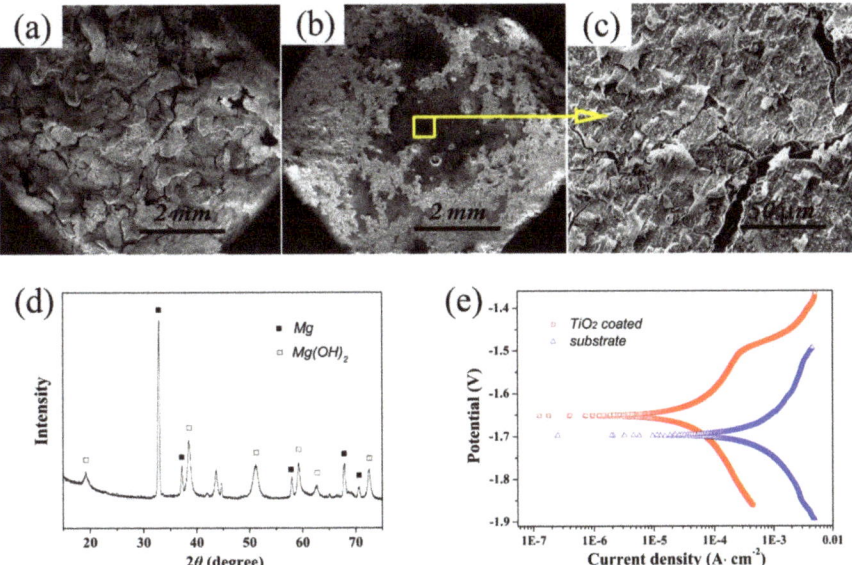

Figure 4. SEM images of (**a**) bare and (**b**,**c**) TiO$_2$-coated MgZn samples after 14 d immersion in simulated body fluids (SBFs); (**d**) XRD pattern of corrosion products and (**e**) potentiodynamic polarization curves in SBF of samples (tested after the coating preparation).

A more quantitative assessment of the corrosion resistance of the MgZn substrate with and without the TiO$_2$ coating was performed using potentiodynamic polarization curve measurements in SBF, as shown in Figure 4e. From the polarization curves, the corrosion potentials (E_{corr}) and corrosion current densities (I_{corr}) were obtained. As is known, good corrosion resistance and low corrosion rate can be reflected in a higher corrosion potential and a lowered corrosion current density. The E_{corr} of the MgZn sample increased from −1.70 to −1.65 V after the TiO$_2$ coating deposition. The coated sample exhibited a more positive corrosion potential than the bare substrate, so the substrate will be corroded more easily than the TiO$_2$-coated sample under the same conditions. In addition, it is found that the I_{corr} of the TiO$_2$-coated sample markedly decreased compared with that of the bare sample (i.e., 49 vs. 1050 µA/cm^2). Hence, the constructed TiO$_2$ coating is a superior protective layer to retard the corrosion rate of the MgZn substrate.

3.3. Biocompatibility

Materials with a poor hemolysis ratio could cause rupture of red blood cells, which may lead to thrombosis and the implantation failure. The hemolysis ratio of biomaterials in contact with blood should be less than 5%. The results in Table 1 show that serious hemolysis (47.23%, hemolysis ratio) occurred in MgZn alloys without surface treatment, while the hemolysis ratio of samples modified by the TiO$_2$ coating was only 0.1%. The anti-hemolytic property of the Mg alloy was significantly improved by TiO$_2$ surface modification. Gao et al. [24] believed that the poor corrosion resistance of the unmodified magnesium alloy increased the pH value of the blood rapidly and promoted the combination of red blood cells and Ca^{2+} in the solution, finally resulting in the rupture of red blood cells and serious hemolytic reaction. The above results demonstrate that the TiO$_2$ coating can effectively delay the corrosion of substrates and thus improve the hemolysis of Mg alloy.

Table 1. List of the results of hemolysis and cytocompatibility tests.

Samples	Hemolysis Ratio (%)	Cell Viability (%)	
		1 d	3 d
Control	–	100	100
Bare MgZn substrate	47.23	94.1	89.5
MgZn substrate with TiO$_2$ coating	0.10	93.4	94.8

Platelets play an important role in promoting blood coagulation. The platelet adhesion is an essential reaction corresponding to the formation of thrombus and occlusion of arterial. Figure 5 provides the morphology of the platelets immobilized on samples. Figure 5a shows the adhesion of platelets to MgZn alloy after 1 h of culture. The magnesium alloy surface was rapidly corroded in plasma; hence, obvious cracks can be seen after the corrosion product layer drying. In respect of the adhered platelets characteristic, a large number and serious aggregation of platelets was observed. The adhesion and aggregation of platelets will be further activated to induce thrombosis. In addition, the agglomerated platelets are likely to become fibrinogen adsorption sites, and the adsorbed fibrinogen may also lead to thrombosis. The results indicate that the unmodified Mg alloy is easy to adsorb platelets and has poor blood compatibility.

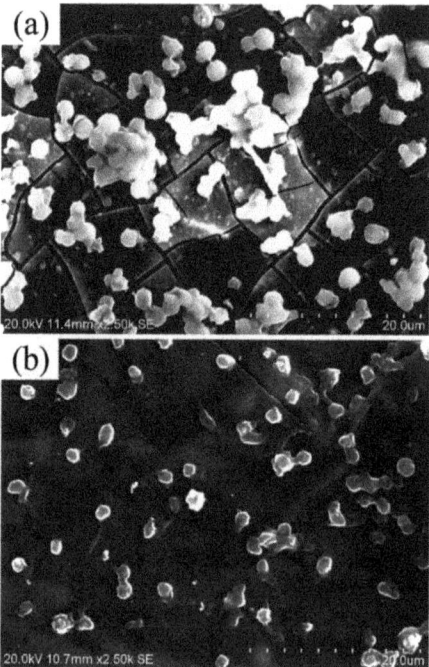

Figure 5. Typical morphology of adherent platelets on surface of (a) MgZn substrate and (b) TiO$_2$ coating.

Figure 5b shows the adhesion of platelets on the surface of the TiO$_2$ coating. The corrosion resistance of the MgZn alloy was enhanced by surface modification, so after soaking in platelet-rich plasma for 1 h, the sample was not corroded. Compared with the case of bare substrate, a remarkable reduced number of adhered platelets could be seen on the surface of TiO$_2$ samples, and no agglomeration occurred. The nearly round shape and well-distributed morphology implied that the fixed platelets were not activated during the culture. The results suggest that the TiO$_2$ coating has a better ability of anti-platelet adhesion.

Accordingly, in consideration of the hemolysis ratio and the adsorbed platelets morphology of different samples, the TiO$_2$-coated MgZn alloy not only possesses excellent properties in cutting down the hemolysis ratio but also has satisfied characteristics of not immobilizing or activating the platelets.

The TiO$_2$-coated magnesium alloys exhibit good cytocompatibility. The viability of endothelial cells reduced in the first 3 days when exposed to the bare magnesium extract. By contrast, the cell viability of the coated group was above 90% at any time point, showing the desirable cytocompatibility, as presented in Table 1. The results could be attributed to the lower values of Mg^{2+} ion concentration, pH value, and osmolality in the extracts of TiO$_2$-coated samples than those of bare magnesium [25]. Figure 6 shows the morphologies of Ea.hy926 cells cultured on the coated and uncoated groups for 1 day. For the uncoated samples, no cell was observed on the surface. As for the TiO$_2$-coated sample, it can be seen that the Ea.hy926 cells attached and proliferated well on the sample surface, and spread in the shape of a spindle.

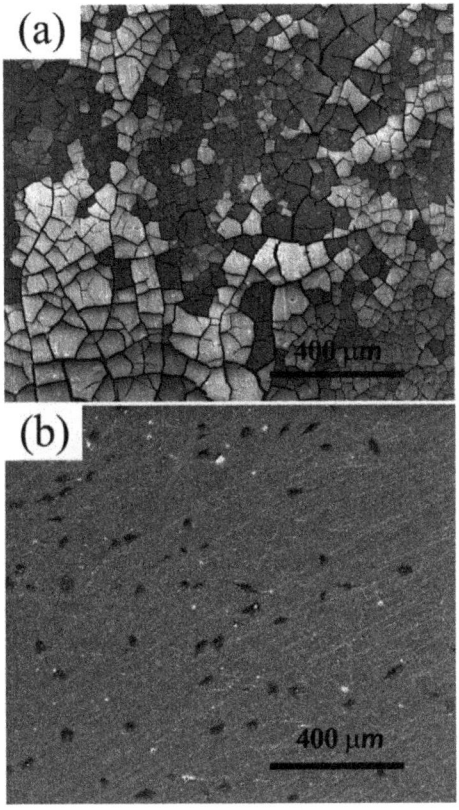

Figure 6. SEM images of Ea.hy926 cells after culturing for 1 d on (**a**) MgZn substrate and (**b**) TiO$_2$ coating.

The endothelial cell plays a key role in constructing vascular tissue, and cell growth and endothelialization can be controlled by the surface on which it attaches [26]. Generally, a smaller contact angle can correspond to a stronger hydrophilicity of materials, which is more conducive to cell adhesion [27]. The contact angle of the TiO$_2$-coated sample is 79.6°, much higher than that of the uncoated MgZn alloy (8.4°, see Figure 3a,b). However, although the uncoated MgZn alloy has the better hydrophilicity, the cell adhesion on the surface is poor. In this paper, the results indicated that the TiO$_2$-coated sample was stable in the physiological environment and conducive for cell growth and proliferation. Therefore, we believe that the effect of the alkaline environment and hydrogen evolution by the rapid corrosion might worsen the cell adherence and spreading on the uncoated Mg alloy surface.

4. Conclusions

In this work, the titanium oxide coating was prepared on the MgZn alloy surface by magnetron sputtering. The corrosion behavior and biocompatibility have been evaluated. The major conclusions of the present work are as follows.

(1) A 400 nm-thick titanium oxide coating with a smooth surface was deposited on the MgZn substrate after 2 h magnetron sputtering at room temperature. The coating was composed of dense amorphous TiO_2 nanoparticles.
(2) The corrosion resistance of MgZn alloy was improved apparently by the TiO_2 coating. After 14 d of immersion in SBF, the surface of the TiO_2-coated sample was less corroded than that of the substrate.
(3) The uncoated Mg alloys caused serious hemolysis and aggregation of platelets, whereas the TiO_2-coated sample had a hemolysis ratio of less than 1% and showed a better ability of anti-platelet adhesion. The TiO_2-coated MgZn alloy exhibited lower cytotoxicity and the endothelial cells attached well on the surface, indicating good cytocompatibility.

Author Contributions: Conceptualization, S.H. and L.Y.; methodology, S.H. and W.Y.; formal analysis, Z.Y. and S.L.; writing—original draft preparation, S.H. and Y.L.; writing—review and editing, S.H. All authors have read and agreed to the published version of the manuscript.

Funding: The research was funded by the Henan Center for Outstanding Overseas Scientists (grant no. GZS2018003), Key Scientific Research Projects of Colleges and Universities in Henan Province (grant no. 19B430008), and National Natural Science Foundation of China (grant no. 51801171).

Conflicts of Interest: The authors declare no conflict of interest.

References

1. Chagnon, M.; Guy, L.G.; Jackson, N. Evaluation of magnesium-based medical devices in preclinical studies: Challenges and points to consider. *Toxicol. Pathol.* **2019**, *47*, 390–400. [CrossRef] [PubMed]
2. Rahim, M.; Ullah, S.; Mueller, P. Advances and challenges of biodegradable implant materials with a focus on magnesium-alloys and bacterial infections. *Metals* **2018**, *8*, 532. [CrossRef]
3. Haude, M.; Ince, H.; Abizaid, A.; Toelg, R.; Lemos, P.A.; von Birgelen, C.; Christiansen, E.H.; Wijns, W.; Neumann, F.; Kaiser, C.; et al. Safety and performance of the second-generation drug-eluting absorbable metal scaffold in patients with de-novo coronary artery lesions (BIOSOLVE-II): 6 month results of a prospective, multicentre, non-randomised, first-in-man trial. *Lancet* **2016**, *387*, 31–39. [CrossRef]
4. Ho, M.; Chen, C.; Wang, C.; Chang, S.; Hsieh, M.; Lee, C.; Wu, V.C.; Hsieh, I. The development of coronary artery stents: From bare-metal to bio-resorbable types. *Metals* **2016**, *6*, 168. [CrossRef]
5. Soleymani, F.; Emadi, R.; Sadeghzade, S.; Tavangarian, F. Bioactivity behavior evaluation of PCL-chitosan-nanobaghdadite coating on AZ91 magnesium alloy in simulated body fluid. *Coatings* **2020**, *10*, 231. [CrossRef]
6. Saadati, A.; Hesarikia, H.; Nourani, M.R.; Taheri, R.A. Electrophoretic deposition of hydroxyapatite coating on biodegradable Mg-4Zn-4Sn-0.6Ca-0.5Mn alloy. *Surf. Eng.* **2020**, *36*, 908–918. [CrossRef]
7. Dong, H.; Li, D.; Mao, D.; Bai, N.; Chen, Y.; Li, Q. Enhanced performance of magnesium alloy for drug-eluting vascular scaffold application. *Appl. Surf. Sci.* **2018**, *435*, 320–328. [CrossRef]
8. Zhang, D.; Liu, Y.; Liu, Z.; Wang, Q. Advances in antibacterial functionalized coatings on Mg and its alloys for medical use—A review. *Coatings* **2020**, *10*, 828. [CrossRef]
9. Elkaiam, L.; Hakimi, O.; Aghion, E. Stress corrosion and corrosion fatigue of biodegradable Mg-Zn-Nd-Y-Zr alloy in in-vitro conditions. *Metals* **2020**, *10*, 791. [CrossRef]
10. Song, C.; Yang, Y.; Zhou, Y.; Wang, L.; Zhu, S.; Wang, J.; Zeng, R.; Zheng, Y.; Guan, S. Electrochemical polymerization of dopamine with/without subsequent PLLA coating on Mg-Zn-Y-Nd alloy. *Mater. Lett.* **2019**, *252*, 202–206. [CrossRef]

11. Liu, X.; Zhen, Z.; Liu, J.; Xi, T.; Zheng, Y.; Guan, S.; Zheng, Y.; Cheng, Y. Multifunctional MgF$_2$/polydopamine coating on mg alloy for vascular stent application. *J. Mater. Sci. Technol.* **2015**, *31*, 733–743. [CrossRef]
12. Liu, J.; Zheng, B.; Wang, P.; Wang, X.; Zhang, B.; Shi, Q.; Xi, T.; Guan, S. Enhanced in vitro and in vivo performance of Mg-Zn-Y-Nd alloy achieved with APTES pretreatment for drug-eluting vascular stent application. *ACS Appl. Mater. Interfaces* **2016**, *8*, 17842–17858. [CrossRef] [PubMed]
13. Yuan, T.; Yu, J.; Cao, J.; Gao, F.; Zhu, Y.; Cheng, Y.; Cui, W. Fabrication of a delaying biodegradable magnesium alloy-based esophageal stent via coating elastic polymer. *Materials* **2016**, *9*, 384. [CrossRef] [PubMed]
14. Wang, P.; Liu, J.; Shen, S.; Li, Q.; Luo, X.; Xiong, P.; Gao, S.; Yan, J.; Cheng, Y.; Xi, T. In vitro and in vivo studies on two-step alkali-fluoride-treated Mg-Zn-Y-Nd alloy for vascular stent application: Enhancement in corrosion resistance and biocompatibility. *ACS Biomater. Sci. Eng.* **2019**, *5*, 3279–3292. [CrossRef]
15. Hou, S.; Mi, L.; Wang, L.; Zhu, S.; Hu, J.; Ding, Q.; Guan, S. Corrosion protection of Mg-Zn-Y-Nd alloy by flower-like nanostructured TiO$_2$ film for vascular stent application. *J. Chem. Technol. Biotechnol.* **2013**, *88*, 2062–2066.
16. Chen, S.; Guan, S.; Hou, S.; Wang, L.; Zhu, S.; Wang, J.; Li, W. Characterization and corrosion properties of Ti-O/HA composite coatings on Mg-Zn alloy. *Surf. Interface Anal.* **2011**, *43*, 1575–1580. [CrossRef]
17. Zhao, A.; Wang, Z.; Zhou, S.; Xue, G.; Wang, Y.; Ye, C.; Huang, N. Titanium oxide films with vacuum thermal treatment for enhanced hemocompatibility. *Surf. Eng.* **2014**, *31*, 898–903. [CrossRef]
18. Ramos-Corella, K.J.; Sotelo-Lerma, M.; Gil-Salido, A.A.; Rubio-Pino, J.L.; Auciello, O.; Quevedo-López, M.A. Controlling crystalline phase of TiO$_2$ thin films to evaluate its biocompatibility. *Mater. Technol.* **2019**, *34*, 455–462. [CrossRef]
19. Lin, Z.; Zhao, Y.; Chu, P.K.; Wang, L.; Pan, H.; Zheng, Y.; Wu, S.; Liu, X.; Cheung, K.M.; Wong, T.; et al. A functionalized TiO$_2$/Mg$_2$TiO$_4$ nano-layer on biodegradable magnesium implant enables superior bone-implant integration and bacterial disinfection. *Biomaterials* **2019**, *219*, 119372. [CrossRef]
20. Huang, N.; Yang, P.; Cheng, X.; Leng, Y.; Zheng, X.; Cai, G.; Zhen, Z.; Zhang, F.; Chen, Y.; Liu, X.; et al. Blood compatibility of amorphors titanium oxide films synthesized by ion beam enhanced deposition. *Biomaterials* **1998**, *19*, 771–776.
21. Hou, S. Solvothermal fabrication of TiO$_2$ nanosheet films on degradable Mg-Zn alloys. *Surf. Eng.* **2016**, *32*, 745–749. [CrossRef]
22. Wang, J.; Wang, L.; Guan, S.; Zhu, S.; Ren, C.; Hou, S. Microstructure and corrosion properties of as sub-rapid solidification Mg-Zn-Y-Nd alloy in dynamic simulated body fluid for vascular stent application. *J. Mater. Sci. Mater. Med.* **2010**, *21*, 2001–2008. [CrossRef]
23. Kokubo, T.; Takadama, H. How useful is SBF in predicting in vivo bone bioactivity? *Biomaterials* **2006**, *27*, 2907–2915. [CrossRef] [PubMed]
24. Gao, F.; Hu, Y.; Li, G.; Liu, S.; Quan, L.; Yang, Z.; Wei, Y.; Pan, C. Layer-by-layer deposition of bioactive layers on magnesium alloy stent materials to improve corrosion resistance and biocompatibility. *Bioact. Mater.* **2020**, *5*, 611–623. [CrossRef] [PubMed]
25. Gu, X.N.; Guo, H.M.; Wang, F.; Lu, Y.; Lin, W.T.; Li, J.; Zheng, Y.F.; Fan, Y.B. Degradation, hemolysis, and cytotoxicity of silane coatings on biodegradable magnesium alloy. *Mater. Lett.* **2017**, *193*, 266–269. [CrossRef]
26. Guo, X.; Wang, X.; Li, X.; Jiang, Y.C.; Han, S.; Ma, L.; Guo, H.; Wang, Z.; Li, Q. Endothelial cell migration on poly(epsilon-caprolactone) nanofibers coated with a nanohybrid shish-kebab structure mimicking collagen fibrils. *Biomacromolecules* **2020**, *21*, 1202–1213. [CrossRef]
27. Yeh, H.I.; Lu, S.K.; Tian, T.Y.; Hong, R.C.; Lee, W.H.; Tsai, C.H. Comparison of endothelial cells grown on different stent materials. *J. Biomed. Mater. Res. A* **2006**, *76*, 835–841. [CrossRef]

Publisher's Note: MDPI stays neutral with regard to jurisdictional claims in published maps and institutional affiliations.

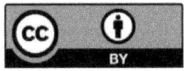

© 2020 by the authors. Licensee MDPI, Basel, Switzerland. This article is an open access article distributed under the terms and conditions of the Creative Commons Attribution (CC BY) license (http://creativecommons.org/licenses/by/4.0/).

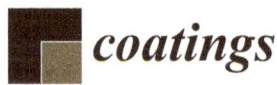

Article

Nanostructured Titanium for Improved Endothelial Biocompatibility and Reduced Platelet Adhesion in Stent Applications

Maria Antonia Llopis-Grimalt [1,2], Maria Antònia Forteza-Genestra [1,2], íctor Alcolea-Rodriguez [1], Joana Maria Ramis [1,2,*] and Marta Monjo [1,2,*]

[1] Group of Cell Therapy and Tissue Engineering, Department of Fundamental Biology and Health Sciences, Research Institute on Health Sciences (IUNICS), University of the Balearic Islands, 07122 Palma, Spain; mantonia.llopis@uib.es (M.A.L.-G.); maria.forteza@ssib.es (M.A.F.-G.); valcolear@gmail.com (V.A.-R.)

[2] Health Research Institute of the Balearic Islands (IdISBa), 07010 Palma, Spain

* Correspondence: joana.ramis@uib.es (J.M.R.); marta.monjo@uib.es (M.M.); Tel.: +34-971259607 (M.M.)

Received: 10 August 2020; Accepted: 18 September 2020; Published: 22 September 2020

Abstract: Although coronary stents have improved the early and long-term consequences of arterial lesions, the prevention of restenosis and late stent thrombosis is key to prevent a new obstruction of the vessel. Here we aimed at improving the tissue response to stents through surface modification. For that purpose, we used two different approaches, the use of nanostructuration by electrochemical anodization and the addition of a quercitrin (QR) coating to the Ti surface. Four surfaces (Ti, NN, TiQR and NNQR) were characterized by atomic force microscopy, scanning electronic microscopy and contact angle analysis and QR content was evaluated by fluorescent staining. Cell adhesion, cytotoxicity, metabolic activity and nitric oxide (NO) production was evaluated on primary human umbilical cord endothelial cells (HUVECs). Platelet adhesion, hemolysis rate and *Staphylococcus epidermidis* CECT 4184 adhesion at 30 min were analyzed. Nanostructuration induced an increase on surface roughness, and QR coating decreased the contact angle. All surfaces were biocompatible, with no hemolysis rate and lower platelet adhesion was found in NN surfaces. Finally, *S. epidermidis* adhesion was lower on TiQR surfaces compared to Ti. In conclusion, our results suggest that NN structuration could improve biocompatibility of bare metal stents on endothelial cells and reduce platelet adhesion. Moreover, QR coating could reduce bacterial adhesion.

Keywords: stents; surface modification; flavonoids; quercitrin; TiO_2 nanostructure; platelet adhesion; in vitro endothelialization; hemolysis; bacterial adhesion

---

1. Introduction

Cardiovascular disease is the leading cause of mortality worldwide and its underlying cause is atherosclerosis; a degenerative progressive disease characterized by the accumulation of lipids and immune cell plaques that affect coronary, carotid and other peripheral arteries. The conjunction of immune cells and inflammation with hyperlipidemia (elevated low-density lipoproteins (LDL) levels) influences the plaque rupture and the development of myocardial infarction and stroke [1–3].

Different materials, such as titanium, nitinol, stainless steel and CoCr alloys have been widely used as bare metal stent materials. However, in most cases the use of bare metal stents causes the development of in-stent restenosis, producing the narrowing of the arterial walls due to the vascular smooth muscle cells (SMCs) proliferation [4]. Restenosis consists of the arterial wall healing response to the injury; and the resulting neointima is a combination of SMCs, the extracellular matrix and macrophages [5]. Another less frequent but serious complication of metal stents is infections. Metal stent infections are associated with an acute inflammation of the arterial wall and vessel thrombosis, and *Staphylococcus aureus* is responsible of about 80% of stent infections. Due to the heterogeneous clinical presentation of stent infections its diagnosis is difficult and there are not many standards for its prevention and treatment [6].

Drug eluting stents (DESs) are used to inhibit the proliferation of smooth muscle cells, decreasing the risk of in-stent restenosis by the delivery of an appropriate concentration of an effective agent locally without systemic toxicity [7]. Usually, this controlled liberation of the therapeutic agent is achieved due to the use of a polymer coating; however, there are some complications associated to the use of polymers, considered as one of the leading causes of late stent thrombosis [8,9]. Thus, the use of a nanostructured surface could provide an alternative for the application of the stent coating without the need of using a polymer.

Titanium oxide (TiO_2) presents an excellent tissue response and although its mechanical properties are not ideal for stents it has been proposed as a surface modification for bare metal stents, providing an hemocompatible surface with improved biocompatibility [10], in which other coatings could also be applied.

Nanoscale topography has shown to control several molecular and cellular processes on its own without the need to change the surface chemical composition. This capacity to modulate cell behavior through topographical features has been observed with different cell types [11,12], showing for example an enhanced endothelial cell attachment and migration on stent surfaces. Furthermore, small pore diameters, less than 100 nm, have proved to promote cell adhesion and differentiation, while bigger diameters promote cell apoptosis [13,14]. Specifically, TiO_2 nanotubes with a 100 nm diameter have shown to decrease HUVEC viability and functionality, highlighting the importance of studying the effect of nanostructures with diameters below 100 nm [15], as the creation of a nanoscale topography on stent surfaces would mimic the vessel structure, improving its biocompatibility [4]. Recent studies suggest that TiO_2 nanotubes improve extracellular matrix secretion and endothelial cell functions while inhibiting vascular smooth muscle cells proliferation, implying that nanostructuration may be a good approach to achieve a faster endothelialization [4].

Another strategy to improve cell differentiation and to avoid bacterial adhesion on implantable devices is to apply a coating with a biomolecule, which can add other beneficial properties to the stent. The coating of TiO_2 with biomolecules, such as fibronectin, has shown to improve HUVEC morphology and nitric oxide (NO) production [15], showing the importance of the evaluation of biomolecule functionalization of stents. Flavonoids are natural phenolic compounds present in the human diet with antioxidant, anti-inflammatory and antimicrobial capacity, with demonstrated beneficial effects on human cells. Quercitrin is a flavonoid that was selected among others in our previous research due to its promotion of gingival cell differentiation and the decrease in *Staphylococcus epidermidis* growth rate [16,17]. In the past years, the potential of poly-phenol (as flavonoids) based coatings in medical devices has risen with applications in different fields such as, cardiovascular stents, dental or orthopedic implants. Titanium surfaces functionalized with quercitrin have shown bone-stimulating, anti-inflammatory and antifibrotic effects in vitro on human bone marrow mesenchymal stem cells and human gingival fibroblasts [18–20].

We aimed to produce a surface that could promote HUVEC function while avoiding platelet and bacterial adhesion. A quercitrin functionalized nanostructured TiO_2 surface was produced and characterized by atomic force microscopy (AFM), scanning electron microscopy (SEM) and contact angle analysis. Then, we analyzed the effect of the surfaces on HUVEC biocompatibility and function, in addition to its hemocompatibility and platelet adhesion. Finally, we evaluated *Staphylococcus epidermidis* adhesion and biofilm formation to the different surfaces.

2. Materials and Methods

2.1. Materials

Machined titanium discs, c.p. grade IV, 6.2 mm diameter and 2 mm height were purchased from Implantmedia (Lloseta, Spain). APTES, quercitrin standard, 2-aminoethyl diphenylborinate (DPBA), polyethylene glycol 4000 (PEG4000) and ammonium fluoride (NH_4F) were purchased from Sigma-Aldrich (St. Louis, MO, USA). Deionized water was obtained from a Millipore system (Billerica, MA, USA). Technical acetone and NaOH were purchased from Fisher Scientific (Madrid, Spain). Reagent grade nitric acid (69.5%), absolute ethanol and anhydrous toluene were purchased from Scharlab (Barcelona, Spain). Hellmanex III solution was purchased from Hellma Hispania (Badalona, Spain).

2.2. Surface Nanostructuration

Titanium discs were polished and cleaned as previously described [21]. Afterwards a nanonet (NN) nanostructure was produced using an Autolab (Metrohm Autolab BV, Utrecht, The Netherlands), the titanium samples as an anode and a platinum electrode (Metrohm Autolab BV, Utrecht, The Netherlands) as a cathode as previously described [22]. Polished titanium discs were anodized in an etilenglycol based electrolyte (0.1 M NH_4F, 8 M H_2O) with a first anodization of 30 min at 35 V and a second one of 10 min at the same voltage. A peeling was done between the first and second anodization using Scotch® MagicTM tape (3M, Maplewood, MN, USA).

2.3. Preparation of Quercitrin-Nanocoated Titanium Surfaces

To obtain the quercitrin-nanocoated titanium surfaces, machined Ti disks and NN-nanostructured Ti disks were used. Machined Ti disks were passivated with 30% HNO_3 for 30 min, rinsed with water until the pH became neutral and left in water for 48 h. NN disks were rinsed with water and left in water for 48 h. Then, all coins were dried under a N_2 flow and aminosilanized with 2% APTES in dry toluene for 24 h under a controlled atmosphere, in order to maintain the relative humidity levels below 10%. After that, the surfaces were chemically functionalized with quercitrin by immersion in a quercitrin hydrate 1 mM aqueous solution (250 µL/coin) at pH 5.5 for 1 h. Then, samples were washed twice with water, dried under a N_2 flow and stored under vacuum at −20 °C until use. The samples were prepared in aseptic conditions.

2.4. Quantification of Quercitrin Grafted to Titanium Surfaces by Fluorescence Spectroscopy

A stock solution of quercitrin standard (500 µM) was prepared in absolute ethanol and stored in aliquots at −80 °C. Standard surfaces with a known amount of quercitrin were prepared by drop casting a volume of stock solution containing a known amount of quercitrin (0.1, 0.25, 0.5, 0.75, 1 or 1.5 nmol) on the surface of passivated Ti coins, which were further allowed to air-dry for 20 min. In a 96-well plate suitable for fluorescence measurements, the samples and standard surfaces were carefully stained with 5 µL of DPBA (22 mM) in methanol and 5 µL of PEG400 (5%, m/v) in ethanol. After 1.5 h, the fluorescence emission spectrum of the samples was acquired, from $\lambda em = 500$ nm to $\lambda em = 700$ nm at an excitation wavelength of $\lambda ex = 480$ nm, using a Varian Cary Eclipse fluorescence spectrophotometer with a microplate reader (Agilent Technologies, Santa Clara, CA, USA). A calibration curve was obtained from the maximum fluorescence intensity at $\lambda em = 570$ nm. Three sample and standard replicates ($n = 3$) were used in each analysis. Fluorescence images ($\lambda ex = 450$–490 nm) were taken with a Leica DM R (Wetzla, Germany) fluorescence microscope and pseudocolored with Leica software.

2.5. Surface Characterization

The morphology of the different surfaces was analyzed using scanning electron microscopy. Samples were sputter gold coated before SEM analysis. Images were acquired using a scanning electron microscope (SEM; Hitachi S-3400 N, Krefeld, Germany) using secondary electrons, vacuum conditions and 15 kV of voltage. Images were analyzed using ImageJ software (version 1.49u, National Institutes of Health, Bethesda, MD, USA) to determine the pore diameter.

Topography of the samples was analyzed using an atomic force microscope (VECCO model multicode, VECCO, Plainview, Oyster Bay, NY, USA) in the air tapping mode with a scan size of 10 µm in combination with HQ: NSC35/Al probes (Mikromasch, Lady's Island, SC, USA) with a nominal spring constant of 16 N/m and resonance frequency of 300 kHz.

The static contact angle was calculated by the sessile drop method using a Nikon D3300 (AF-P DX 18-55 mm lent). The contact angle measurements were performed using four samples of each group using 2 µL ultrapure water as the wetting agent. Image analysis was performed using ImageJ software (National Institutes of Health, Bethesda, MD, USA).

2.6. Cell Culture

A pool of human umbilical vein endothelial cells (HUVECs) from different donors (Lonza, Clonetics, Basilea, Switzerland) was used. Lonza assured that cells were ethically and legally obtained, and all donors provided written informed consent. Cells were cultured at 37 °C, 5% CO_2 and maintained in basal medium EBMTM (Lonza, Clonetics, Basilea, Switzerland) supplemented with EGM™ SingleQuots™ (Lonza, Clonetics, Basilea, Switzerland). Cells were seeded in 96-well plates at a density of 7.0×10^3 cells per well for 7 days.

2.7. Bioactivity of Nanostructured Surfaces on HUVEC

Cell adhesion: HUVECs were allowed to adhere for 30 min to the different surfaces. Unbounded cells were removed by washing twice with PBS and cell adhesion was analyzed using the Presto Blue reagent following the manufacturer's protocol (Life Technologies, Carlsbad, CA, USA). Briefly, 10 µL of Presto Blue was added to all samples containing 100 µL of the culture medium. Samples were incubated at 37 °C overnight and then the absorbance of the medium was read at 570 and 600 nm.

Cytotoxicity assay: after 48 h of culture, the presence of lactate dehydrogenase (LDH) in the culture media was used as an index of cell death. Following the manufacturer's instructions (Cytotoxicity Detection kit, Roche Diagnostics, Manheim, Germany), LDH activity was determined spectrophotometrically after 30 min of incubation at room temperature of 50 µL of culture media and 50 µL of the reaction mixture by measuring the oxidation of nicotinamide adenine dinucleotide (NADH) at 490 nm in the presence of pyruvate. Results were presented relative to the LDH activity in the medium of cells cultured in tissue culture plastic (TCP) (low control, 0% of cell death) and of cells growing on TCP treated with surfactant triton X-100 1% (high control, 100% of cell death).

Metabolic activity: total metabolic activity was analyzed at 48 h and 7 days of HUVECs culture using the Presto Blue reagent (Life Technologies, Carlsbad, CA, USA) following the manufacturer's protocol. Presto Blue was added to all samples containing 100 µL of the culture medium. Samples were incubated at 37 °C for 1 h and then the absorbance of the medium was read at 570 and 600 nm.

NO production: NO production was analyzed by measuring the amount of nitrate and nitrite present in the culture media after 48 h and 7 days of incubation using the Nitrate/Nitrite Colorimetric Assay Kit (Cayman Chemical, Ann Arbor, MI, USA). NO production values were normalized by the metabolic activity of each sample.

2.8. Hemocompatibility of the Modified Surfaces

To study the hemocompatibility of the modified surfaces the hemolysis rate was analyzed. In order to do this, 15 mL tubes with 10 mL of PBS were prepared and incubated with the samples for 24 h at 37 °C in orbital agitation at 180 rpm. In addition, tubes with only PBS and no samples were incubated as a negative control, and tubes with MilliQ water as positive control. After the incubation time, 2 mL of blood samples were collected from two different donors and diluted with 2.5 mL of NaCl 0.9%. Then, 200 µL of the diluted samples were added to the 15 mL tube prepared the day before. Samples were then incubated at 37 °C for 1 h and then centrifuged at 1590× g for 5 min. After that, 100 µL of the supernatant were collected and absorbance at 540 nm was read, calculating the hemolysis rate as % versus positive control.

2.9. Platelet Adhesion on the Modified Surfaces

To study platelet adhesion on the modified surfaces, blood from three different donors was collected and centrifuged at 390× g for 10 min. Supernatants were collected and mixed to create a platelet pool. After that, 100 µL of the platelet pool were seeded on the implants and cultured for 2 h at 37 °C, 5% CO_2. Then, samples were washed twice with PBS and fixed with a 4% glutaraldehyde solution for 2 h. Finally, samples were washed with MilliQ water and stored at 4 °C with water until use. Samples were dehydrated before the analysis with scanning electron microscopy. Images were acquired using a scanning electron microscope (SEM; Hitachi S-3400 N, Krefeld, Germany) using secondary electrons, vacuum conditions and 15 kV of voltage. Images were analyzed using ImageJ software (version 1.49u) National Institutes of Health, Bethesda, MD, USA) to determine platelet number per implant.

2.10. Bacterial Culture

The bacterial strain used in this study was *Staphylococcus epidermidis* 4184 (CECT, Valencia, Spain; *S. epidermidis*). The strain was maintained in Luria-Bertani (LB) agar plates (Scharlab, Sentmenat, Spain) and cultured in LB broth (Scharlab, Sentmenat, Spain) for 24 h at 37 °C under aerobic conditions in an orbital shaker (180 rpm).

2.11. Bacterial Adhesion and Biofilm Formation on the Modified Surfaces

S. epidermidis adhesion was analyzed after 30 min of incubation with the different surfaces. A bacterial suspension with a 600 nm absorbance of 0.2 corresponding to 7.9×10^7 CFU/mL, estimated from the plates that present between 25 and 300 CFUs, was prepared and 200 µL were seeded on the implants. This bacterial suspension was incubated for 30 min at 37 °C under aerobic conditions. After that, samples were washed twice with PBS in order to eliminate not attached bacteria and then they were sonicated in 500 µL of PBS for 15 min at a frequency of 42 kHz using an ultrasonic bath BRANSON 5510 (Emerson Industrial Automation, Soest, The Netherlands). After sonication, samples were agitated by vortex to detach the bacteria from the surface and serial dilutions were made. These dilutions were seeded in LB agar plates and incubated at 37 °C under aerobic conditions for 48 h. Finally, bacterial colony forming units (CFUs) were estimated from the plates that presented between 25 and 300 CFUs. The results were expressed as CFU/cm^2 of the implant surface.

To analyze the biofilm formation, the same procedure was followed but the samples were incubated with the bacterial suspension for 24 h instead of 30 min. Results were also expressed as CFU/cm^2 of the implant surface.

2.12. Statistical Analysis

All data are presented as the mean value ± standard error of the mean (SEM). A Shapiro–Wilk test was done to assume parametric or non-parametric distributions. Variance homogeneity was analyzed using Levene's test. Parametric data was analyzed by a one-way ANOVA using as post hoc Bonferroni for data with homogeneous variance or Games Howell for data with non-homogeneous variance. Non-parametric data was analyzed by Kruskal–Wallis. To evaluate the effect of nanostructuration or quercitrin functionalization a Student's *t*-test (parametric) or Mann Whitney (non-parametric) was used. Results were considered statistically significant at $p < 0.05$. SPSS software (version 18.0, Chicago, IL, USA) and GraphPad Prism (version 7, La Jolla, CA, USA) were used.

3. Results

3.1. Characterization of Surface Topography and Wettability

An NN surface was obtained with the anodization conditions used, as demonstrated by the SEM images (Figure 1). In addition, coating of the Ti and NN surfaces with quercitrin did not affect its morphology or the pore size, calculated measuring both the length and the width of the pore, since it did not present a circular morphology (Table 1). The data obtained using AFM showed that nanostructured surfaces presented higher Ra and Rq values compared to the non nanostructured ones ($p < 0.001$). No differences on the roughness parameters were added by QR functionalization. In contrast, water contact angle (CA) measurements indicated that although all surfaces were hydrophilic (CA lower than 90°), the contact angle of QR coated samples (TiQR and NNQR) was lower compared to Ti and NN, respectively (QR coated versus non-coated groups; $p < 0.001$).

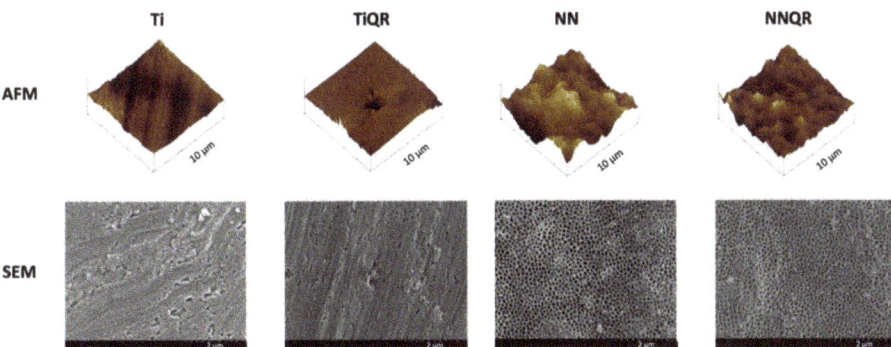

Figure 1. Physical characterization of nanostructured surfaces. Representative AFM (atomic force microscopy) and SEM (scanning electron microscopy) images of the different nanostructured titanium surfaces. Scale bars for each image are shown.

Table 1. Physical characterization of the different titanium surfaces. Values represent the mean ± S.E.M. ° = water contact angle, ↔ = pore width, ↕ = pore length, Ra = average roughness, Rq = root mean square. Results were statistically compared by an ANOVA and Bonferroni as post hoc: * $p < 0.05$ versus Ti; $ $p < 0.05$ versus TiQR and # $p < 0.05$ versus NN.

Parameter	Ti	TiQR	NN	NNQR
Contact angle (°)	68.4 ± 1.4	61.3 ± 1.6 *	66.6 ± 0.6	60.5 ± 0.7 *,#
Pore size (nm) ↔	-	-	84.2 ± 4.2	79.8 ± 2.5
Pore size (nm) ↕	-	-	55.8 ± 2.8	51.0 ± 1.13
Ra (nm)	37.2 ± 5.9	25.0 ± 3.6	61.8 ± 5.3 *, $	46.8 ± 7.2 $
Rq (nm)	46.8 ± 7.2	34.7 ± 4.2	78.4 ± 6.6 *, $	70.6 ± 8.8 $

3.2. Physical Characterization of Quercitrin Nanocoated Surfaces

A homogeneous quercitrin coating was obtained on both Ti and NN surfaces as demonstrated by the fluorescence coating. The fluorescence microscope images showed higher fluorescence in NN-QR surfaces compared to TiQR, indicating a higher amount (2.5-fold) of quercitrin linked to the nanostructured surfaces, as shown in Figure 2.

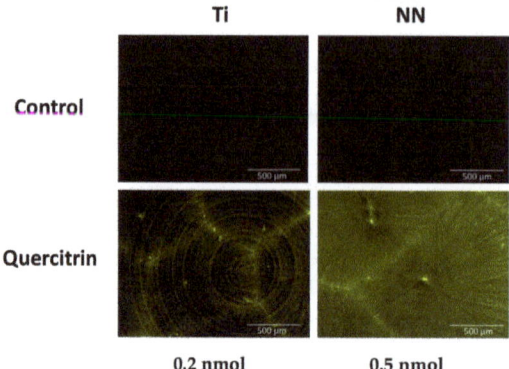

Figure 2. Quercitrin functionalized titanium surfaces staining. Representative fluorescence images of the quercitrin functionalized titanium surfaces after a fluorescence staining. 0.2 ± 0.1 nmol of QR were immobilized for the TiQR group while up to 0.5 ± 0.2 nmol of QR could be detected for the NNQR group.

3.3. Bioactivity of the Quercitrin Functionalized Nanostructured Surfaces on HUVEC

HUVECs were used as a vascular endothelial cell in vitro model to determine the potential effects of the nanostructuration and quercitrin coating of surfaces on endothelial cells.

HUVEC adhesion on the different surfaces was analyzed 30 min after seeding (Figure 3A), showing a higher adhesion on the NN surface compared to TiQR (24.7% increase) and a lower adhesion on NNQR compared to NN surfaces (34.4% decrease). After 48 h of culture, cytotoxicity levels of cells cultured on all surfaces were lower than 30% (Figure 3B), which is the limit for biological evaluation of medical devices (ISO 10993-5:2009). Furthermore, all the modified surfaces showed improved biocompatibility compared to Ti, though for the NNQR statistical significance was not reached. Next, we evaluated the effect of the surfaces on HUVEC metabolic activity at 48 h and 7 days of culture (Figure 3C,D). An effect of quercitrin functionalization was observed on metabolic activity, being higher on cells cultured on the quercitrin coated surfaces (TiQR and NNQR) compared to Ti after 48 h (15.6% and 46.7% increase respectively) and 7 days of incubation (57.2% and 78.1% increase respectively).

Furthermore, NO production was analyzed to study the effect of the surface modification on HUVEC differentiation after 48 h and 7 d of incubation (Figure 4). NO levels in the cell culture media were corrected by the metabolic activity levels of each specific sample. After 48 h of incubation lower NO production was observed in cells cultured on the quercitrin coated surfaces, being significant for both the TiQR and NNQR group compared to Ti (42.72% and 42.72% decrease respectively), and an effect of quercitrin was observed. After 7 days of incubation a decrease in NO production can be observed in all groups (TiQR, NN and NNQR) compared to Ti, although statistical significance was only achieved in NNQR compared to Ti and TiQR. In addition, an effect of nanostructuration and quercitrin was observed, showing a lower NO production in cells cultured onto nanostructured and quercitrin coated surfaces.

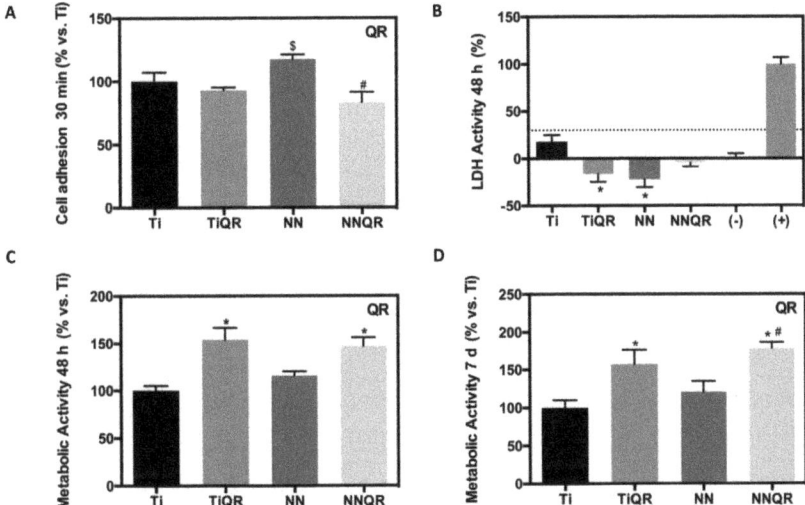

Figure 3. Surface bioactivity on human umbilical vein endothelial cells (HUVECs). (**A**) Cell adhesion to the surfaces after 30 min of incubation, expressed as % vs. Ti ($n = 6$). (**B**) Cytotoxicity of cells cultured on the different surfaces, measured as LDH activity; cells cultured on (TCP) are considered (−) an cells treated with Triton 100X 1% are considered (+; $n = 7$). (**C**) Metabolic activity of cells cultured on the different surfaces for 48 h; results are expressed as % vs. Ti ($n = 7$). (**D**) Metabolic activity of cells cultured on the different surfaces for 7 days ($n = 7$). Values represent the mean ± S.E.M. Results were statistically compared by an ANOVA and Bonferroni as a post hoc for LDH activity and metabolic activity 7 d, by ANOVA and Games Howell as a post hoc for cell adhesion and by Kruskal–Wallis for metabolic activity 48 h. * $p < 0.05$ versus Ti; # $p < 0.05$ versus NN and $ $p < 0.05$ versus TiQR. QR indicates the effect of quercitrin functionalization ($p < 0.05$), as assessed by Student's t-test for cell adhesion, LDH activity and metabolic activity 7 d and by Mann–Whitney for metabolic activity 48 h.

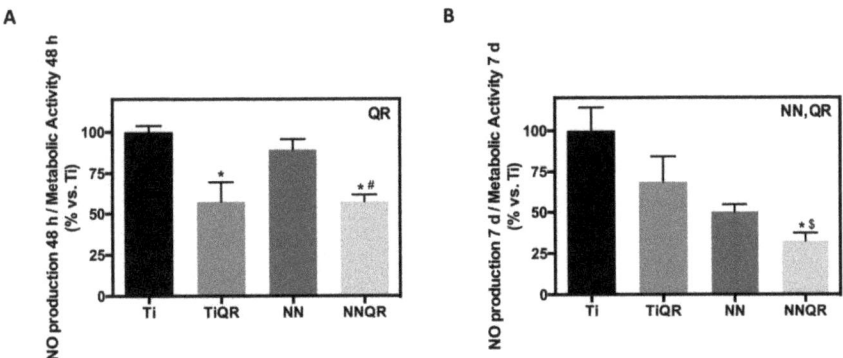

Figure 4. HUVEC NO production corrected by metabolic activity levels. (**A**) NO production corrected by metabolic activity levels after 48 h of incubation; results are expressed as % vs. Ti ($n = 7$). (**B**) NO production corrected by metabolic activity after 7 d of incubation; results are expressed as % vs. Ti. Values represent the mean ± S.E.M ($n = 7$). Results were statistically compared by an ANOVA and Bonferroni as a post hoc for NO production 48 h and Kruskal–Wallis for NO production 7d. * $p < 0.05$ versus Ti; $ $p < 0.05$ versus TiQR; # $p < 0.05$ versus NN. QR indicates effect of quercitrin functionalization ($p < 0.05$); NN indicates effect of nanostructuration ($p < 0.05$) as assessed by a Student's t-test for NO production 48 h or Mann–Whitney for NO production 7 d.

3.4. Hemocompatibility of the Nanostructured Quercitrin Functionalized Nanostructured Surfaces

To test the hemocompatibility of the surfaces, a hemolysis rate test and a platelet adhesion experiment were performed (Figure 5). All the surfaces tested showed no hemolysis rate when tested using blood collected from different donors. In addition, platelet adhesion was lower in nanostructured surfaces (NN and NNQR) compared to Ti (77.1% and 48.1% decrease respectively) and TiQR (93.9% and 64.9% decrease respectively). Quercitrin coating of the surfaces did not decrease platelet adhesion, in contrast, NNQR surface showed a higher platelet adhesion than NN, although this did not reach statistical significance. In this case, the nanostructuration of the surfaces had a greater impact than the quercitrin coating on the hemocompatibility of the surfaces.

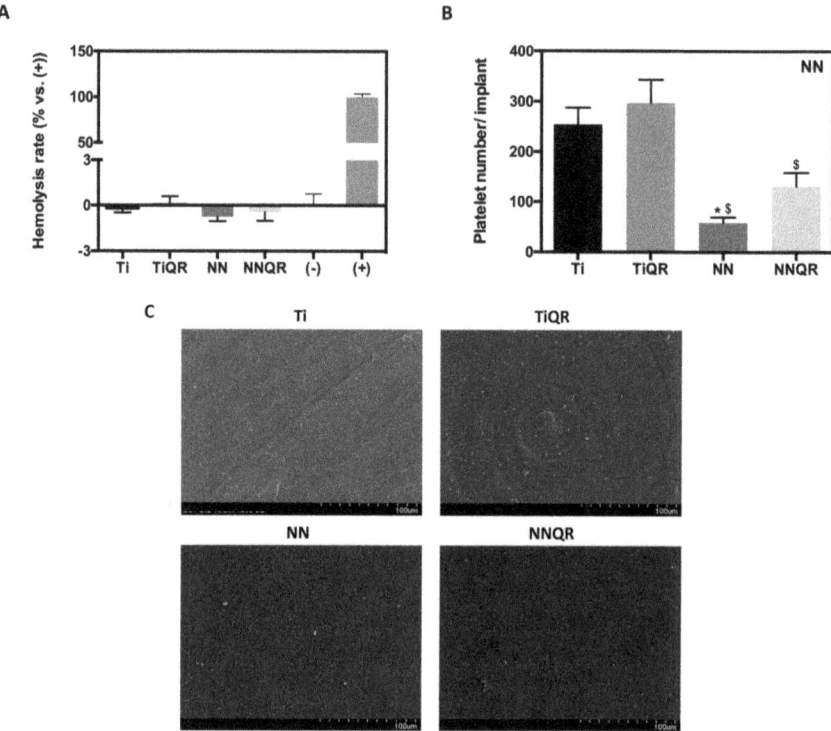

Figure 5. Hemocompatibility and platelet adhesion. (**A**) Hemolysis rate induced by the surfaces after 1 h of incubation, expressed as % vs. (+) that was set to 100%. Blood incubated with water is considered (+), and blood incubated with PBS is considered (−) ($n = 6$). (**B**) Platelet adhesion after 2 h on the different surfaces ($n = 8$). (**C**) Representative SEM images of human platelets adhered to the different surfaces. Values represent the mean ± S.E.M. Results were statistically compared by Kruskal–Wallis. * $p < 0.05$ versus Ti; $ $p < 0.05$ versus TiQR. NN indicates the effect of nanostructuration ($p < 0.05$) as assessed by Mann–Whitney.

3.5. Bacterial Adhesion and Biofilm Formation on the Nanostructured Quercitrin Functionalized Surfaces

S. epidermidis adhesion on the different surfaces was tested after 30 min of seeding (Figure 6A). Bacterial adhesion was lower on TiQR surfaces compared to Ti (50.2% decrease) and there was no difference between NN and NNQR compared to Ti. Although there was no decrease of bacterial adhesion on these surfaces, it is important to mention the fact that there was no increase despite their higher surface roughness on nanostructured groups. No differences were observed in the ability of the bacteria to create a biofilm after 24 h among the groups (Figure 6B).

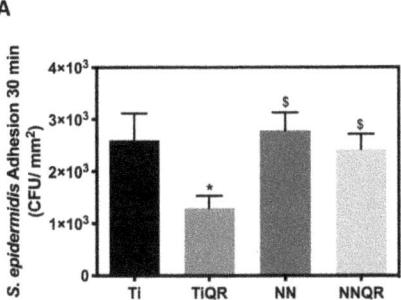 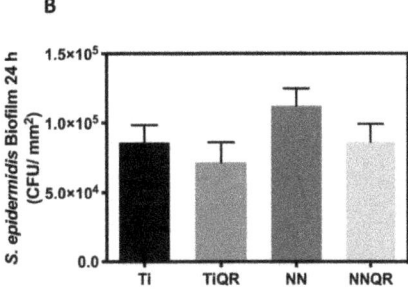

Figure 6. *Staphylococcus epidermidis* adhesion and biofilm formation. (**A**) *S. epidermidis* adhesion after 30 min of incubation. (**B**) *S. epidermidis* biofilm formation after 24 h of incubation on the surfaces. Values represent the mean ± S.E.M., ($n = 6$). Three different experiments were performed in duplicate. Results were statistically compared by Kruskal–Wallis for bacterial adhesion and an ANOVA and Bonferroni as a post hoc for biofilm formation. * $p < 0.05$ versus Ti; $ $p < 0.05$ versus TiQR.

4. Discussion

Cardiovascular diseases represent one of the leading causes of premature death and bring a tremendous economic burden [23]. Ti and its alloys are widely used for biomedical implants, such coronary bare metal stents, which usually fail due to in-stent restenosis. In this work, we tried two different approaches to improve the outcome of this material: the use of nanostructuration and the addition of a quercitrin coating to the Ti surface. Although we failed to find a synergic effect, we found on one hand that nanostructuration decreased platelet adhesion and in turn decreased the risk of thrombosis, while improving the biocompatibility of endothelial cells; and on the other hand we found that QR coating decreased bacterial adhesion, thus decreasing the risk of infection.

The characterization of the nanostructures produced in the present study allowed the determination of roughness, contact angle and geometry of the pores that could influence the cell and bacterial response. Roughness was similar when compared to other studies [24], but geometry and hydrophilicity of these surfaces showed some differences. Thus, our nanonet structure differed in morphology and geometry compared to nanopores in other studies [25], showing also a higher hydrophilicity compared to our study. The use of a nanostructured TiO_2 surface of the stent allows the creation of a surface that mimics the vascular walls, as it possesses nanostructured features, such as collagen and elastin of the endothelial cellular matrix. Previous studies have described that the presence of nanostructures on the surface enhances stent endothelialization preventing thrombosis [26–28]. However, in other studies nanostructuration of Ti surfaces did not show any effect on platelet aggregation compared with Ti before endothelialization [10,29]. In our study, all surfaces tested were hemocompatible, showing a low hemolysis rate, and nanostructured surfaces (NN and NNQR) presented significantly lower platelet adhesion compared to the non-nanostructured ones (Ti and TiQR). This result supports that our nanostructured surface could help prevent stent related thrombosis, as nanostructuration prevents platelet aggregation on the surface.

Another important aspect when developing new high-risk medical devices such as coronary stents is the biocompatibility, which follows ISO 10993:5. All our new surfaces tested were biocompatible, and the nanostructured surface (NN) showed the best biocompatibility results on endothelial cells of all the groups, proving that TiO_2 coatings possess excellent biocompatibility, in agreement with other reports [22]. In regard to cell adhesion, some studies have shown a lower cell count after one day of culture on Ti nanotubular surfaces with a 110 nm diameter [15], showing the importance of evaluating nanostructured surfaces with smaller diameters, like the ones produced in this study, with an average size of 84.2 ± 4.2 nm × 55.8 ± 2.8 nm. Although our results show a higher cell adhesion in the NN group, we failed to find a significant difference with nanostructuration.

Another aspect evaluated in this work is related to the differentiation of the HUVEC cells, which can be measured with the release of nitric oxide. Nitric oxide synthase (NOS-3) is present in the vascular endothelium and synthetizes nitric oxide (NO) from L-arginine. NO has an atheroprotective, thromboresistant and vasodilator role in the endothelium. Therefore, the dysfunction of this pathway contributes to various cardiovascular disorders such as hypertension, atherosclerosis, intimal hyperplasia or restenosis [30,31]. Different studies have reported an increase in NO production of HUVEC cultured on nanostructured surfaces compared to cells cultured on Ti [10,15]. However, we observe a decrease in NO production of cells cultured on NNQR surfaces after 48 h and 7 d compared to Ti, and after 7 days an effect of nanostructuration and QR coating was observed, leading to a decrease in NO production, which could be related to a higher cell proliferation and a lower cell differentiation. It should be kept in mind that both, micro and nanostructuration may affect the cellular response to the surfaces, in fact, in a previous study, we could demonstrate that NN surfaces induced an oriented alignment of both human gingival fibroblasts and human bone marrow mesenchymal stem cells, leading in turn to an improved expression of differentiation markers [22,32]. In a previous paper, we also showed that gingival fibroblast cells grew aligned to machined surfaces and disorderly on the polished ones [32].

Finally, bacterial adhesion to the modified surfaces was studied. Infections following the placement of cardiovascular devices is rare but it can be life-threatening and difficult to treat [6,33], and the increase of surface roughness induced by the nanostructuration process could favor bacterial adhesion, as reported in other studies [34]. Nevertheless, *S. epidermidis* adhesion was equal in nanostructured and Ti surfaces.

In regard to the second strategy with the addition of a quercitrin coating, we have previously fully characterized the coating and demonstrated that the flavonoid quercitrin could be an excellent choice for implant coating due to its multifunctional properties [18,19,35,36]. Most flavonoids are considered nontoxic and are present in plant-derived foods and present anti-inflammatory, antimutagenic and anticarcinogenic properties [37]. In previous studies, we have demonstrated that quercitrin coating presents good biocompatibility, osteopromotive, anti-inflammatory and antibacterial activity [18,19,35,36]. Here, we proved that quercitrin could also be applied as a coating for bare metal stents, and combined with the nanostructured surface, to overcome the main drawbacks of DES. In fact, the coating procedure was adapted and proved to perform successfully on the nanostructured surfaces, showing a higher amount of linked flavonoid. In addition, it is important to mention that the QR coating did not alter the nanostructure morphology or topography, in agreement with previous studies where it was demonstrated that the coating did not affect surface roughness [18,19]. The water contact angle was the only parameter affected by the QR coating, and this decrease was expected due to the presence of the biomolecule on the implant surface. The use of a coating that is covalently linked to the surface, as demonstrated by FTIR spectroscopy and XPS in previous studies [18,19], could provide an alternative to the use of a polymer, which is considered as one of the leading causes of late stent thrombosis in DES [8,9]. Similar to previous reports [19,35], QR coated surfaces were also biocompatible on HUVEC cells, and remarkably showed higher metabolic activity in all evaluated time points, similar to other studies with mesenchymal stem cells [18,19]. This result is promising since a rapid endothelialization of the stent surface is very important in order to avoid thrombosis, a major complication of DES. After 48 h of incubation with the surfaces, NO production levels show an opposite profile compared to the metabolic activity. This could indicate that the QR coating is promoting cell proliferation rather than initiating cell differentiation. However, after 7 days of incubation a tendency of lower NO production in the nanostructured surfaces (NN and NNQR) was found. In the case of NNQR surface, this result correlated again with the metabolic activity profile, being this surface the one that stimulated a higher cell proliferation and a lower cell differentiation.

On the other hand, QR coating did not seem to have an important impact on hemocompatibility of the different surfaces, as no differences were observed on the hemolysis rate and platelet adhesion, despite flavonoids having been reported to present antiplatelet effects and to be able to inhibit platelet aggregation [38,39].

Last, due to the clinical implications of implant-related infections and with the rising of antimicrobial resistance, there is a need to develop antibacterial coatings with other molecules rather than antibiotics. Plants synthesize flavonoids in response to microbial infection and they have also been proposed as resistance-modifying agents that can act synergically with antibiotics against resistant bacterial strains [37]. In previous studies in our research group, TiQR surfaces significantly decreased *Streptococcus mutans* adhesion compared to Ti [20], similar to the present results with *S. epidermidis*. Therefore, this type of surface could help to prevent intravascular bare metal stent infections, which are rare but a serious complication, and often leads to emergency surgery. Moreover, bacteria commonly found in skin flora such as *S. aureus* and *S. epidermidis* are the most common bacterial causes of both vascular graft and stent infections [40], from which we reported an effect. However, future studies in elucidating the effects of QR on different bacterial may be useful for optimizing the efficiency and feasibility of the QR-coated biomaterials in biomedical applications.

The fact that these studies were performed using Ti discs represent a limitation in the study, together with the fact that HUVEC behavior and hemocompatibility were tested in vitro in conditions that are far from the in vivo situation. In future studies, nanostructuration or quercitrin coating should be performed on a final medical device using coronary Ti stents, and including mechanical testing in the studies using various modes of failing such as bending, torsion, tensile, crushing, abrasion and fatigue to analyze if any of these modifications are affecting the mechanical properties and durability. Finally, an in vivo study with a validated animal model under aseptic and infected conditions is necessary to determine the histological effects of the coatings and its hemocompatibility in an in vivo environment.

5. Conclusions

Nanostructuration of Ti surfaces has shown improved biocompatibility on endothelial cells and hemocompatibility, which could represent a good option as a surface modification for bare metal stents to produce a rapid re-endothelialization and prevent thrombosis. Moreover, the use of quercitrin functionalization on Ti implants has shown lower bacterial adhesion, which could reduce the risk of bacterial infection.

Author Contributions: Conceptualization, M.M., J.M.R., and M.A.L.-G.; methodology, M.M., J.M.R., and M.A.L.-G.; validation, M.M. and J.M.R.; formal analysis, M.M., J.M.R., and M.A.L.-G.; investigation, M.A.L.-G., M.A.F.-G., and V.A.-R.; resources, M.M. and J.M.R.; data curation, M.A.L.-G.; writing—original draft preparation, M.A.L.-G.; writing—review and editing, M.M., J.M.R., and M.A.L.-G.; supervision, M.M. and J.M.R.; project administration, M.M. and J.M.R.; funding acquisition, M.M. and J.M.R. All authors have read and agreed to the published version of the manuscript.

Funding: This research was funded by a grant from the Osteology Foundation (Switzerland; 13-069), by the Ministerio de Educación Cultura y Deporte (contract to M.A. L.G; FPU15/03412), by Instituto de Salud Carlos III, co-funded by the ESF European Social Fund and the ERDF European Regional Development Fund (contract to J.M.R.; MS16/00124), Ministerio de Economía y Competividad (contract to M.M.; IEDI-2017-00941), and the Institut d'Investigació Sanitària de les Illes Balears (ITS2018-002-TALENT PLUS JUNIOR PROGRAM, JUNIOR18/01)

Acknowledgments: The authors thank Ferran Hierro and Joan Cifre, (UIB) for their technical contribution with SEM and AFM, respectively.

Conflicts of Interest: The authors declare no conflict of interest.

References

1. Lusis, A.J. Atherosclerosis Aldons. *Nature* **2010**, *407*, 233–241. [CrossRef] [PubMed]
2. Schaftenaar, F.; Frodermann, V.; Kuiper, J.; Lutgens, E. Atherosclerosis: The interplay between lipids and immune cells. *Curr. Opin. Lipidol.* **2016**, *27*, 209–215. [CrossRef] [PubMed]
3. O'Connell, B.M.; McGloughlin, T.M.; Walsh, M.T. Factors that affect mass transport from drug eluting stents into the artery wall. *Biomed. Eng. Online* **2010**, *9*, 6–8. [CrossRef] [PubMed]

4. Mohan, C.C.; Sreerekha, P.R.; Divyarani, V.V.; Nair, S.; Chennazhi, K.; Menon, D. Influence of titania nanotopography on human vascular cell functionality and its proliferation in vitro. *J. Mater. Chem.* **2012**, *22*, 1326–1340. [CrossRef]
5. Costa, M.A.; Simon, D.I. Molecular basis of restenosis and drug-eluting stents. *Circulation* **2005**, *111*, 2257–2273. [CrossRef]
6. Zhang, K.; Liu, T.; Li, J.-A.; Chen, J.-Y.; Wang, J.; Huang, N. Surface modification of implanted cardiovascular metal stents: From antithrombosis and antirestenosis to endothelialization. *J. Biomed. Mater. Res. Part A* **2014**, *102*, 588–609. [CrossRef]
7. Htay, T.; Liu, M.W. Drug-eluting stent: A review and update. *Vasc. Health Risk Manag.* **2005**, *1*, 263–276. [CrossRef]
8. Bedair, T.M.; Min, I.J.; Park, W.; Joung, Y.K.; Han, D.K. Sustained drug release using cobalt oxide nanowires for the preparation of polymer-free drug-eluting stents. *J. Biomater. Appl.* **2018**, *33*, 352–362. [CrossRef]
9. Lee, C.H.; Hsieh, M.J.; Liu, K.S.; Cheng, C.W.; Chang, S.H.; Liu, S.J.; Wang, C.J.; Hsu, M.Y.; Hung, K.C.; Yeh, Y.H.; et al. Promoting vascular healing using nanofibrous ticagrelor-eluting stents. *Int. J. Nanomed.* **2018**, *13*, 6039–6048. [CrossRef]
10. Mohan, C.C.; Chennazhi, K.P.; Menon, D. In vitro hemocompatibility and vascular endothelial cell functionality on titania nanostructures under static and dynamic conditions for improved coronary stenting applications. *Acta Biomater.* **2013**, *9*, 9568–9577. [CrossRef]
11. Dobbenga, S.; Fratila-Apachitei, L.E.; Zadpoor, A.A. Nanopattern-induced osteogenic differentiation of stem cells—A systematic review. *Acta Biomater.* **2016**, *46*, 3–14. [CrossRef]
12. Metavarayuth, K.; Sitasuwan, P.; Zhao, X.; Lin, Y.; Wang, Q. Influence of Surface Topographical Cues on the Differentiation of Mesenchymal Stem Cells in Vitro. *ACS Biomater. Sci. Eng.* **2016**, *2*, 142–151. [CrossRef]
13. Park, J.; Bauer, S.; Von Der Mark, K.; Schmuki, P. Nanosize and Vitality: TiO_2 Nanotube Diameter Directs Cell Fate. *Nano Lett.* **2007**, *7*, 1686–1691. [CrossRef] [PubMed]
14. Park, J.; Bauer, S.; Schlegel, K.A.; Neukam, F.W.; von der Mark, K.; Schmuki, P. TiO_2 Nanotube Surfaces: 15 nm-An Optimal Length Scale of Surface Topography for Cell Adhesion and Differentiation. *Small* **2009**, *5*, 666–671. [CrossRef] [PubMed]
15. Jin, Z.; Yan, X.; Liu, G.; Lai, M. Fibronectin modified TiO_2 nanotubes modulate endothelial cell behavior. *J. Biomater. Appl.* **2018**, *33*, 44–51. [CrossRef]
16. Gómez-Florit, M.; Monjo, M.; Ramis, J.M. Identification of quercitrin as a potential therapeutic agent for periodontal applications. *J. Periodontol.* **2014**, *85*, 966–974. [CrossRef] [PubMed]
17. Satué, M.; Arriero, M.D.M.; Monjo, M.; Ramis, J.M. Quercitrin and Taxifolin stimulate osteoblast differentiation in MC3T3-E1 cells and inhibit osteoclastogenesis in RAW 264.7 cells. *Biochem. Pharmacol.* **2013**, *86*, 1476–1486. [CrossRef]
18. Córdoba, A.; Monjo, M.; Hierro-Oliva, M.; González-Martín, M.L.; Ramis, J.M. Bioinspired Quercitrin Nanocoatings: A Fluorescence-Based Method for Their Surface Quantification, and Their Effect on Stem Cell Adhesion and Differentiation to the Osteoblastic Lineage. *ACS Appl. Mater. Interfaces* **2015**, *7*, 16857–16864. [CrossRef]
19. Córdoba, A.; Satué, M.; Gómez-Florit, M.; Hierro-Oliva, M.; Petzold, C.; Lyngstadaas, S.P.; González-Martín, M.L.; Monjo, M.; Ramis, J.M. Flavonoid-Modified Surfaces: Multifunctional Bioactive Biomaterials with Osteopromotive, Anti-Inflammatory, and Anti-Fibrotic Potential. *Adv. Healthc. Mater.* **2015**, *4*, 540–549. [CrossRef]
20. Gomez-Florit, M.; Pacha-Olivenza, M.A.; Fernández-Calderón, M.C.; Córdoba, A.; González-Martín, M.L.; Monjo, M.; Ramis, J.M. Quercitrin-nanocoated titanium surfaces favour gingival cells against oral bacteria. *Sci. Rep.* **2016**, *6*, 22444. [CrossRef]
21. Lamolle, S.F.; Monjo, M.; Lyngstadaas, S.P.; Ellingsen, J.E.; Haugen, H.J. Titanium implant surface modification by cathodic reduction in hydrofluoric acid: Surface characterization and in vivo performance. *J. Biomed. Mater. Res. Part A* **2009**, *88*, 581–588. [CrossRef] [PubMed]
22. Llopis-Grimalt, M.A.; Amengual-Tugores, A.M.; Monjo, M.; Ramis, J.M. Oriented cell alignment induced by a nanostructured titanium surface enhances expression of cell differentiation markers. *Nanomaterials* **2019**, *9*, 1661. [CrossRef] [PubMed]

23. Heidenreich, P.A.; Trogdon, J.G.; Khavjou, O.A.; Butler, J.; Dracup, K.; Ezekowitz, M.D.; Finkelstein, E.A.; Hong, Y.; Johnston, S.C.; Khera, A.; et al. Forecasting the future of cardiovascular disease in the United States: A policy statement from the American Heart Association. *Circulation* **2011**, *123*, 933–944. [CrossRef]
24. Kulkarni, M.; Patil-Sen, Y.; Junkar, I.; Kulkarni, C.V.; Lorenzetti, M.; Iglič, A. Wettability studies of topologically distinct titanium surfaces. *Colloids Surf. B Biointerfaces* **2015**, *129*, 47–53. [CrossRef]
25. Liu, G.; Du, K.; Wang, K. Surface wettability of TiO_2 nanotube arrays prepared by electrochemical anodization. *Appl. Surf. Sci.* **2016**, *388*, 313–320. [CrossRef]
26. Karagkiozaki, V.; Karagiannidis, P.G.; Kalfagiannis, N.; Kavatzikidou, P.; Patsalas, P.; Georgiou, D.; Logothetidis, S. Novel nanostructured biomaterials: Implications for coronary stent thrombosis. *Int. J. Nanomed.* **2012**, *7*, 6063–6076.
27. Choudhary, S.; Berhe, M.; Haberstroh, K.M.; Webster, T.J. Increased endothelial and vascular smooth muscle cell adhesion on nanostructured titanium and CoCrMo. *Int. J. Nanomed.* **2006**, *1*, 41–49. [CrossRef] [PubMed]
28. Maguire, P.D.; McLaughlin, J.A.; Okpalugo, T.I.T.; Lemoine, P.; Papakonstantinou, P.; McAdams, E.T.; Needham, M.; Ogwu, A.A.; Ball, M.; Abbas, G.A. Mechanical stability, corrosion performance and bioresponse of amorphous diamond-like carbon for medical stents and guidewires. *Diam. Relat. Mater.* **2005**, *14*, 1277–1288. [CrossRef]
29. Achneck, H.E.; Jamiolkowski, R.M.; Jantzen, A.E.; Haseltine, J.M.; Lane, W.O.; Huang, J.K.; Galinat, L.J.; Serpe, M.J.; Lin, F.H.; Li, M.; et al. The biocompatibility of titanium cardiovascular devices seeded with autologous blood-derived endothelial progenitor cells. EPC-seeded antithrombotic Ti Implants. *Biomaterials* **2011**, *32*, 10–18. [CrossRef]
30. O'Connor, D.M.; O'Brien, T. Nitric oxide synthase gene therapy: Progress and prospects. *Expert Opin. Biol. Ther.* **2009**, *9*, 867–878. [CrossRef]
31. Vallance, P.; Hingorani, A. Endothelial nitric oxide in humans in health and disease. *Int. J. Exp. Pathol.* **1999**, *80*, 291–303. [CrossRef] [PubMed]
32. Gómez-Florit, M.; Ramis, J.M.; Xing, R.; Taxt-Lamolle, S.; Haugen, H.J.; Lyngstadaas, S.P.; Monjo, M. Differential response of human gingival fibroblasts to titanium- and titanium-zirconium-modified surfaces. *J. Periodontal Res.* **2014**, *49*, 425–436. [CrossRef] [PubMed]
33. Lejay, A.; Koncar, I.; Diener, H.; Vega de Ceniga, M.; Chakfé, N. Post-operative Infection of Prosthetic Materials or Stents Involving the Supra-aortic Trunks: A Comprehensive Review. *Eur. J. Vasc. Endovasc. Surg.* **2018**, *56*, 885–900. [CrossRef]
34. Teughels, W.; Van Assche, N.; Sliepen, I.; Quirynen, M. Effect of material characteristics and/or surface topography on biofilm development. *Clin. Oral Implants Res.* **2006**, *17* (Suppl. S2), 68–81. [CrossRef]
35. Llopis-Grimalt, M.A.; Arbós, A.; Gil-Mir, M.; Mosur, A.; Kulkarni, P.; Salito, A.; Ramis, J.M.; Monjo, M. Multifunctional Properties of Quercitrin-Coated Porous Ti-6Al-4V Implants for Orthopaedic Applications Assessed In Vitro. *J. Clin. Med.* **2020**, *9*, 855. [CrossRef] [PubMed]
36. Córdoba, A.; Manzanaro-Moreno, N.; Colom, C.; Rønold, H.J.; Lyngstadaas, S.P.; Monjo, M.; Ramis, J.M. Quercitrin Nanocoated Implant Surfaces Reduce Osteoclast Activity In Vitro and In Vivo. *Int. J. Mol. Sci.* **2018**, *19*, 3319. [CrossRef]
37. Górniak, I.; Bartoszewski, R.; Króliczewski, J. Comprehensive review of antimicrobial activities of plant flavonoids. *Phytochem. Rev.* 2019; *18*, 241–272.
38. Faggio, C.; Sureda, A.; Morabito, S.; Sanches-Silva, A.; Mocan, A.; Nabavi, S.F.; Nabavi, S.M. Flavonoids and platelet aggregation: A brief review. *Eur. J. Pharmacol.* **2017**, *807*, 91–101. [CrossRef]
39. Guerrero, J.A.; Lozano, M.L.; Castillo, J.; Benavente-García, O.; Vicente, V.; Rivera, J. Flavonoids inhibit platelet function through binding to the thromboxane A2 receptor. *J. Thromb. Haemost.* **2005**, *3*, 369–376. [CrossRef]
40. Bosman, W.M.P.F.; Borger Van Der Burg, B.L.S.; Schuttevaer, H.M.; Thoma, S.; Hedeman Joosten, P.P. Infections of intravascular bare metal stents: A case report and review of literature. *Eur. J. Vasc. Endovasc. Surg.* **2014**, *47*, 87–99. [CrossRef]

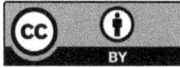

© 2020 by the authors. Licensee MDPI, Basel, Switzerland. This article is an open access article distributed under the terms and conditions of the Creative Commons Attribution (CC BY) license (http://creativecommons.org/licenses/by/4.0/).

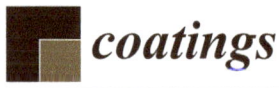

Review

Role of Melatonin in Bone Remodeling around Titanium Dental Implants: Meta-Analysis

Nansi López-Valverde [1], Beatriz Pardal-Peláez [1], Antonio López-Valverde [1,*] and Juan Manuel Ramírez [2]

[1] Department of Surgery, Instituto de Investigación Biomédica de Salamanca (IBSAL), University of Salamanca, 37007 Salamanca, Spain; nlovalher@usal.es (N.L.-V.); bpardal@usal.es (B.P.-P.)
[2] Department of Morphological Sciences, University of Cordoba, Avenida Meneéndez Pidal S/N, 14071 Cordoba, Spain; jmramirez@uco.es
* Correspondence: alopezvalverde@usal.es

Abstract: The theory, known as the "brain-bone axis" theory, involves the central nervous system in bone remodeling. The alteration of the nervous system could lead to abnormal bone remodeling Melatonin produced by the pineal gland is a hormone that is characterized by its antioxidant properties. The aim of this meta-analysis was to examine the role of melatonin in the growth of new bone around titanium dental implants in vivo. A manual search of the PubMed and Web of Science databases was conducted to identify scientific studies published until November 2020. We included randomized clinical trials (RCTs) and animal studies where melatonin was used with titanium implants. Fourteen studies met the inclusion criteria. Quality was assessed using the Jadad scale and SYRCLE's risk of bias tool. Our meta-analysis revealed that the use of melatonin during implant placement improves bone-to-implant contact percentages in animals (difference of means, random effects: 9.59 [95% CI: 5.53–13.65]), reducing crestal bone loss in humans (difference of means, random effects: −0.55 [95% CI: 1.10–0.00]). In animals, titanium implants using melatonin increase bone-to-implant contact surface 2–6 weeks after their placement and reduce crestal bone loss in humans following six months. The results of this meta-analysis should be taken with caution, due to the small samples and the large heterogeneity among studies.

Keywords: melatonin; bone formation; titanium dental implants; systematic review; meta-analysis

Citation: López-Valverde, N.; Pardal-Peláez, B.; López-Valverde, A.; Ramírez, J.M. Role of Melatonin in Bone Remodeling around Titanium Dental Implants: Meta-Analysis. *Coatings* **2021**, *11*, 271. https://doi.org/10.3390/coatings11030271

Academic Editors: Devis Bellucci and Toshiyuki Kawai

Received: 15 January 2021
Accepted: 20 February 2021
Published: 25 February 2021

Publisher's Note: MDPI stays neutral with regard to jurisdictional claims in published maps and institutional affiliations.

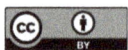

Copyright: © 2021 by the authors. Licensee MDPI, Basel, Switzerland. This article is an open access article distributed under the terms and conditions of the Creative Commons Attribution (CC BY) license (https://creativecommons.org/licenses/by/4.0/).

1. Introduction

The first description of osseointegration was provided by Brånemark and colleagues [1] more than 50 years ago, and to date, this process still remains unexplored. One of the theories posed in recent years, referred to as the "brain-bone axis theory" by certain authors [2], has drawn particular interest. It suggests the involvement of the sympathetic nervous system (SNS) in bone remodeling, claiming the need for the autonomic nervous system to be undamaged in order to contribute to the maintenance of healthy bone tissue, with its alteration leading to possible anomalies in bone remodeling [3,4]. This remodeling process would be mainly controlled by neurotransmitters (noradrenaline, serotonin and dopamine), and growth hormones secreted by the pituitary gland could stimulate osteoblast and osteoclast proliferation, which plays a crucial part in the bone formation-destruction balance [5,6].

It has been proven that the group of glucose-sensing neurons in the hypothalamic arcuate nucleus makes control of the skeleton by the brain possible [7], and that long-term use of certain central nervous depressant drugs causes a reduction in bone mass that results in osteoporosis, and therefore in high rates of dental implant failure in patients under treatment with such drugs [8].

The biofunctionalization of a certain biomaterial consists of modifying the physicochemical characteristics of its surface, which improves a body's biological response when it comes into contact with it, despite the fact that there are other factors that influence the creation of an adequate surface bone-implant contact, such as bone quality or proper surgical technique [9–11].

In recent decades, different techniques to improve titanium (Ti) surface topography and promote osseointegration have been developed, since Ti surfaces have no antioxidant properties and the cells that grow on the surface may be under permanent oxidative stress [12]. Current research is focused on obtaining surfaces that may achieve better and faster osseointegration through morphological or biochemical modification [13,14].

Melatonin (MT) (Melatonin, N-acetyl 5-methoxytryptamine) is a hormone that is mainly synthetized in the pineal gland. It is regarded as a relevant mediator of angiogenesis and bone formation due to its antioxidant effects, its production being precisely modulated under the influence of the hypothalamus [15–17]. Previous studies have assessed its anti-inflammatory properties, as well as its relevant role in peri-implant bone formation [18–21], all due to its extraordinary capacity to destroy reactive oxygen species [22]. In this regard, the benefits of its topical application on post-extraction sockets and before dental surgery to prevent bisphosphonate-related osteonecrosis have also been noted [23]. However, it should be noted that despite this knowledge, the clinical application of antioxidant therapies and surface biofunctionalization in this respect to enhance dental-implant surgery is very limited.

The purpose of our study was to carry out a systematic review of the literature related to bone growth and remodeling around Ti dental implants, combined with MT.

2. Materials and Methods

Eligible studies were selected according to the Preferred Reporting Items for Systematic Review and Meta-Analysis (PRISMA) guidelines for systematic reviews and meta-analysis [24] (Table S1, Checklist).

2.1. Protocol

The Population, Intervention, Comparison and Outcome framework (PICO) was used as a basis to formulate the research question, which was: "The inclusion of melatonin in dental implant surgery: does it influence osseointegration?".

(P) Participants: the subjects received endo-bone implant placement. (I) Interventions: implants including melatonin. (C) Control: implants without melatonin. (O) Outcome: Bone-to-Implant Contact (BIC) (in animal studies) and Marginal Bone Level (MBL) in randomized clinical trials (RCTs).

2.2. Data Sources and Search Strategy

The PubMed and Web of Science electronic databases were searched for findings published in the last 15 years until November 2020. The search terms used were: "titanium dental implants AND melatonin surface"; "melatonin AND dental implants"; and "melatonin AND dental implants AND bone formation". The Boolean operator "AND" was used to combine the searches.

2.3. Inclusion and Exclusion Criteria

The inclusion criteria for the study selection were:

- Randomized clinical trials and animal studies on Ti implants, with and without the incorporation of melatonin.
- Randomized clinical trials and animal studies that reported bone-implant contact percentages, with and without the incorporation of melatonin.
- Studies with a minimum of six implants/group.

The exclusion criteria for the study selection were:

- In vitro studies.
- Narrative and systematic reviews.
- Clinical cases.

- Studies that assessed the effectiveness of melatonin in bone regeneration without including dental implants, duplicates and those that failed to meet the inclusion criteria.

2.4. Data Extraction and Analysis

Those articles that failed to address the research question were removed. The corresponding titles and abstracts of the eligible articles were taken, and two reviewers (NL-V and AL-V) separately drew up a selection of them. The reviewers discussed and solved the discrepancies over the choice of articles that arose. The full versions of the chosen articles were then obtained for review and inclusion.

2.5. Risk of Bias (RoB) of the Selected Articles

The methodology of the scientific evidence gathered in the selected studies was assessed using SYRCLE's risk of bias tool (an adapted version of the Cochrane RoB tool, with specific biases in animal studies) [25].

2.6. Quality of the Reports of the Selected Articles

This assessment was based on the provided ARRIVE (Animal Research: Reporting of In Vivo Experiments) guidelines [26], with a total of 23 items. The reviewers, N.L.-V. and A.L.-V., allocated each item a score of 0 (not reported) or 1 (reported), including an overall inventory of all the selected studies.

2.7. Quality of the Reports of the Included Randomized Clinical Trials

The assessment was carried out using the Jadad scale [27], which reveals the methodological quality of a study based on how it describes randomization, blinding and dropouts (withdrawals). The scale goes from 0 to 5, with a score of ≤ 2 meaning poor quality and a score of ≥ 3 meaning that the report meets high quality standards.

2.8. Statistical Analysis

The meta-analysis was conducted using the RevMan 5 program (Review Manager (RevMan) [Computer program]. Version 5.4. Copenhagen, Denmark: The Nordic Cochrane Centre, The Cochrane Collaboration, London, UK, 2014). Animal studies were assessed for BIC [28–30] between 2 and 6 weeks after placement, and crestal bone loss or MBL of implants was assessed in RCTs 6 months after placement [31,32]. Mean difference (MD) and standard deviation (SD) were used for the assessment of continuous variables (BIC and crestal bone loss), weighting by inverse variance with a 95% confidence interval (CI). The threshold for statistical significance was established at $p < 0.05$. Heterogeneity was assessed by calculating I2 and Chi-square, using a random effects model in both cases. The sensitivity analysis was conducted by excluding one study at a time to check whether there were changes in the results. A funnel plot graph was used to assess publication bias.

3. Results

3.1. Characteristics of the Studies

Until November 2020, a total of 135 studies were identified for subsequent assessment by the reviewers. After a first screening, 41 duplicate studies were removed. In a second screening, 26 studies that did not clearly meet the inclusion criteria, and were therefore considered inadequate, were removed (Figure 1, Flowchart). Table 1 provide the evaluation of the ARRIVE criteria in animal studies. Tables 2 and 3 provide a general description of the details corresponding to the RCTs and experimental animal studies, respectively. Table 4 provides the Jadad quality score in RCTs.

Table 1. Checklist of ARRIVE criteria reported by the included studies.

Studies	Palin et al., 2018 [33]	Salomó-Coll et al., 2016 [34]	Dundar et al., 2016 [35]	Calvo-Guirado et al., 2015 [36]	Tresguerres et al., 2012 [37]	Muñoz et al., 2012 [38]	Guardia et al., 2011 [39]	Calvo-Guirado et al., 2010 [40]	Calvo-Guirado et al., 2009 [41]	Cutando et al., 2008 [42]	Takechi et al., 2008 [43]
1. Title	1	1	1	1	1	1	1	1	1	1	1
Abstract	-	-	-	-	-	-	-	-	-	-	-
2. Species	1	1	1	1	1	1	1	1	1	1	1
3. Key finding	1	1	1	1	1	1	1	1	1	1	1
Introduction	-	-	-	-	-	-	-	-	-	-	-
4. Background	1	1	1	1	1	1	1	1	1	1	1
5. Reasons for animal models	0	0	0	0	0	0	0	0	0	0	0
6. Objectives	1	1	1	1	1	1	1	1	1	1	1
Methods	-	-	-	-	-	-	-	-	-	-	-
7. Ethical statement	1	1	1	1	1	1	1	1	1	1	1
8. Study design	1	1	1	1	1	1	1	1	1	1	1
9. Experimental procedures	1	1	1	1	1	1	1	1	1	1	1
10. Experimental animals	1	1	1	1	1	1	1	1	1	1	1
11. Accommodation and handling of animals	0	1	0	1	0	0	1	1	1	1	0
12. Sample size	1	1	1	1	1	1	1	1	1	1	1
13. Assignment of animals to experimental groups	1	1	1	1	1	0	0	1	0	0	0
14. Anaesthesia	1	1	1	1	1	1	1	1	1	1	1
15. Stadistical methods	1	1	1	1	1	1	1	1	1	1	1
Results	-	-	-	-	-	-	-	-	-	-	-
16. Experimental results	1	1	1	1	1	1	1	1	1	1	1
17. Results and estimation	0	1	0	1	1	1	1	1	1	1	1
Discussion	-	-	-	-	-	-	-	-	-	-	-
18. Interpretation and Scientific implications	1	1	1	1	1	1	1	1	1	1	1
19. 3Rs reported	0	0	0	0	0	0	0	0	0	0	0
20. Adverse events	0	0	0	0	0	0	0	0	0	0	0
21. Study limitations	0	0	0	0	0	0	0	0	0	0	0
22. Generalization/applicability	0	0	0	0	0	0	1	0	0	0	0
23. Funding	0	0	0	0	0	1	1	0	0	1	1
Total Score	15	17	15	17	16	16	18	17	16	17	16

Mode Value: 16.36 ± 0.88 (Mean value and standard deviation); Each item was allocated a score of "0" (not reported) or "1" (reported). The total score of each of the included studies was also recorded.

FLOWCHART

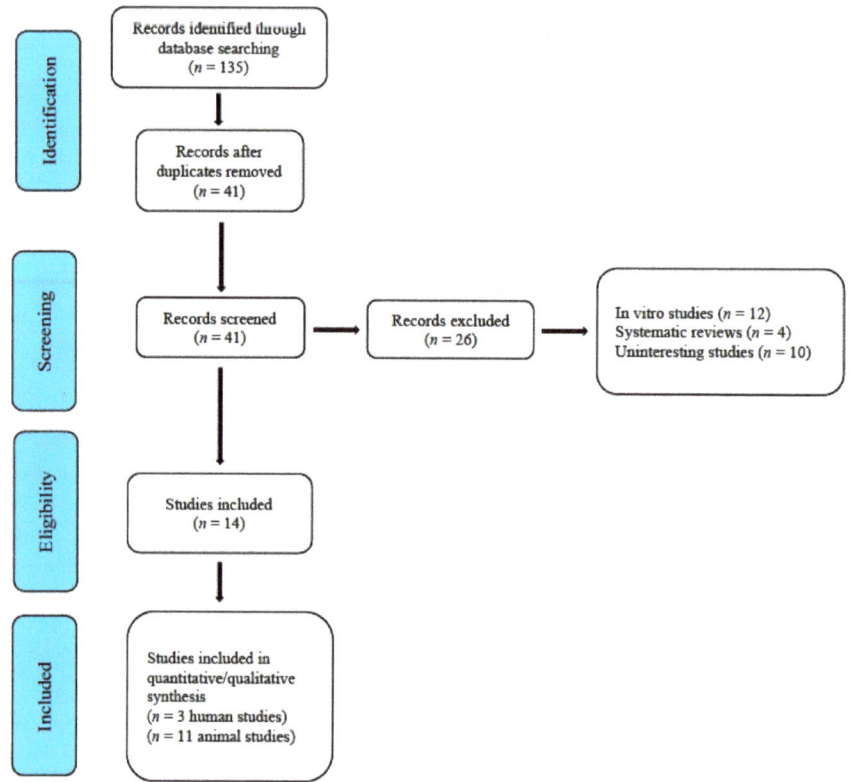

Figure 1. Flowchart.

3.2. Risk of Bias and Quality Assessment of Animals Included Studies

The risk of bias assessment results for the animal studies are shown in Figure 2. Although allocation to blinding was mentioned in several articles, the lack of information resulted in a high and unclear risk of bias for most of the items. The ARRIVE checklist criteria for the animal studies [26] included are shown in Table 1. The mean score of the studies was 16.36 ± 0.88. All the studies provided adequate information in terms of title, abstract, introduction, ethical declaration, species, surgical procedure, assessment of results and statistical analysis. None of the studies reported items 5 (Reasons for animal models), 19 (3Rs, Replace, Reduce and Refine), 20 (Adverse events), 21 (Study limitations) or 22 (Generalization/applicability).

Table 2. Characteristics of randomized clinical trials (RCTs).

Study, Year	Participants Number	Interventions Number	Implants Number	Outcomes	Test Group p-Values	Conclusions
Hazzaa et al., 2020. [44].	23	46 sites for dental implants.	46	- Radiographic evaluation: MBL and BL - PPD - PIST	$p = 0.000$	The combined use of ABG with MLN is a promising alternative for early loading.
Hazzaa et al., 2019. [45].	26	26 sites for dental implants.	52	- Radiographic evaluation: MBL and BD - GI	$p = 0.001$	Application of melatonin with ABG around immediate implants is a valuable option for replacing missing teeth in the esthetic zone in terms of soft and hard tissues.
El-Gammal et al., 2016. [46].	14	14 sites for dental implants.	14	Periotest; MPD; DPD; and MBL	$p = 0.2$	The topical application of melatonin could be a good treatment option for dental implants in the posterior maxilla.

MBL (Marginal Bone Loss); BD (Bone Density); PPD (Pre-implant Probing Depth); PIST (Peri-implant soft tissue); GI (Gingival Index); MPD (Mesial Probing Depth); DDP (Distal Probing Depth); ABG (Autogenous Bone Graft); MT (Melatonin).

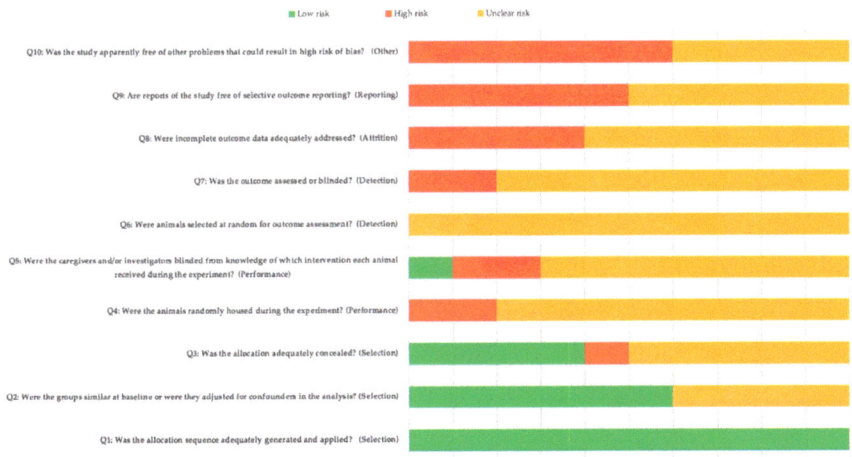

Figure 2. SYRCLE's risk of bias tool.

Table 3. Characteristics of Animal Studies.

Studies, Year	Animals	Melatonin Administration Form	Implants Number	Implantation Sites	Tracing (Weeks)	Conclusions
Palin et al., 2018 [33]	Rat model	Melatonin in saline solution; orally	36	Tibia	60 days	The use of melatonin restores the bone repair process during the osseointegration phase.
Salomó-Coll et al., 2016 [34]	American foxhound dog model	Implants submerged in melatonin at 5% in solution	36	Jaw, premolars area	12 weeks	Topical applications of melatonin to implants placed immediately after extraction improved osseointegration and reduced bone resorption.
Dúndar et al., 2016 [35]	New Zealand rabbit model	Locally (powder melatonin) into the dental implant socket before implant placement	24	Tibia	4 weeks	Local melatonin administration at the osteotomy site during surgical implant insertion may stimulate more BIC.
Calvo-Guirado et al., 2015 [36]	New Zealand rabbit model	Local application of melatonin (Titanium dental implant with melatonin doping surface)	20	Tibia	1 week and 4 weeks	The use of melatonin improves the formation of new bone around the implants.
Tresguerres et al., 2012 [37]	New Zealand rabbit model	3 mg of melatonin administered locally at the osteotomy site as a lyophilizate powder before implant placement	20	Jaw, molars area	4 weeks	Local melatonin administered in the osteoctomy site at the time of implant placement may induce more trabecular bone to implant contact and more trabecular area density.
Muñoz et al., 2012 [38]	Beagle dog model	Topical administration. Prior to implanting, a layer of 1.2 mg lyophilized powdered melatonin was applied to the bone hole	48	Jaw, premolars area.	2, 5 and 8 weeks	Melatonin has stimulating effects on osteogenesis and enhances the formation of new bone around titanium implants in the early stages of healing.
Guardia et al., 2011 [39]	Beagle dog model	Prior to implanting, a layer of 1.2 mg lyophilized powdered melatonin was applied to the bone hole	48	Jaw, premolars and molars area	5 and 8 weeks	Melatonin may bring about a reduction in bone resorption and an increase in bone mass because of its repression of osteoclast activation.
Calvo-Guirado et al., 2010 [40]	Beagle dog model	Implants covered with 5 mg lyophilized powdered melatonin	36	Femur	2 and 4 weeks	Melatonin-coated implants increase BIC and reduce crestal bone loss.
Calvo-Guirado et al., 2009 [41]	Beagle dog model	Prior to implanting, a layer of 5 mg lyophilized powdered melatonin was applied to the bone hole	24	Jaw, premolars area	2, 4 and 12 weeks	Melatonin increases BIC and reduces crestal bone loss.
Cutando et al., 2008 [42]	Beagle dog model	Topical administration. Prior to implanting, a layer of 1.2 mg lyophilized powdered melatonin was applied to the bone hole	48	Jaw, premolars area	2 weeks	Topical application of melatonin may act as a biomimetic agent in the placement of endoosseous dental implants.
Takechi et al., 2008 [43]	Rat model	Locally injected around the implant sites 5 days after implantation	48	Tibia	4 weeks	Melatonin has effects on osteogenesis and enhances the formation of new bone around titanium implants.

3.3. Methodological Quality of the Included Randomized Studies

The mean score of the studies was 3.3 ± 1.2. Two of the included studies [44,46] scored ≥3; the study by Hazzaa et al. [45] obtained the lowest score (Table 4).

Table 4. Jadad quality score of randomized controlled trial, included in the meta-analysis.

Study and Year	Randomization	Blinding	Dropouts	Total Score
Hazzaa et al., 2020. [44]	3	0	0	3
Hazzaa et al., 2019. [45]	1	0	0	2
El-Gammal et al., 2016. [46]	3	1	1	5

Each study was assigned a score of 0–5; Mode value: 3.3 ± 1.2 (Mean value and standard deviation).

3.4. Meta-Analysis Results

The meta-analysis for bone-implant contact was carried out between 2 and 6 weeks after implant placement in animal studies [34–37,39,41–43], while that of crestal bone loss was performed six months after placement in RCTs [44–46].

Three animal studies were excluded from the quantitative analysis: that by Palin et al. [33], as it did not measure bone-implant contact; the study by Muñoz et al. [38], which combined melatonin with growth hormone; and the study conducted by Calvo-Guirado et al. in 2010 [40], where melatonin was combined with pig bone.

Heterogeneity in the results was very high (I^2 = 96%; Chi-square = 193.87; 95% CI), which is why a random effects model was chosen, assuming that the differences among studies were due to heterogeneity, and that the effect of small studies on the result of the meta-analysis was relevant. The results of the sensitivity analysis did not suggest the exclusion of any study to be the cause for heterogeneity, the latter being always above 90%; however, it appeared to be the cause for significant changes in the direction or size of the effect. Since in this case the large effect size suggested a positive result (higher percentage of bone-implant contact), the forest plot's labels were inverted.

The study of the forest plot (Figure 3) revealed no significant differences between the two groups (melatonin vs. placebo) in the studies of Guardia et al. [39], Calvo-Guirado et al. en 2015 [36] and Salomó-Coll et al. [34], since confidence intervals at 95% overlap and cross the line of no effect. In the remaining studies [33,35,37,38,40–43], the experimental group (melatonin) achieves significantly better results than the placebo group. There were also no noticeable differences among studies, since the confidence intervals of the selected studies overlap, except in the case of Takechi et al. [43], where results were more favorable to melatonin than in the other studies.

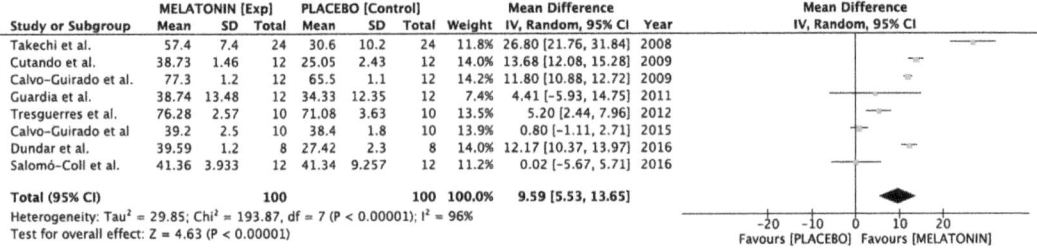

Figure 3. Forest plot for the meta-analysis of animal studies assessing bone-implant contact between 2 to 6 weeks after placement, taking the mean difference as the effect size index, weighting by inverse variance and assuming a random effects model. CI = Confidence Interval.

The meta-analysis revealed that treatment with melatonin is associated with greater contact between the implant's surface and the bone in the assessment carried out between 2 and 6 months after implant placement (difference in means, random effects: 9.59 [95% CI: 5.53–13.65]).

As regards RCTs, three studies [44–46] assessed crestal bone loss 6 months after placement were selected.

Heterogeneity was high ($I^2 = 95\%$; Chi-square = 41, 50; 95% CI), so a random effects model was chosen, assuming that the differences among studies were due to heterogeneity rather than chance. The study of the forest plot (Figure 4) revealed that the difference between the two study groups (melatonin vs. placebo) was not significant in the study by El-Gammal et al. [46], while in the two studies by Hazzaa et al. [44,45], the experimental group (melatonin) achieved better results than the placebo group.

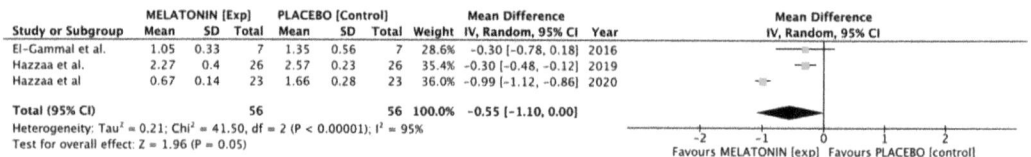

Figure 4. Forest plot for the meta-analysis of the human clinical trials assessing crestal bone loss 6 months after placement, taking the mean difference as the effect size index, weighting by inverse variance and assuming a random effects model. CI = Confidence Interval.

The meta-analysis also proved that, after 6 months, the implants placed in the experimental group (melatonin) presented less marginal bone loss than those placed in the control group (difference in means, random effects: −0.55 [95% CI: 1.10–0.00]). The load increase in the study by El-Gammal et al. [46] led to a widening of the confidence interval for the overall effect size. Nevertheless, because of the small size of the sample and the large heterogeneity among studies, the results of this meta-analysis should be taken with caution

3.5. Publication Bias and Heterogeneity

The experimental studies show graphical signs of publication bias, as can be observed in the Funnel Plot (Figure 5).

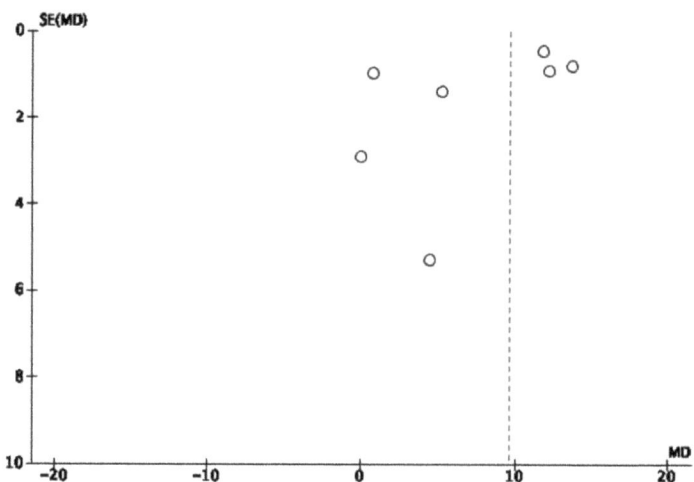

Figure 5. Funnel plot for animal studies. The asymmetry proves publication bias.

4. Discussion

The purpose of this study was to explore the role of MT in bone growth and remodeling around Ti dental implants, both in RCTs and in experimental animal trials.

Bone remodeling involves hormones, cytokines, growth factors and other molecules [47] with MT being one of the hormones that modulates bone formation and absorption.

Certain studies have reported that MT stimulates the osteogenic activity of bone tissue, increasing human osteoblast differentiation in vitro and inducing the formation of cortical bone in mice in [48].

The relationship between MT and bone metabolism has been demonstrated in several studies [37,41,45], with evidence of its effect as a precursor of bone cells in rat bone marrow [49]. Koyama and colleagues [50] were the first to prove that the administration of MT in young rats during their growth period increased spongy bone mass and inhibited bone resorption. If such findings were to be confirmed using adult animals with no endogenous MT, they could be useful to explain the concept of osseointegration. Satomura and colleagues proved that MT accelerates osteoblastic differentiation in humans and rodents, suggesting its possible application as pharmaceutical agent to promote bone regeneration [51]. Nevertheless, in an in vitro study on the effect of melatonin on adipogenesis and osteogenesis in human mesenchymal stem cells, Zhang and colleagues [52] reported an early increase in adhesion and proliferation but found no differences in extended culture periods.

The experimental studies included in our meta-analysis [34–37,39,41–43] show the beneficial effects of MT as regards bone regeneration around Ti dental implants, be it topically applied on implant beds [34,37,39,41,42], coating the implant [35,36], or injected around the implants at the time of placement [43]. However, although certain studies reported a reduction in osteoclastogenesis [53] when topically applied to the alveolar socket after extraction prior to surgery [23], Cobo-Vázquez and colleagues [54], in a pilot study using a sample of 10 patients, found no differences regarding bone density when MT was applied to post-extraction alveolar sockets of retained mandibular third molars. According to our systematic review, Tresguerres and colleagues [37] presented the most thorough histological results, reporting changes in the cortical and medullary regions, and a larger amount of trabecular tissue in contact with the implants in the group treated with MT. The remaining studies only reported histomorphometric results [34–36,39,40,42,43].

Current studies regard the skeleton as a true endocrine organ controlled by the hypothalamus [55]. Protein degradation mediated by the ubiquitin-proteasome pathway is essential to regulate the balance between bone formation and bone resorption through certain signal transduction pathways, which regulate the activity of mature osteoblasts and osteoclasts [56].

Apart from contributing to synchronize biological rhythms and its antioxidant and inflammatory effects, among others, MT has immunomodulatory effects and induces apoptosis [57]. However, the role of MT in the formation of new bone is not fully defined, its reduction being regarded as proportional to skeletal maturation and with contraindications concerning its function, such as the fact that certain individuals with different defects in osteoblast function are at a greater risk for osteosarcoma. Conversely, MT can improve the normal functions of osteoblasts, and would therefore play a protective role against bone cancer [58,59].

Because of the ethical implications associated with histopathological examinations, the RCTs included in our meta-analysis exclusively reported macroscopic and radiologic results; nevertheless, the reduced number of included studies prevented an adequate and conclusive meta-analysis. Moreover, the study by Hazzaa and colleagues [45] presented certain limitations in its design and in how it was conducted, such as group randomization, implant location, reason for removal, demographic characteristics of the participants and the degree to which they balanced between groups that reduce the reliability of its results [60]. Nonetheless, our meta-analysis found that MT stimulates the formation of new bone and increases bone density around Ti dental implants, although it presented serious limitations, mainly associated with the heterogeneity among the selected studies and the scarcity of RCTs. On the other hand, there were significant discrepancies among animal studies regarding measurement of the parameters of bone surface in contact with the implant, as had been observed in the radiologic measurements in the RCTs. There were also major differences regarding the amounts, preparation, forms of application, concentrations and application timing of MT. Another important limitation was that none of the included studies considered factors such as bone quality or the surgical technique used—these factors would provide biases in obtaining results.

The study by Takechi and colleagues [43], which is consistent with that of Satomura and colleagues [51], was the only one where melatonin was used systemically (intraperitoneal, 100 mg/Kg weight) until the animals were sacrificed (4 weeks after implant placement): this form of administration and dosage conflicts with those used by the other authors included in the review [33–43]. The systemic administration of MT requires large doses of the drug, which increases the possibility of side effects; therefore, the topical application of MT is preferred over its systemic administration [61]. This same discrepancy in form of administration and dosage could be observed in the RCTs, while Hazzaa and colleagues and El-Gammal and colleagues [44,46] used MT in the form of topical gel, in doses of 1.2 mg., and Hazzaa and colleagues [45] used it in powder form, not specifying the dosage. Hence, there is no consensus as to the best route of administration for this molecule, and the dosage required to achieve the desired effect.

5. Conclusions

Bearing in mind the limitations of most of the studies, all of those included in this meta-analysis reported that the topical application of MT on the ostectomy site at the time of implant placement can induce greater bone-to-implant contact, as well as greater bone mass and density around Ti dental implants, especially in the earliest stages of healing, thus favoring osseointegration. Nevertheless, to clearly confirm such affirmations, further research using broader, well-designed samples with long-term monitoring and standardized protocols for application, MT dosage and assessment of bone parameters is required; all with the purpose of ensuring predictable and reliable outcomes.

Supplementary Materials: The following are available online at https://www.mdpi.com/2079-6412/11/3/271/s1, Table S1: PRISMA Checklist.

Author Contributions: Study concept, N.L.-V. and A.L.-V.; literature search, N.L.-V. and J.M.R.; data analysis, B.P.-P.; drafting of the manuscript, N.L.-V. and A.L.-V.; critical revision of the manuscript, A.L.-V. and J.M.R. All authors have read and agreed to the published version of the manuscript.

Funding: This research received no external funding.

Institutional Review Board Statement: Not applicable.

Informed Consent Statement: Not applicable.

Data Availability Statement: Not applicable.

Conflicts of Interest: The authors declare no conflict of interest.

Abbreviations

MT	Melatonin
Ti	Titanium
RCTs	Randomized Clinical Trials
BIC	Bone Implant Contact
MLB	Marginal Bone Loss
BD	Bone Density
PPD	Pre-Implant Probing Depth
PIST	Peri-Implant Soft Tissue
GI	Gingival Index
MPD	Mesial Probing Depth
DDP	Distal Probing Depth
ABG	Autogenous Bone Graft

References

1. Brånemark, P.I.; Adell, R.; Breine, U.; Hansson, B.O.; Lindström, J.; Ohlsson, A. Intra-osseous anchorage of dental prostheses. I. Experimental studies. *Scand. J. Plast. Reconstr. Surg.* **1969**, *3*, 81–100.
2. Naveau, A.; Shinmyouzu, K.; Moore, C.; Avivi-Arber, L.; Jokerst, J.; Koka, S. Etiology and Measurement of Peri-Implant Crestal Bone Loss (CBL). *J. Clin. Med.* **2019**, *8*, 166. [CrossRef]
3. He, J.-Y.; Zheng, X.-F.; Jiang, L.-S. Autonomic control of bone formation: Its clinical relevance. *Handb. Clin. Neurol.* **2013**, *117*, 161–171. [PubMed]
4. He, J.-Y.; Jiang, L.-S.; Dai, L.-Y. The Roles of the Sympathetic Nervous System in Osteoporotic Diseases: A Review of Experimental and Clinical Studies. *Ageing Res. Rev.* **2011**, *10*, 253–263.
5. Olney, R.C. Regulation of bone mass by growth hormone. *Med. Pediatric Oncol.* **2003**, *41*, 228–234. [CrossRef] [PubMed]
6. López-Valverde, N.; Flores-Fraile, J.; López-Valverde, A. The Unknown Process Osseointegration. *Biology* **2020**, *9*, 168. [CrossRef] [PubMed]
7. Shi, H.; Sorrell, J.E.; Clegg, D.J.; Woods, S.C.; Seeley, R.J. The Roles of Leptin Receptors on POMC Neurons in the Regulation of Sex-Specific Energy Homeostasis. *Physiol. Behav.* **2010**, *11*, 165–172. [CrossRef]
8. Gupta, B.; Acharya, A.; Pelekos, G.; Gopalakrishnan, D.; Kolokythas, A. Selective serotonin reuptake inhibitors and dental implant failure-a significant concern in elders? *Gerodontology* **2017**, *34*, 505–507. [CrossRef]
9. Pellegrino, G.; Grande, F.; Ferri, A.; Pisi, P.; Gandolfi, M.G.; Marchetti, C. Three-Dimensional Radiographic Evaluation of the Malar Bone Engagement Available for Ideal Zygomatic Implant Placement. *Methods Protoc.* **2020**, *3*, 52. [CrossRef] [PubMed]
10. Buser, D.; Sennerby, L.; De Bruyn, H. Modern implant dentistry based on osseointegration: 50 years of progress, current trends and open questions. *Periodontology* **2017**, *73*, 7–21. [CrossRef]
11. Piatelli, A. *Bone Response to Dental Implant Materials*, 1st ed.; Woodhead Publishing: Cambridge, UK, 2016.
12. Iwai-Yoshida, M.; Shibata, Y.; Wurihan; Suzuki, D.; Fujisawa, N.; Tanimoto, Y.; Kamijo, R.; Maki, K.; Miyazaki, T. Antioxidant and osteogenic properties of anodically oxidized titanium. *J. Mech. Behav. Biomed. Mater.* **2012**, *13*, 230–236. [CrossRef]
13. Coelho, P.G.; Granjeiro, J.M.; Romanos, G.E.; Suzuki, M.; Silva, N.R.F.; Cardaropoli, G.; Thompson, V.P.; Lemons, J.E. Basic research methods and current trends of dental implant surfaces. *J. Biomed. Mater. Res. Part B Appl. Biomater.* **2009**, *88*, 579–596. [CrossRef]
14. López-Valverde, N.; Flores-Fraile, J.; Ramírez, J.M.; Sousa, B.M.; Herrero-Hernández, S.; López-Valverde, A. Bioactive Surfaces vs. Conventional Surfaces in Titanium Dental Implants: A Comparative Systematic Review. *J. Clin. Med.* **2020**, *9*, 2047. [CrossRef]
15. Ramírez-Fernández, M.P.; Calvo-Guirado, J.L.; Maté Sánchez de-Val, J.E.; Delgado-Ruiz, R.A.; Negri, B.; Pardo-Zamora, G.; Peñarrocha, D.; Barona, C.; Granero, J.M.; Alcaraz-Baños, M. Melatonin promotes angiogenesis during repair of bone defects: A radiological and histomorphometric study in rabbit tibiae. *Clin. Oral Investig.* **2013**, *17*, 147–158.
16. Tordjman, S.; Chokron, S.; Delorme, R.; Charrier, A.; Bellissant, E.; Jaafari, N.; Fougerou, C. Melatonin: Pharmacology, Functions and Therapeutic Benefits. *Curr. Neuropharmacol.* **2017**, *15*, 434–443. [CrossRef] [PubMed]
17. Amaral, F.G.D.; Cipolla-Neto, J. A brief review about melatonin, a pineal hormone. *Arch. Endocrinol. Metab.* **2018**, *62*, 472–479. [CrossRef]
18. Najafi, M.; Shirazi, A.; Motevaseli, E.; Rezaeyan, A.H.; Salajegheh, A.; Rezapoor, S. Melatonin as an anti-inflammatory agent in radiotherapy. *Inflammopharmacology* **2017**, *25*, 403–413. [CrossRef]
19. Mauriz, J.L.; Collado, P.S.; Veneroso, C.; Reiter, R.J.; González-Gallego, J. A review of the molecular aspects of melatonin's anti-inflammatory actions: Recent insights and new perspectives. *J. Pineal Res.* **2013**, *54*, 1–14. [CrossRef]
20. Liu, J.; Huang, F.; He, H.W. Melatonin effects on hard tissues: Bone and tooth. *Int. J. Mol. Sci.* **2013**, *14*, 10063–10074. [CrossRef] [PubMed]
21. Salomó-Coll, O.; de Maté-Sánchez, J.E.V.; Ramírez-Fernandez, M.P.; Hernández-Alfaro, F.; Gargallo-Albiol, J.; Calvo-Guirado, J.L. Osseoinductive elements around immediate implants for better osseointegration: A pilot study in foxhound dogs. *Clin. Oral Implants Res.* **2018**, *29*, 1061–1069. [CrossRef] [PubMed]
22. Manchester, L.C.; Coto-Montes, A.; Boga, J.A.; Andersen, L.P.H.; Zhou, Z.; Galano, A.; Vriend, J.; Tan, D.X.; Reiter, R.J. Melatonin: An ancient molecule that makes oxygen metabolically tolerable. *J. Pineal Res.* **2015**, *59*, 403–419. [CrossRef] [PubMed]
23. Rodríguez-Lozano, F.J.; García-Bernal, D.; de los Ros-Roca, M.; del Carmen Alguero, M.; Oñate-Sánchez, R.E.; Camacho-Alonso, F.; Moraleda, J.M. Cytoprotective effects of melatonin on zoledronic acid-treated human mesenchymal stem cells in vitro. *J. Craniomaxillofac. Surg.* **2015**, *43*, 855–862. [CrossRef]
24. Hutton, B.; Ferrán Catalá-López, F.; Moher, D. The PRISMA statement extension for systematic reviews incorporating network meta-analysis: PRISMA-NMA. *Med. Clin.* **2016**, *16*, 262–266. [CrossRef] [PubMed]
25. Hooijmans, C.R.; Rovers, M.M.; de Vries, R.B.; Leenaars, M.; Ritskes-Hoitinga, M.; Langendam, M.W. SYRCLE's risk of bias tool for animal studies. *BMC Med. Res. Methodol.* **2014**, *14*, 43. [CrossRef]
26. Stadlinger, B.; Pourmand, P.; Locher, M.C.; Schulz, M.C. Systematic review of animal models for the study of implant integration, assessing the influence of material, surface and design. *J. Clin. Periodontol.* **2012**, *39*, 28–36. [CrossRef]
27. Jadad, A.R.; Moore, R.A.; Carroll, D.; Jenkinson, C.; Reynolds, D.J.; Gavaghan, D.J.; McQuay, H.J. Assessing the quality of reports of randomized clinical trials: Is blinding necessary? *Control Clin. Trials* **1996**, *17*, 1–12. [CrossRef]

28. Degidi, M.; Perrotti, V.; Piattelli, A.; Iezzi, G. Mineralized bone-implant contact and implant stability quotient in 16 human implants retrieved after early healing periods: A histologic and histomorphometric evaluation. *Int. J. Oral Maxillofac. Implant.* **2010**, *25*, 45–48.
29. Bornstein, M.M.; Valderrama, P.; Jones, A.A.; Wilson, T.G.; Seibl, R.; Cochran, D.L. Bone apposition around two different sandblasted and acid-etched titanium implant surfaces: A histomorphometric study in canine mandibles. *Clin. Oral Implant. Res.* **2008**, *19*, 233–241. [CrossRef]
30. Froum, S.J.; Simon, H.; Cho, S.C.; Elian, N.; Rohrer, M.D.; Tarnow, D.P. Histologic evaluation of bone-implant contact of immediately loaded transitional implants after 6 to 27 months. *Int. J. Oral Maxillofac. Implant.* **2005**, *20*, 54–60.
31. Cosola, S.; Marconcini, S.; Boccuzzi, M.; Menchini-Fabris, G.B.; Covani, U.; Peñarrocha-Diago, M.; Peñarrocha-Oltra, D. Radiological Outcomes of Bone-Level and Tissue-Level Dental Implants: Systematic Review. *Int. J. Environ. Res. Public Health* **2020**, *17*, 6920. [CrossRef] [PubMed]
32. Laurell, L.; Lundgren, D. Marginal bone level changes at dental implants after 5 years in function: A meta-analysis. *Clin. Implant. Dent. Relat. Res.* **2011**, *13*, 19–28. [CrossRef] [PubMed]
33. Palin, L.P.; Polo, T.O.B.; Batista, F.R.; Gomes-Ferreira, P.H. Garcia Junior, I.R.; Rossi, A.C.; Freire, A.; Faverani, L.P.; Sumida, D.H.; Okamoto, R. Daily melatonin administration improves osseointegration in pinealectomized rats. *J. Appl. Oral Sci.* **2018**, *26*, e20170470. [CrossRef]
34. Salomó-Coll, O.; Maté-Sánchez de Val, J.E.; Ramírez-Fernández, M.P.; Satorres-Nieto, M.; Gargallo-Albiol, J.; Calvo-Guirado, J.L. Osseoinductive elements for promoting osseointegration around immediate implants: A pilot study in the foxhound dog. *Clin. Oral Implant. Res.* **2016**, *27*, e167–e175. [CrossRef] [PubMed]
35. Dundar, S.; Yaman, F.; Saybak, A.; Ozupek, M.F.; Toy, V.E.; Gul, M.; Ozercan, I.H. Evaluation of Effects of Topical Melatonin Application on Osseointegration of Dental Implant: An Experimental Study. *J. Oral Implantol.* **2016**, *42*, 386–389. [CrossRef]
36. Calvo-Guirado, J.L.; Aguilar Salvatierra, A.; Gargallo-Albiol, J.; Delgado-Ruiz, R.A.; Maté Sanchez, J.E.; Satorres-Nieto, M. Zirconia with laser-modified microgrooved surface vs. titanium implants covered with melatonin stiulates bone formation. Experimental study in tibia rabbits. *Clin. Oral Implant. Res.* **2015**, *26*, 1421–1429. [CrossRef]
37. Tresguerres, I.F.; Clemente, C.; Blanco, L.; Khraisat, A.; Tamimi, F.; Tresguerres, J.A. Effects of local melatonin application on implant osseointegration. *Clin. Implant. Dent. Relat. Res.* **2012**, *14*, 395–399. [CrossRef]
38. Muñoz, F.; López-Peña, M.; Miño, N.; Gómez-Moreno, G.; Guardia, J.; Cutando, A. Topical application of melatonin and growth hormone accelerates bone healing around dental implants in dogs. *Clin. Implant. Dent. Relat. Res.* **2012**, *14*, 226–235. [CrossRef] [PubMed]
39. Guardia, J.; Gómez-Moreno, G.; Ferrera, M.J.; Cutando, A. Evaluation of effects of topic melatonin on implant surface at 5 and 8 weeks in Beagle dogs. *Clin. Implant. Dent. Relat. Res.* **2011**, *13*, 262–268. [CrossRef] [PubMed]
40. Calvo-Guirado, J.L.; Gómez-Moreno, G.; López-Marí, L.; Guardia, J.; Marínez-González, J.M.; Barone, A.; Tresguerres, I.F.; Paredes, S.D.; Fuentes-Breto, L. Actions of melatonin mixed with collagenized porcine bone versus porcine bone only on osteointegration of dental implants. *J. Pineal Res.* **2010**, *48*, 194–203. [CrossRef] [PubMed]
41. Calvo-Guirado, J.L.; Gómez-Moreno, G.; Barone, A.; Cutando, A.; Alcaraz-Baños, M.; Chiva, F.; López-Marí, L.; Guardia, J. Melatonin plus porcine bone on discrete calcium deposit implant surface stimulates osteointegration in dental implants. *J. Pineal Res.* **2009**, *47*, 164–172. [CrossRef] [PubMed]
42. Cutando, A.; Gómez-Moreno, G.; Arana, C.; Muñoz, F.; Lopez-Peña, M.; Stephenson, J.; Reiter, R.J. Melatonin stimulates osteointegration of dental implants. *J. Pineal Res.* **2008**, *45*, 174–179. [CrossRef] [PubMed]
43. Takechi, M.; Tatehara, S.; Satomura, K.; Fujisawa, K.; Nagayama, M. Effect of FGF-2 and melatonin on implant bone healing: A histomorphometric study. *J. Mater. Sci. Mater. Med.* **2008**, *19*, 2949–2952. [CrossRef]
44. Hazzaa, H.H.A.; Shawki, N.A.; Abdelaziz, L.M.; Shoshan, H.S. Early Loading of Dental Implant Grafted with Autogenous Bone Alone or Combined with Melatonin Gel: A Randomized Clinical Trial. *Austin J. Dent.* **2020**, *7*, 1137.
45. Hazzaa, H.H.A.; El-Kilani, N.S.; Elsayed, S.A.; Abd El Massieh, P.M. Evaluation of Immediate Implants Augmented with Autogenous Bone/Melatonin Composite Graft in the Esthetic Zone: A Randomized Controlled Trial. *J. Prosthodont.* **2019**, *28*, e637–e642. [CrossRef]
46. El-Gammal, M.Y.; Salem, A.S.; Anees, M.M.; Tawfik, M.A. Clinical and Radiographic Evaluation of Immediate Loaded Dental Implants with Local Application of Melatonin: A Preliminary Randomized Controlled Clinical Trial. *J. Oral Implantol.* **2016**, *42*, 119–125. [CrossRef]
47. Ostrowska, Z.; Kos-Kudla, B.; Nowak, M.; Swietochowska, E.; Marek, B.; Gorski, J.; Kajdaniuk, D.; Wolkowska, K. The relationship between bone metabolism, melatonin and other hormones in sham-operated and pinealectomized rats. *Endocr. Regul.* **2003**, *37*, 211–224. [PubMed]
48. Roth, J.A.; Kim, B.G.; Lin, W.L.; Cho, M.I. Melatonin promotes osteoblast differentiation and bone formation. *J. Biol. Chem.* **1999**, *274*, 22041–22047. [CrossRef] [PubMed]
49. Witt-Enderby, P.; Radio, N.M.; Doctor, J.S.; Davis, V.L. Therapeutic treatments potentially mediated by melatonin receptors: Potential clinical uses in the prevention of osteoporosis, cancer and as an adjuvant therapy. *J. Pineal Res.* **2006**, *41*, 297–305. [CrossRef] [PubMed]

50. Koyama, H.; Nakade, O.; Takada, Y.; Kaku, T.; Lau, K.H. Melatonin at pharmacologic doses increases bone mass by suppressing resorption through down-regulation of the RANKL-mediated osteoclast formation and activation. *J. Bone Miner. Res.* **2002**, *17*, 1219–1229. [CrossRef]
51. Satomura, K.; Tobiume, S.; Tokuyama, R.; Yamasaki, Y.; Kudoh, K.; Maeda, E.; Nagayama, M. Melatonin at pharmacological doses enhances human osteoblastic differentiation in vitro and promotes mouse cortical bone formation in vivo. *J. Pineal Res.* **2007**, *42*, 231–239. [CrossRef] [PubMed]
52. Zhang, L.; Su, P.; Xu, C.; Chen, C.; Liang, A.; Du, K.; Peng, Y.; Huang, D. Melatonin inhibits adipogenesis and enhances osteogenesis of human mesenchymal stem cells by suppressing PPARγ expression and enhancing Runx2 expression. *J. Pineal Res.* **2010**, *49*, 364–372. [CrossRef] [PubMed]
53. Cutando, A.; López-Valverde, A.; Gómez-de-Diego, R.; Arias-Santiago, S.; de Vicente-Jiménez, J. Effect of gingival application of melatonin on alkaline and acid phosphatase, osteopontin and osteocalcin in patients with diabetes and periodontal disease. *Med. Oral Patol. Oral Cir. Bucal* **2013**, *18*, e657–e663. [CrossRef] [PubMed]
54. Cobo-Vázquez, C.; Fernández-Tresguerres, I.; Ortega-Aranegui, R.; López-Quiles, J. Effects of local melatonin application on post-extraction sockets after third molar surgery. A pilot study. *Med. Oral Patol. Oral Cir. Bucal* **2014**, *19*, e628–e633. [CrossRef] [PubMed]
55. Tyrovola, J.B. The "Mechanostat" Principle and the Osteoprotegerin-OPG/RANKL/RANK System PART II. The Role of the Hypothalamic-Pituitary Axis. *J. Cell Biochem.* **2017**, *118*, 962–966. [CrossRef] [PubMed]
56. Vriend, J.; Reiter, R.J. Melatonin, bone regulation and the ubiquitin-proteasome connection: A review. *Life Sci.* **2016**, *145*, 152–160. [CrossRef]
57. Carlberg, C. Gene regulation by melatonin. *Ann. N. Y. Acad. Sci.* **2000**, *917*, 387–396. [CrossRef]
58. Gupta, D. How important is the pineal gland in children? In *Advances in Pineal Research*; Reiter, R.J., Pang, S.F., Eds.; John Libbey: London, UK, 1989; pp. 291–297.
59. Lu, K.H.; Su, S.C.; Lin, C.W.; Hsieh, Y.H.; Lin, Y.C.; Chien, M.H.; Reiter, R.J.; Yang, S.F. Melatonin attenuates osteosarcoma cell invasion by suppression of c-c motif chemokine ligand 24 through inhibition of the c-jun n-terminal kinase pathway. *J. Pineal Res.* **2018**, *65*, e12507. [CrossRef]
60. Brignardello-Petersen, R. Melatonin as an adjunct to autogenous bone grafts may result in small benefits in probing depth, marginal bone loss, and gingival index of sites with immediate implants. *J. Am. Dent. Assoc.* **2018**, *149*, e85. [CrossRef]
61. Xiao, L.; Lin, J.; Chen, R.; Huang, Y.; Liu, Y.; Bai, J.; Ge, G.; Shi, X.; Chen, Y.; Shi, J.; et al. Sustained Release of Melatonin from GelMA Liposomes Reduced Osteoblast Apoptosis and Improved Implant Osseointegration in Osteoporosis. *Oxid. Med. Cell. Longev.* **2020**, *2020*, 6797154. [CrossRef]

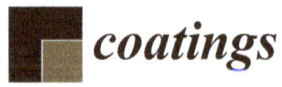

Article

Evaluation of Antithrombogenic pHPC on CoCr Substrates for Biomedical Applications

Catrin Bannewitz [1,*], Tim Lenz-Habijan [1], Jonathan Lentz [2], Marcus Peters [3], Volker Trösken [1], Sabine Siebert [2], Sebastian Weber [2], Werner Theisen [2], Hans Henkes [4] and Hermann Monstadt [1]

[1] phenox GmbH, Lise-Meitner-Allee 31, 44801 Bochum, Germany; tim.habijan@rub.de (T.L.-H.); volker.troesken@phenox.info (V.T.); hermann.monstadt@phenox.info (H.M.)
[2] Lehrstuhl Werkstofftechnik, Ruhr-Universität Bochum, Universitätsstrasse 150, 44801 Bochum, Germany; lentz@wtech.rub.de (J.L.); siebert@wtech.rub.de (S.S.); weber@wtech.rub.de (S.W.); theisen@wtech.rub.de (W.T.)
[3] Department of Molecular Immunology, Ruhr-Universität Bochum, Universitätsstrasse 150, 44801 Bochum, Germany; marcus.peters@rub.de
[4] Neuroradiologische Klinik, Klinikum Stuttgart, Kriegsbergstraße 60, 70174 Stuttgart, Germany; hhhenkes@aol.com
* Correspondence: catrin.bannewitz@rub.de

Abstract: Bare metal endovascular implants pose a significant risk of causing thrombogenic complications. Antithrombogenic surface modifications, such as phenox's "Hydrophilic Polymer Coating" (pHPC), which was originally developed for NiTi implants, decrease the thrombogenicity of metal surfaces. In this study, the transferability of pHPC onto biomedical CoCr-based alloys is examined. Coated surfaces were characterized via contact-angle measurement and atomic force microscopy. The equivalence of the antithrombogenic effect in contact with whole human blood was demonstrated in vitro for CoCr plates compared to NiTi plates on a platform shaker and for braided devices in a Chandler loop. Platelet adhesion was assessed via scanning electron microscopy and fluorescence microscopy. The coating efficiency of pHPC on CoCr plates was confirmed by a reduction of the contact angle from 84.4° ± 5.1° to 36.2° ± 5.2°. The surface roughness was not affected by the application of pHPC. Platelet adhesion was significantly reduced on pHPC-coated specimens. The platelet covered area was reduced by 85% for coated CoCr plates compared to uncoated samples. Uncoated braided devices were completely covered by platelets, while on the pHPC-coated samples, very few platelets were visible. In conclusion, the antithrombogenic effect of pHPC coating can be successfully applied on CoCr plates as well as stent-like CoCr braids.

Keywords: antithrombogenic; endovascular implants; surface modifications; platelet adhesion; hydrophilic polymer coating; shape memory alloys; biomaterials; CoCr alloys; medical devices

Citation: Bannewitz, C.; Lenz-Habijan, T.; Lentz, J.; Peters, M.; Trösken, V.; Siebert, S.; Weber, S.; Theisen, W.; Henkes, H.; Monstadt, H. Evaluation of Antithrombogenic pHPC on CoCr Substrates for Biomedical Applications. *Coatings* **2021**, *11*, 93. https://doi.org/10.3390/coatings11010093

Received: 18 December 2020
Accepted: 13 January 2021
Published: 15 January 2021

Publisher's Note: MDPI stays neutral with regard to jurisdictional claims in published maps and institutional affiliations.

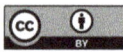

Copyright: © 2021 by the authors. Licensee MDPI, Basel, Switzerland. This article is an open access article distributed under the terms and conditions of the Creative Commons Attribution (CC BY) license (https://creativecommons.org/licenses/by/4.0/).

1. Introduction

Ischemic and hemorrhagic vascular diseases (e.g., myocardial infarct, stroke, atherosclerosis) are among the most frequent causes of death in Western countries [1]. Today, metallic implants are the mainstay of endovascular therapy, which is true for peripheral, cardiological, and neurovascular interventions. For the purpose of vessel occlusion, device-induced thrombus formation is desired, but when it comes to vessel reconstruction, the inherent thrombogenicity of stents and their derivates is an issue [2,3].

Extended research in the field of endovascular treatments of diseases has brought forth a large variety of devices designed for many purposes. While the designs of stents and flow diverters vary significantly, the most commonly used materials today are NiTi alloys, CoCr alloys, or medical-grade steel due to their excellent biocompatibility and mechanical properties [4].

However, once exposed to blood, endovascular implants with a bare metal surface trigger the adhesion of plasma proteins and activate both the coagulation cascade and surrounding thrombocytes. Thrombus formation may result, eventually causing local and distal vessel occlusion [5–8].

The previous paradigm for dealing with this issue comprised the modification of the coagulation system and the platelet function of the patient who is supposed to receive the device implant. Medications that interfere with the various platelet receptors are given according to complex regimens. Typically, the standard of care to prevent thrombus formation on vascular implants is a dual antiplatelet therapy (DAPT) with acetylsalicylic acid (ASA) and Clopidogrel, followed by monotherapy with ASA only, which is often continued for the rest of the patient's life [9,10].

DAPT was and remains, for the time being, the cornerstone of stenting. However, its action is, to a certain degree, unpredictable, subject to several interactions, and difficult to test [11]. Clinical complications may result from hypo- or hyperresponse of patients to the same standard dosage. While DAPT does effectively lower the risk of vessel occlusion in most patients, it simultaneously increases the risk of hemorrhagic events, especially in the first year after implantation [7,8,12–17]. Finally, the emergency treatment of endovascular diseases is severely limited, as effective platelet inhibition should ideally start a few days prior to treatment. Especially in the case of hemorrhagic emergency (e.g., subarachnoid hemorrhage after rupture of an intracranial aneurysm), early treatment is necessary to prevent cerebral infarction, meaning that the application of antiplatelet agents might not be recommended due to the increased risk of rebleeding [18].

Many attempts have been made to avoid this dilemma. There is a large variety of biodegradable or drug-eluting stents with promising results that improved the situation, but did not make DAPT obsolete [19,20].

Some more recent approaches have aimed to reduce the thrombogenicity of the implant surface itself with coatings or surface modifications that disguise the foreign material as endogenous. Efforts to develop such a surface modification have existed for many years. Promising results were obtained in vitro, but most of these were limited to ideal substrates like glass or carefully polished metal or polymer slides. Technical surfaces and the highly complex forms of medical implants seem to hold more challenges regarding antithrombogenicity [21–24]. Other approaches have managed to shorten the time that DAPT is necessary by inducing faster endothelialization (e.g., the COBRA coronary stent with Polyzene-F coating), but do not solve the problems with non-responders or when emergency treatment is required [25].

Currently, only two coatings seem to follow a "bio-mimicry" approach on actual devices: Medtronic's "Shield" technology and phenox's "Hydrophilic Polymer Coating" (pHPC). The Shield technology is available on Medtronic's Pipeline Flex Embolization Device (PED) with Shield Technology (PED Shield). pHPC is currently available on the pCONUS HPC Bifurcation Aneurysm Implant and on the p48 MW HPC and p64 MW HPC flow diverters. All devices are indicated for the treatment of intracranial aneurysms.

The Shield technology is a synthetic phosphorylcholine polymer that is naturally present on the surface of erythrocytes [26,27].

PED Shield implants have been shown to cause fewer thrombogenic effects compared to other uncoated flow diverters in vitro and ex vivo. However, clinical data do not show successful usage of the PED Shield under monotherapy [27–30].

pHPC is a coating technology developed by phenox GmbH, Bochum, Germany, and has demonstrated effective antithrombogenic properties in vitro and in human approaches when applied to NiTi surfaces of laser-cut or braided implants [31,32].

The successful and effective antithrombogenic "disguise" of devices would be a significant advancement for all applications where foreign materials come in contact with blood. That is why it is of utmost interest if pHPC can be applied to materials other than NiTi that are commonly used for devices in blood contact. While NiTi exhibits a surface oxide mainly consisting of TiO_2, for CoCr alloys, the high amount of Cr is responsible for the formation of a thick oxide layer that mostly consists of Cr_2O_3 [33].

Therefore, the purpose of this study was to evaluate the compatibility of pHPC with CoCr-alloy substrates. The coating efficiency, quality, and (anti)thrombogenicity of pHPC on CoCr substrates was examined by means of dynamic contact-angle (CA) measurement, atomic force microscopy (AFM), in vitro testing, fluorescence microscopy, and scanning electron microscopy (SEM).

2. Materials and Methods

2.1. Specimens and Coating

Coated and uncoated specimens that were manufactured from two commercially pure, biomedical-grade CoCr-based alloys were analyzed. In particular, plates made from L-605 (CoCr-based alloy, ASTM F90) and flow-diverter-like braids made from 35NLT wires (CoCr-based alloy, ASTM F562) served as substrates for different tests. L-605 is a Co-based-alloy with chromium (Cr), tungsten (W), and nickel (Ni) as the main alloying elements. The 35NLT braid resembles the design of the p48 MW (HPC), and was used to compare the coating efficiency and antithrombogenicity of pHPC on a flow diverter made of CoCr wires. 35NLT is a Co-based-alloy with Ni, Cr, and molybdenum (Mo) as the main alloying elements [34]. Both CoCr alloys are standard materials for medical applications and are already in use for stents, flow diverters, or artificial heart valves [35,36].

NiTi plates and p48 MW or p48 MW HPC implants (provided by phenox GmbH, Bochum, Germany) were used as references to compare the performance of the antithrombogenic pHPC coating on CoCr and NiTi alloys. The test plates (9 × 9 × 0.5 mm) were laser-cut, pickled, electropolished, and passivated to create a homogenous, shiny surface resembling that of laser-cut stents made of CoCr or NiTi alloys. Subsequently, the specimens were coated with the antithrombogenic pHPC by phenox GmbH.

pHPC is a newly developed glycan-based multilayer polymer mimicking the glycocalyx from the natural outer layer on cells. As the outer layer of endothelial cells, the glycocalyx forms the inner lining of blood vessels. On NiTi surfaces, the pHPC's thickness ranges between 5 and 20 nm, as estimated by X-ray photoelectron spectroscopy [31,37]. The application process and the thin nature of the coating do not influence the physical and mechanical properties of the devices that it is applied to.

2.2. Coating Efficiency—Wettability

In the literature, the antithrombogenic pHPC coating is known to change the wettability of NiTi surfaces, and can therefore be used as an indicator for the coating efficiency [31]. Thus, in this study, the wettability and hydrophilicity of the plates were measured using a modified Wilhelmy Plate method in a tensiometer (DCAT 21, DataPhysics Instruments GmbH, Stuttgart, Germany) through immersion of the sample plates in pure water. The dynamic contact angle was derived from the weight change during immersion, as water will form a larger lamella when the specimens are more hydrophilic. The CAs of the NiTi ($n = 10$) and CoCr ($n = 10$) plates were measured before and after the coating of the samples.

2.3. Atomic Force Microscopy

AFM of coated and uncoated NiTi and CoCr plates was performed on a Dimension FastScan AFM (Bruker, Billerica, MA, USA) to characterize the topographic nature of the plates before and after coating. An area of 1 × 1 µm was scanned on each sample, and the surface analysis was assessed through determination of the mean arithmetic roughness value, Ra, from three randomly chosen line scans (length of 1 µm each).

2.4. In Vitro Blood Contact

Blood sampling was performed under the approval of the ethics commission of the Faculty of Medicine of the Ruhr Universität Bochum, Germany (registration number: 16-5991). Informed consent was obtained from all individual participants included in the study. All procedures performed in studies involving human participants were in accordance with the ethical standards of the institutional and/or national research committee and with the 1964 Helsinki Declaration and its later amendments or comparable ethical standards.

For in vitro testing, the plates were incubated under dynamic conditions on a shaker in heparinized human venous blood. The blood was collected from 10 voluntary and healthy donors. An abnormal blood count measured via a hematology analyzer (KM-21 N, Sysmex, Nordersted, Germany) and the intake of drugs interfering with blood coagulation were exclusion criteria for participation in the study. All steps were performed under sterile conditions. The plates were rinsed twice in phosphate-buffered saline (PBS) before blood contact. Afterwards, they were incubated under dynamic conditions in 24-well plates in 2 mL blood on a shaker (speed level 4; Titramax 100, Heidolph Instruments, Schwabach, Germany). After 10 min of incubation, non-adherent cells were removed by rinsing the specimens with PBS.

The stent devices were incubated in a modified Chandler loop flow model. Blood was collected with the "S-Monovette Blood collection system" (Sarsted, Nümbrecht, Germany). An abnormal blood count measured via a hematology analyzer (KM-21 N, Sysmex, Nordersted, Germany) and the intake of drugs interfering with blood coagulation were exclusion criteria for participation in the study. The devices were deployed in PVC tubes (Rehau, Erlangen, Germany) with an inner diameter of 3 mm. The tubes were first rinsed with PBS and filled with 2 mL of blood, leaving an air bubble of 1 mL inside the tube; then, the tube's ends were interconnected, forming loops. The loops were then rotated at a rate of 30 rotations per minute in a water bath at 37 °C for 120 min. The rotation speed resulted in a flow volume of 60 mL/min and a flow velocity of 90 mL/min (due to the air bubble), thereby resembling typical flow rates in the vertebral artery [38]. The blood count was again performed after incubation.

2.5. CD61 Immunohistochemistry

CD61 (integrin b-3) is a glycoprotein found on the surface of platelets. CD61+ adherent platelets were stained using CD61-PE antibody (BD Pharmingen, Heidelberg, Germany) fluorescence staining. After incubation in whole blood, the specimens were rinsed with PBS twice in order to remove non-adherent cells. The antibody was diluted 1:5 in PBS and added to the specimens. After 15 min incubation in the dark, specimens were rinsed with PBS twice, fixed with 1% paraformaldehyde (Sigma-Aldrich, Taufkirchen, Germany) in PBS, and analyzed using a fluorescence microscope (Olympus BX40, Olympus, Hamburg, Germany) equipped with a digital camera (Moticam 5, Motic, Wetzlar, Germany).

2.6. Semi-Quantitative Phase Analyses

Platelet adherence was assessed by analyzing the platelet-covered area of the plates using ImageJ software (National Institutes of Health, Bethesda, MD, USA). Four defined areas of interest per plate (0.06 mm^2 each, total 0.24 mm^2) were examined. The results were reported as the percentage of positively stained area by relating the positively stained area (CD61+ stained cells) with the absolute area of the regions of interest.

2.7. Scanning Electron Microscopy

To examine the level of platelet activation and clot formation on the stent devices, SEM examinations were performed after incubation in the Chandler loop on the same specimens used for fluorescence imaging.

After incubation, the specimens were prepared for SEM examination by rinsing with PBS twice, fixing with 3.7% glutaraldehyde (Sigma-Aldrich, Taufkirchen, Germany) in PBS for 15 min, dehydrating with an ascending series of alcohols, drying for 24 h at room temperature, and, finally, sputtering with gold (Edwards Sputter Coater S150B9, Edwards Limited, Crawley, UK).

SEM was performed on an LEO 1530 Gemini (Carl Zeiss AG, Jena, Germany).

2.8. Statistical Analysis

Data from platelet activation were analyzed with the Mann–Whitney test. If a significant difference was found, treated groups were compared with the control group by using Dunn's post-test. GraphPad Prism software (version 3.03; GraphPad Software Inc., La Jolla, CA, USA) was used for the analysis. p-values of less than 0.05 were considered statistically significant. The data of the surface roughness was assessed by determining the average Ra for three individual lines per scan. Results are presented as 'mean ± standard error of the mean' (mean ± SE).

3. Results

3.1. Surface Analysis—Wettability and Surface Topography

The results of the CA measurement are given in Table 1. The CAs were 78.1° ± 4.8° for the uncoated NiTi specimens and 84.4° ± 5.1° for the uncoated CoCr specimens. After functionalization with pHPC, the CAs of CoCr and NiTi plates were decreased by roughly 45°–50° (CA of 31.6° ± 2.2° for the NiTi plates, 36.2° ± 5.2° for the CoCr plates).

Table 1. Contact angle (CA) and arithmetic roughness of coated and uncoated NiTi and CoCr specimens.

Specimen	NiTi Plate Uncoated	NiTi Plate pHPC Coated	CoCr Plate Uncoated	CoCr Plate pHPC Coated
Contact Angle (CA) [°]	78.1 ± 4.8	31.6 ± 2.2	84.4 ± 5.1	36.2 ± 5.2
Average roughness (Ra) [nm]	0.383 ± 0.094	0.214 ± 0.020	0.029 ± 0.002	0.036 ± 0.001

Figure 1 shows representative AFM images of the uncoated (Figure 1a,c) and coated specimens (Figure 1b,d). Microscopically, the surface of the NiTi plates had a homogeneous surface with a honeycomb-like structure and minimal waviness. The evenly distributed peaks were about 50 nm apart and had an altitude of about 8 nm. The CoCr plates had a homogenous surface profile with peaks of less than 0.2 nm height and a spacing of less than 10 nm, with some slight waviness. The corresponding results of a nanoscopic analysis of the mean arithmetic roughness values (Ra) are given in Table 1. The coating of the specimens did not alter the homogenous surface profile compared to the corresponding uncoated specimens.

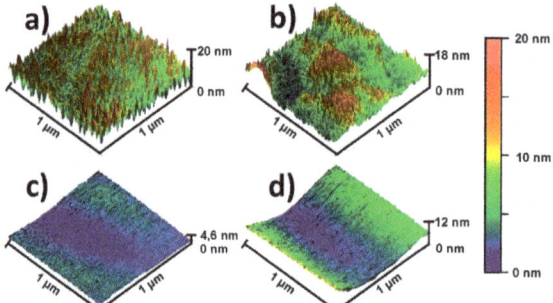

Figure 1. Representative atomic force microscopy (AFM) images of the uncoated (**a**) and coated (**b**) NiTi plates and the uncoated (**c**) and coated (**d**) CoCr plates.

3.2. Thrombogenicity—Fluorescence and SEM Imaging

Figure 2 shows the representative fluorescence microscopic images of pHPC-coated (Figure 2b,d) and uncoated (Figure 2a,c) NiTi and CoCr plates, which were incubated in vitro in human blood and stained with CD61 antibody. Few CD61+ platelets were detected on the coated specimens (yellow fluorescence), whereas the uncoated specimens were homogenously covered with cells in each experiment.

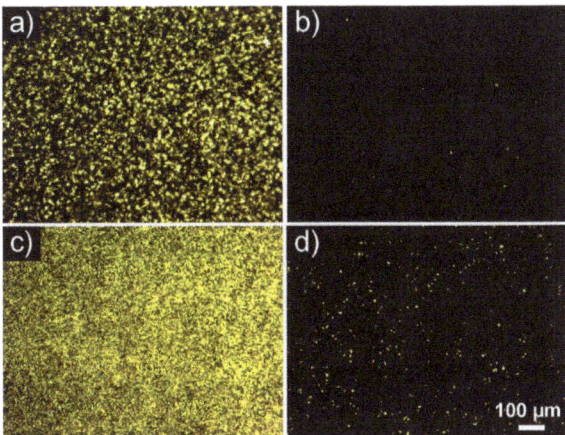

Figure 2. Representative fluorescence micrographs of uncoated (**a,c**) and phenox's "Hydrophilic Polymer Coating" (pHPC)-coated (**b,d**) NiTi (**a,b**) and CoCr (**c,d**) specimens. The plates were incubated in whole human blood for 10 min under dynamic conditions. Adherent platelets were stained with a CD61 antibody (yellow fluorescence). (Scale bar for all images 100 µm.)

Figure 3 shows the results of the quantitative phase analysis of the platelet-covered area on the plates. The amount of surface area covered with adhering thrombocytes was significantly lower on the pHPC-coated NiTi and CoCr plates compared to the uncoated ones. Overall, the CoCr plates did elicit more platelet activation than the NiTi plates. Uncoated CoCr specimens were covered with CD61+ platelets by 85.5% ± 10.7%, while the uncoated NiTi specimens were covered by 66.9% ± 21.5%. The pHPC-coated CoCr plates were covered by 12.8% ± 9.4% and the coated NiTi plates by 6.7% ± 8.8%. On average, the platelet adherence was reduced by 90% on coated NiTi and by 85% on the pHPC-coated CoCr specimens.

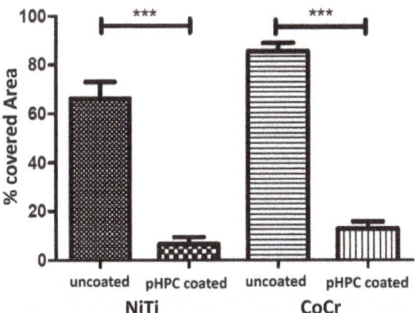

Figure 3. Quantitative phase analysis of the area coated with CD61+ cells from experiments with ten different donors (mean ± SE; asterisks denote significance at *** $p \leq 0.001$; Mann–Whitney and Dunn's post-test; sample size uncoated vs. coated $n = 10$). While significantly fewer CD61+ platelets adhered to the coated specimens than to the uncoated ones, there is no significant difference between the NiTi and the CoCr specimens.

Additionally, stent devices were incubated in a modified Chandler loop flow model with whole human blood for 120 min, and adherent cells were again stained with a CD61 antibody and analyzed using fluorescence microscopy.

Figure 4 shows representative fluorescence micrographs of uncoated and pHPC-coated p48 MW (NiTi) and CoCr braids. While the uncoated devices were completely covered with adherent platelets, there were considerably fewer fluorescent cells on the pHPC-coated braids. On both the p48 MW HPC and the coated CoCr braids, the adherent cells tended to adhere to contact points where the wires of the braids crossed over each other.

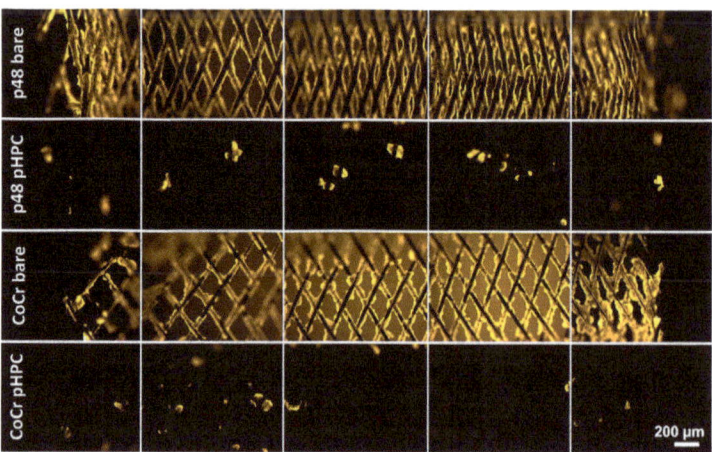

Figure 4. Representative fluorescence micrographs of uncoated and pHPC-coated p48 MW and CoCr specimens. The devices were incubated in whole human blood in a modified Chandler loop flow model under dynamic conditions at 37 °C for 120 min. Adherent platelets were stained with a CD61 antibody (yellow fluorescence). Though the uncoated devices were completely covered with adherent platelets, there were considerably fewer fluorescent cells on the pHPC-coated braids. (Scale bar for all images 200 μm.)

Figure 5 shows representative SEM images of the respective stent devices after incubation in the Chandler loop. The wires of the uncoated devices (Figure 5a,c,e,g) were completely covered by a dense layer of fibrin and embedded platelets. In contrast, only a few platelets were visible on the pHPC-coated samples (Figure 5b,d,f,h). Again, the predominant adherence of platelets at the crossings of the wires on the coated devices was observed.

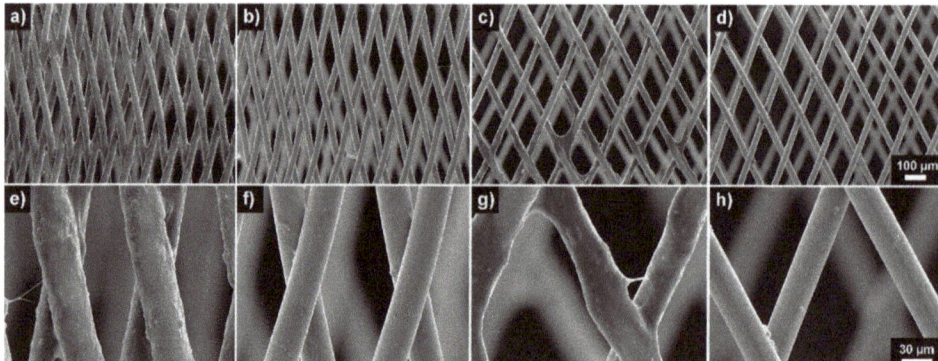

Figure 5. Representative scanning electron microscopy (SEM) images (in secondary electron contrast) of coated (**b,d,f,h**) and uncoated (**a,c,e,g**) NiTi (**a,b,e,f**) and CoCr (**c,d,g,h**) devices after incubation in whole human blood in a modified Chandler loop flow model under dynamic conditions at 37 °C for 120 min. The uncoated devices were completely covered with adherent platelets and fibrin clots, while only a few cells adhered to the pHPC-coated devices. (Scale bar for the upper row 100 μm, scale bar for the lower row 30 μm.)

4. Discussion

pHPC was originally developed for surface modification of NiTi devices and is approved and available on endovascular stent devices made from NiTi. However, the most commonly used materials for similar applications, apart from NiTi alloys, are CoCr alloys and medical-grade steel [4]. While NiTi exhibits a surface oxide that mainly consists of TiO_2, for CoCr alloys, the high amount of Cr is responsible for the formation of a thick oxide layer that mostly consists of Cr_2O_3 [33]. Hence, the purpose of this study was to evaluate the compatibility of pHPC with CoCr-alloy substrates to expand the range of antithrombogenic biomaterials that are commonly used in blood contact. Therefore, the coating efficiency, quality, and (anti)thrombogenicity of pHPC on CoCr substrates was examined by means of dynamic contact-angle (CA) measurement, atomic force microscopy (AFM), in vitro testing, fluorescence microscopy, and scanning electron microscopy (SEM).

The platelet activation and adhesion were significantly reduced on pHPC-coated CoCr specimens compared to the corresponding uncoated specimens (Figures 2–4). The surface area covered by adherent platelets was reduced by 85% on the pHPC-coated CoCr plates compared to a reduction by 90% on coated NiTi (Figure 3). This is also true for pHPC-coated NiTi and CoCr braids when tested under dynamic conditions in a Chandler loop experiment (Figures 4 and 5). It is known that the thrombogenicity of a surface depends on the preceding adhesion of proteins [39]. In turn, the adhesion of proteins depends on the surface topography and wettability [40].

The surface topography of a biomaterial's surface has been shown to have a great impact on the adherence and proliferation of proteins and, thereby, cells; therefore, it is of interest regarding platelet activation and endothelialization of vascular implants [40]. The microscopic and nanoscopic surface structure was apparently unaffected by the coating (Table 1, Figure 1). The NiTi plates were very smooth and had a consistent surface structure, typical for electropolished NiTi [41], while the CoCr plates were even smoother. The surface structures of the NiTi and CoCr samples were not microscopically or macroscopically affected by the coating. The coating is known to be extremely thin (<10 nm) on NiTi [31] and apparently formed the same way on CoCr, as the coating procedure did not affect the original surface. The smooth surfaces of the plates resembled those of typical bare metal stents, which are also usually electropolished to deburr the edges and to create a smooth surface finish after laser cutting, thereby lowering the likelihood of a foreign body response by blood or vessel cells [42,43].

While the pHPC coating does not affect the topography of the NiTi and CoCr plates, it certainly does affect the wettability (Table 1).

The CAs of the uncoated plates can be considered as weakly hydrophilic, with 78.1° ± 4.8° for the NiTi surface and 84.4° ± 5.1° for the CoCr surface (Table 1) [44]. After functionalization of the surfaces using the pHPC coating, the decrease of the CA by roughly 45° to 50° resulted in a moderately hydrophilic surface (CA of 36.2° ± 5.2° for the CoCr plates and 31.6° ± 2.2° for the NiTi plates—see Table 1), thereby indicating successful coating of both materials.

A biomaterial's wettability is known to influence the adhesion of proteins and, thereby, to influence the interaction with cells [45]. However, the wettability of devices is of interest for further reasons. The adhesion of proteins is known to be the start of cell-surface interaction [46]. Firstly, thrombocyte activation and adhesion might be affected by a changed wettability on the surface of implants designed to treat vascular disease, and secondly, the proliferation of endothelial cells might be enhanced or decreased due to the same effect. A moderate wettability with CAs of around 35° can be considered optimal for devices that are in contact with blood. Protein adsorption to surfaces is the beginning of all cell-surface interactions. Extremely hydrophilic (CA < 25°) or hydrophobic surfaces (CA > 85°) do reduce protein adsorption and, thereby, reduce cell-surface interaction in general [45]. Platelet activation and adherence are known to be decreased by increasing wettability [47–49]. However, endothelialization, which is important for the long-term biocompatibility of endovascular devices, is decreased on extremely hydrophilic or hydrophobic surfaces due to the reduced adhesion of extracellular matrix proteins (EMPs). Moderately hydrophilic surfaces, like pHPC-coated NiTi or CoCr surfaces, however, do allow the adherence of extracellular matrix proteins (and, therefore, endothelialization), with a maximum endothelial cell adhesion occurring at a CA of 35° to 50° [45,50].

This is in line with the observations from our three animal studies. In those studies, pHPC-coated and uncoated specimens were implanted in the carotid arteries of New Zealand white rabbits for 30 and 120 d. It was shown that pHPC coating of NiTi surfaces does not delay the ingrowth of stent devices into the vessel wall [51,52]. The antithrombogenic effect of pHPC has been shown to last long enough after implantation to keep patients under ASA monotherapy until the device is completely incorporated by endothelial cells [32]. If this is true for CoCr substrates as well still needs to be examined in further research.

Overall, the antithrombogenic effect of pHPC was successfully applied to two different medical CoCr alloys (plates from L-605 and flow-diverter-like stent devices from 35NLT wires). The transfer onto other materials for biomedical applications might be of interest for further research. The remaining platelets on the coated stent devices were predominantly observed at the contact points of the crossings of wires. This has been observed before on braided devices after implantation in animals and humans, and is mainly caused by additional turbulence at these points, as platelets are activated by additional sheer stress [53–55].

However, the surfaces of medical-grade CoCr alloys and stainless steels are effectively alike. While NiTi exhibits a surface oxide mainly consisting of TiO_2, for CoCr alloys and stainless steel, the high amount of Cr is responsible for the formation of a thick oxide layer that mostly consists of Cr_2O_3 [33]. pHPC might, therefore, be effortlessly transferred onto stainless steel devices as well.

Even though the results are promising, further experiments regarding the coating's mechanical and biological durability on CoCr surfaces might be of further interest. However, these properties need to be evaluated under consideration of the actual application because, e.g., different implant designs might generate different loads, have different surface properties, or hold other challenges.

5. Conclusions

The conducted experiments demonstrate the transferability of the pHPC technology onto two different CoCr alloys for biomedical applications. The coating was successfully applied to plates and braided wires without negatively affecting the materials' surface quality. Furthermore, the platelet adhesion was significantly reduced on coated NiTi and CoCr devices compared to uncoated devices. The results of this study show that antithrombogenic pHPC coating is a promising candidate for the development of endovascular devices of different materials with antithrombogenic surface properties.

6. Patents

Patent "Beschichtung für Medizinprodukte" pending under the application numbers DE 10 2017 111 486 A1, DE 10 2017 011 956 A1, and WO 00 2018 210 989 A1.

Author Contributions: Conceptualization, C.B., T.L.-H. and H.H.; Formal analysis, C.B. and M.P.; Investigation, C.B. and M.P.; Project administration, T.L.-H.; Resources, W.T. and H.M.; Supervision, V.T., S.S., S.W., W.T., H.H. and H.M.; Validation, C.B., T.L.-H. and M.P.; Visualization, C.B. and T.L.-H.; Writing—original draft, C.B.; Writing—review and editing, C.B., T.L.-H., J.L., H.H. and H.M. All authors have read and agreed to the published version of the manuscript.

Funding: This research received no external funding.

Institutional Review Board Statement: The study was conducted according to the guidelines of the Declaration of Helsinki and approved by the Ethics Committee of the Faculty of Medicine of the Ruhr Universität Bochum, Germany (protocol code 16-5991, 06.04.2017).

Informed Consent Statement: Informed consent was obtained from all subjects involved in the study.

Data Availability Statement: The data that support the findings of this study are available from the corresponding author, C.B., upon reasonable request.

Conflicts of Interest: C.B., T.L.-H., and V.T.: Employee in the R&D department of phenox GmbH; Dr.-Ing. J.L.: Consultant of phenox; PD Dr. rer. nat. M.P.: Institution received research grants from phenox GmbH; Dr.-Ing. S.S., Prof. Dr.-Ing. S.W., and Prof. Dr.-Ing. W.T.: No conflict of interest declared; Prof. Dr. med. Dr. h.c. H.H.: Co-founder and shareholder of phenox GmbH; Prof. Dr.-Ing. H.M.: Co-founder, shareholder, and CEO of phenox GmbH.

References

1. Bundesamt, S. *Gesundheit—Todesursachen in Deutschland*; Statistisches Bundesamt: Wiesbaden, Germany, 2015.
2. Leon, M.B.; Baim, D.S.; Popma, J.J.; Gordon, P.C.; Cutlip, D.E.; Ho, K.K.; Giambartolomei, A.; Diver, D.J.; Lasorda, D.M.; Williams, D.O.; et al. A clinical trial comparing three antithrombotic-drug regimens after coronary-artery stenting. Stent anticoagulation restenosis study investigators. *N. Engl. J. Med.* **1998**, *339*, 1665–1671. [CrossRef] [PubMed]
3. Dotter, C.T. Transluminally-placed coilspring endarterial tuve grafts: Long term patency in canine popliteal artery. *Investig. Radiol.* **1969**, *4*, 329–332. [CrossRef] [PubMed]
4. Machraoui, A.; Grewe, P.; Fischer, A. *Koronarstenting. Werkstofftechnik, Pathomorphologie, Therapie*; Steinkopff: Heidelberg, Germany, 2001; ISBN 978-3-642-57637-9.
5. Gorbet, M.B.; Sefton, M.V. Biomaterial-associated thrombosis: Roles of coagulation factors, complement, platelets and leukocytes. *Biomaterials* **2004**, *25*, 5681–5703. [CrossRef] [PubMed]
6. Mikhalovska, L.I.; Santin, M.; Denyer, S.P.; Lloyd, A.W.; Teer, D.G.; Field, S.; Mikhalovsky, S.V. Fibrinogen adsorption and platelet adhesion to metal and carbon coatings. *Thromb. Haemost.* **2004**, *92*, 1032–1039. [CrossRef]
7. Versteeg, H.H.; Heemskerk, J.W.M.; Levi, M.; Reitsma, P.H. New fundamentals in hemostasis. *Physiol. Rev.* **2013**, *93*, 327–358. [CrossRef] [PubMed]
8. Reininger, A.J. Function of von Willebrand factor in haemostasis and thrombosis. *Haemophilia* **2008**, *14*, 11–26. [CrossRef]
9. Honda, Y.; Fitzgerald, P.J. Stent thrombosis: An issue revisited in a changing world. *Circulation* **2003**, *108*, 2–5. [CrossRef]
10. Kastrati, A.; Schühlen, H.; Hausleiter, J.; Zitzmann-Roth, E. Restenosis after coronary stent placement and randomization to a 4-week combined antiplatelet or anticoagulant therapy: Six-month angiographic follow-up of the intracoronary stenting and antithrombotic regimen (ISAR) trial. *Circulation* **1997**, *96*, 462–467.
11. Martinez-Moreno, R.; Aguilar, M.; Wendl, C.; Bäzner, H.; Ganslandt, O.; Henkes, H. Fatal thrombosis of a flow diverter due to ibuprofen-related antagonization of acetylsalicylic acid. *Clin. Neuroradiol.* **2016**, *26*, 355–358. [CrossRef]
12. Berger, P.B.; Bhatt, D.L.; Fuster, V.; Steg, P.G.; Fox, K.A.A.; Shao, M.; Brennan, D.M.; Hacke, W.; Montalescot, G.; Steinhubl, S.R.; et al. Bleeding complications with dual antiplatelet therapy among patients with stable vascular disease or risk factors for vascular disease: Results from the clopidogrel for high atherothrombotic risk and ischemic stabilization, management, and avoidance (CHARISMA) trial. *Circulation* **2010**, *121*, 2575–2583. [CrossRef]
13. Hankey, G.J.; Eikelboom, J.W. Aspirin resistance. *Lancet* **2006**, *367*, 606–617. [CrossRef]
14. Nguyen, T.A.; Diodati, J.G.; Pharand, C. Resistance to clopidogrel: A review of the evidence. *J. Am. Coll. Cardiol.* **2005**, *45*, 1157–1164. [CrossRef] [PubMed]
15. Farid, N.A.; Kurihara, A.; Wrighton, S.A. Metabolism and disposition of the thienopyridine antiplatelet drugs ticlopidine, clopidogrel, and prasugrel in humans. *J. Clin. Pharmacol.* **2010**, *50*, 126–142. [CrossRef] [PubMed]
16. Dobesh, P.P.; Oestreich, J.H. Ticagrelor: Pharmacokinetics, pharmacodynamics, clinical efficacy, and safety. *Pharmacotherapy* **2014**, *34*, 1077–1090. [CrossRef] [PubMed]
17. Neubauer, H.; Kaiser, A.F.C.; Endres, H.G.; Krüger, J.C.; Engelhardt, A.; Lask, S.; Pepinghege, F.; Kusber, A.; Mügge, A. Tailored antiplatelet therapy can overcome clopidogrel and aspirin resistance–the BOchum CLopidogrel and Aspirin Plan (BOCLA-Plan) to improve antiplatelet therapy. *BMC Med.* **2011**, *9*, 3. [CrossRef] [PubMed]
18. Steiner, T.; Juvela, S.; Unterberg, A.; Jung, C.; Forsting, M.; Rinkel, G. European Stroke Organization guidelines for the management of intracranial aneurysms and subarachnoid haemorrhage. *Cerebrovasc. Dis.* **2013**, *35*, 93–112. [CrossRef]
19. Pan, C.J.; Tang, J.J.; Weng, Y.J.; Wang, J.; Huang, N. Preparation, characterization and anticoagulation of curcumin-eluting controlled biodegradable coating stents. *J. Control. Release* **2006**, *116*, 42–49. [CrossRef]
20. Kufner, S.; Joner, M.; Thannheimer, A.; Hoppmann, P.; Ibrahim, T.; Mayer, K.; Cassese, S.; Laugwitz, K.-L.; Schunkert, H.; Kastrati, A.; et al. Ten-year clinical outcomes from a trial of three limus-eluting stents with different polymer coatings in patients with coronary artery disease. *Circulation* **2019**, *139*, 325–333. [CrossRef]
21. Lopez-Donaire, M.L.; Santerre, J.P. Surface modifying oligomers used to functionalize polymeric surfaces: Consideration of blood contact applications. *J. Appl. Polym. Sci.* **2014**, *131*, 40328:1–40328:15. [CrossRef]
22. Muramatsu, T.; Onuma, Y.; Zhang, Y.-J.; Bourantas, C.V.; Kharlamov, A.; Diletti, R.; Farooq, V.; Gogas, B.D.; Garg, S.; García-García, H.M.; et al. Progress in treatment by percutaneous coronary intervention: The stent of the future. *Rev. Esp. Cardiol.* **2013**, *66*, 483–496. [CrossRef]
23. Kaplan, O.; Hierlemann, T.; Krajewski, S.; Kurz, J.; Nevoralová, M.; Houska, M.; Riedel, T.; Riedelová, Z.; Zárubová, J.; Wendel, H.P.; et al. Low-thrombogenic fibrin-heparin coating promotes in vitro endothelialization. *J. Biomed. Mater. Res. A* **2017**, *105*, 2995–3005. [CrossRef]

24. Shuvalova, Y.A.; Shirokov, R.O.; Kaminnaya, V.I.; Samko, A.N.; Kaminnyi, A.I. Two-year follow-up of percutaneous coronary intervention using EucaTax or Cypher. *Cardiovasc. Revasc. Med.* **2013**, *14*, 284–288. [CrossRef] [PubMed]
25. Cutlip, D.E.; Garratt, K.N.; Novack, V.; Barakat, M.; Meraj, P.; Maillard, L.; Erglis, A.; Jauhar, R.; Popma, J.J.; Stoler, R.; et al 9-month clinical and angiographic outcomes of the COBRA polyzene-f nanocoated coronary stent system. *JACC Cardiovasc. Interv.* **2017**, *10*, 160–167. [CrossRef] [PubMed]
26. Girdhar, G.; Li, J.; Kostousov, L.; Wainwright, J.; Chandler, W.L. In-vitro thrombogenicity assessment of flow diversion and aneurysm bridging devices. *J. Thromb. Thrombolysis* **2015**, *40*, 437–443. [CrossRef]
27. Martínez-Galdámez, M.; Lamin, S.M.; Lagios, K.G.; Liebig, T.; Ciceri, E.F.; Chapot, R.; Stockx, L.; Chavda, S.; Kabbasch, C.; Farago, G.; et al. Periprocedural outcomes and early safety with the use of the Pipeline Flex Embolization Device with Shield Technology for unruptured intracranial aneurysms: Preliminary results from a prospective clinical study. *J. Neurointerv. Surg.* **2017**, *9*, 772–776. [CrossRef]
28. Girdhar, G.; Ubl, S.; Jahanbekam, R.; Thinamany, S.; Belu, A.; Wainwright, J.; Wolf, M.F. Thrombogenicity assessment of Pipeline, Pipeline Shield, Derivo and P64 flow diverters in an in vitro pulsatile flow human blood loop model. *eNeurologicalSci* **2019**, *14*, 77–84. [CrossRef] [PubMed]
29. Martínez-Galdámez, M.; Gil, A.; Caniego, J.L.; Gonzalez, E.; Bárcena, E.; Perez, S.; Garcia-Bermejo, P.; Ortega-Gutierrez, S. Preliminary experience with the Pipeline Flex Embolization Device: Technical note. *J. Neurointerv. Surg.* **2015**, *7*, 748–751. [CrossRef]
30. Hanel, R.A.; Aguilar-Salinas, P.; Brasiliense, L.B.; Sauvageau, E. First US experience with Pipeline Flex with Shield Technology using aspirin as antiplatelet monotherapy. *BMJ Case Rep.* **2017**, *2017*. [CrossRef] [PubMed]
31. Lenz-Habijan, T.; Bhogal, P.; Peters, M.; Bufe, A.; Martinez Moreno, R.; Bannewitz, C.; Monstadt, H.; Henkes, H. Hydrophilic stent coating inhibits platelet adhesion on stent surfaces: Initial results in vitro. *Cardiovasc. Intervent. Radiol.* **2018**, *41*, 1779–1785. [CrossRef]
32. Colgan, F.; Aguilar Pérez, M.; Hellstern, V.; Reinhard, M.; Krämer, S.; Bäzner, H; Henkes, H. *Vertebral Artery Aneurysm: Ruptured Dissecting Aneurysm, Implantation of Telescoping p48_HPC Flow Diverter Stents under Antiaggregation with ASA only: The Aneurysm Casebook: A Guide to Treatment Selection and Technique*; Springer International Publishing: Cham, Switzerland, 2018; pp. 1–16.
33. Roos, E.; Maile, K.; Seidenfuß, M. *Werkstoffkunde für Ingenieure. Grundlagen, Anwendung, Prüfung, 6., Ergänzte und bearbeitete Auflage*; Springer Vieweg: Berlin/Heidelberg, Germany, 2017; ISBN 9783662495322.
34. Murphy, W.; Black, J.; Hastings, G. *Handbook of Biomaterial Properties*; Springer: New York, NY, USA, 2016; ISBN 978-1-4939-3303-7.
35. Williams, D.F. On the mechanisms of biocompatibility. *Biomaterials* **2008**, *29*, 2941–2953. [CrossRef]
36. Wintermantel, E.; Ha, S.-W. *Medizintechnik. Life Science Engineering*; Interdisziplinarität, Biokompatibilität, Technologien, Implantate, Diagnostik, Werkstoffe, Zertifizierung, Business, 5., überarb. und erw. Aufl.; Springer: Berlin/Heidelberg, Germany, 2009; ISBN 9783540939351.
37. Henkes, H.; Bhogal, P.; Aguilar Pérez, M.; Lenz-Habijan, T.; Bannewitz, C.; Peters, M.; Sengstock, C.; Ganslandt, O.; Lylyk, P.; Monstadt, H. Anti-thrombogenic coatings for devices in neurointerventional surgery: Case report and review of the literature. *Interv. Neuroradiol.* **2019**, *25*, 619–627. [CrossRef] [PubMed]
38. Kaps, M. *Sonografie in der Neurologie*; 3. Auflage; Georg Thieme Verlag: New York, NY, USA, 2017.
39. Horbett, T.A. The role of adsorbed proteins in animal cell adhesion. *Colloids Surf. B Biointerfaces* **1994**, *2*, 225–240. [CrossRef]
40. Xu, L.-C.; Bauer, J.W.; Siedlecki, C.A. Proteins, platelets, and blood coagulation at biomaterial interfaces. *Colloids Surf. B Biointerfaces* **2014**, *124*, 49–68. [CrossRef] [PubMed]
41. Maxisch, M.; Ebbert, C.; Torun, B.; Fink, N.; de los Arcos, T.; Lackmann, J.; Maier, H.J.; Grundmeier, G. PM-IRRAS studies of the adsorption and stability of organophosphonate monolayers on passivated NiTi surfaces. *Appl. Surf. Sci.* **2011**, *257*, 2011–2018. [CrossRef]
42. de Scheerder, I.; Verbeken, E.; van Humbeeck, J. Metallic surface modification. *Semin. Interv. Cardiol.* **1998**, *3*, 139–144. [PubMed]
43. Sojitra, P.; Engineer, C.; Kothwala, D.; Raval, A.; Kotadia, H.; Mehta, G. Investigation of material removal, surface roughnessand corrosion behaviour: Surface roughnessand corrosion behaviour. *Trends Biomater. Artif. Organs* **2010**, *23*, 115–121.
44. Bracco, G.; Holst, B. *Surface Science Techniques*; Springer: Berlin/Heidelberg, Germany, 2013; ISBN 9783642342431.
45. Faucheux, N.; Schweiss, R.; Lützow, K.; Werner, C.; Groth, T. Self-assembled monolayers with different terminating groups as model substrates for cell adhesion studies. *Biomaterials* **2004**, *25*, 2721–2730. [CrossRef]
46. Harnett, E.M.; Alderman, J.; Wood, T. The surface energy of various biomaterials coated with adhesion molecules used in cell culture. *Colloids Surf. B Biointerfaces* **2007**, *55*, 90–97. [CrossRef]
47. Wan, G.J.; Huang, N.; Yang, P.; Fu, R.K.Y.; Ho, J.P.Y.; Xie, X.; Zhou, H.F.; Chu, P.K. Platelet activation behavior on nitrogen plasma-implanted silicon. *Mater. Sci. Eng. C* **2007**, *27*, 928–932. [CrossRef]
48. Yang, P.; Huang, N.; Leng, Y.X.; Yao, Z.Q.; Zhou, H.F.; Maitz, M.; Leng, Y.; Chu, P.K. Wettability and biocompatibility of nitrogen-doped hydrogenated amorphous carbon films: Effect of nitrogen. *Nucl. Instrum. Methods Phys. Res. Sect. B Beam Interact. Mater. At.* **2006**, *242*, 22–25. [CrossRef]
49. Tzoneva, R.; Groth, T.; Altankov, G.; Paul, D. Remodeling of fibrinogen by endothelial cells in dependence on fibronectin matrix assembly. Effect of substratum wettability. *J. Mater. Sci. Mater. Med.* **2002**, *13*, 1235–1244. [CrossRef] [PubMed]
50. Arima, Y.; Iwata, H. Effect of wettability and surface functional groups on protein adsorption and cell adhesion using well-defined mixed self-assembled monolayers. *Biomaterials* **2007**, *28*, 3074–3082. [CrossRef] [PubMed]

51. Bhogal, P.; Lenz-Habijan, T.; Bannewitz, C.; Hannes, R.; Monstadt, H.; Simgen, A.; Mühl-Benninghaus, R.; Reith, W.; Henkes, H. The pCONUS HPC: 30-day and 180-day in vivo biocompatibility results. *Cardiovasc. Intervent. Radiol.* **2019**, *42*, 1008–1015. [CrossRef]
52. Lenz-Habijan, T.; Bhogal, P.; Bannewitz, C.; Hannes, R.; Monstadt, H.; Simgen, A.; Mühl-Benninghaus, R.; Reith, W.; Henkes, H. Prospective study to assess the tissue response to HPC-coated p48 flow diverter stents compared to uncoated devices in the rabbit carotid artery model. *Eur. Radiol. Exp.* **2019**, *3*, 47. [CrossRef] [PubMed]
53. Beythien, C.; Terres, W.; Hamm, C.W. In vitro model to test the thrombogenicity of coronary stents. *Thromb. Res.* **1994**, *75*, 581–590. [CrossRef]
54. Miyazaki, Y.; Nomura, S.; Miyake, T.; Kagawa, H.; Kitada, C.; Taniguchi, H.; Komiyama, Y.; Fujimura, Y.; Ikeda, Y.; Fukuhara, S. High shear stress can initiate both platelet aggregation and shedding of procoagulant containing microparticles. *Blood* **1996**, *88*, 3456–3464. [CrossRef] [PubMed]
55. van Beusekom, H.M.M.; van der Giessen, W.J.; van Suylen, R.J.; Bos, E.; Bosman, F.; Serruys, P.W. Histology after stenting of human saphenous vein bypass grafts: Observations from surgically excised grafts 3 to 320 days after stent implantation. *J. Am. Coll. Cardiol.* **1993**, *21*, 45–54. [CrossRef]

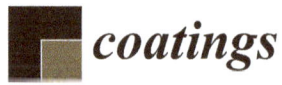

Article

Bone Density around Titanium Dental Implants Coating Tested/Coated with Chitosan or Melatonin: An Evaluation via Microtomography in Jaws of Beagle Dogs

Nansi López-Valverde [1], Antonio López-Valverde [1,*], Juan Manuel Aragoneses [2], Francisco Martínez-Martínez [3], María C. González-Escudero [4] and Juan Manuel Ramírez [5]

[1] Department of Surgery, Instituto de Investigación Biomédica de Salamanca (IBSAL), University of Salamanca, 37007 Salamanca, Spain; nlovalher@usal.es
[2] Dean of The Faculty of Dentistry, Universidad Alfonso X El Sabio, 28691 Madrid, Spain; jaraglam@uax.es
[3] Orthopaedic and Trauma Service, Virgen de la Arrixaca University Hospital, El Palmar, 30120 Murcia, Spain; fcomtnez@um.es
[4] Faculty of Health Sciences, Universidad Católica San Antonio de Murcia (UCAM), 30107 Murcia, Spain; mcgonzalez@ucam.edu
[5] Department of Morphological Sciences, University of Cordoba, Avenida Menéndez Pidal s/n, 14071, 14004 Cordoba, Spain; jmramirez@uco.es
* Correspondence: alopezvalverde@usal.es

Citation: López-Valverde, N.; López-Valverde, A.; Aragoneses, J.M.; Martínez-Martínez, F.; González-Escudero, M.C.; Ramírez, J.M. Bone Density around Titanium Dental Implants Coating Tested/Coated with Chitosan or Melatonin: An Evaluation via Microtomography in Jaws of Beagle Dogs. *Coatings* 2021, *11*, 777. https://doi.org/10.3390/coatings11070777

Academic Editor: Toshiyuki Kawai

Received: 5 June 2021
Accepted: 28 June 2021
Published: 29 June 2021

Publisher's Note: MDPI stays neutral with regard to jurisdictional claims in published maps and institutional affiliations.

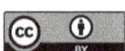

Copyright: © 2021 by the authors. Licensee MDPI, Basel, Switzerland. This article is an open access article distributed under the terms and conditions of the Creative Commons Attribution (CC BY) license (https://creativecommons.org/licenses/by/4.0/).

Abstract: Peri-implant bone density plays an important role in the osseointegration of dental implants. The aim of the study was to evaluate via micro-CT, in Hounsfield units, the bone density around dental implants coated with chitosan and melatonin and to compare it with the bone density around implants with a conventional etched surface after 12 weeks of immediate post-extraction placement in the jaws of Beagle dogs. Six dogs were used, and 48 implants were randomly placed: three groups—melatonin, chitosan, and control. Seven 10 mm × 10 mm regions of interest were defined in each implant (2 in the crestal zone, 4 in the medial zone, and 1 in the apical zone). A total of 336 sites were studied with the AMIDE tool, using the Norton and Gamble classification to assess bone density. The effect on bone density of surface coating variables (chitosan, melatonin, and control) at the crestal, medial, and apical sites and the implant positions (P2, P3, P4, and M1) was analyzed at bivariate and multivariate levels (linear regression). Adjusted effects on bone density did not indicate statistical significance for surface coatings ($p = 0.653$) but did for different levels of ROIs ($p < 0.001$) and for positions of the implants ($p = 0.032$). Micro-CT, with appropriate software, proved to be a powerful tool for measuring osseointegration.

Keywords: titanium dental implants; chitosan coating; melatonin coating; bone density; Hounsfield unity; micro-computed tomography

1. Introduction

Due to its excellent mechanical and biological properties, pure titanium (Ti) and different alloys have been widely used in the fields of orthopedics and dentistry. The use of Ti dental implants has revolutionized the field of dentistry, with implant treatments being performed all over the world, with exponential growth over the years [1,2].

Current dental implant surfaces (SLA, sandblasted, large-grain, acid-etched) require periods of 3 to 6 months to achieve adequate osseointegration [3]. On the other hand, such surfaces are prone to certain bacterial infections, and it is not known whether this propensity is due to the dubious antibacterial properties of Ti, or to the compromised defenses of a certain type of host [4]. For all these reasons, the surfaces of Ti implants are under constant study and evolution, with the aim of shortening waiting times and ensuring osseointegration.

Chitosan (Ch) is a cationic polysaccharide derived from chitin, composed of N-acetylglucosamine and D-glucosamine [5]. It is a biopolymer with interesting properties such as biodegradability, biocompatibility, nontoxicity, and low allergenicity, which, together with other antimicrobial and antifungal properties, make Ch one of the most widely used polymers in the study of antimicrobial chemotherapies in therapeutic development [6–9]. Its favorable biological properties, together with its availability and variety of forms, have made it a good candidate for medical applications, such as periodontal and bone regeneration [10]. Several studies have demonstrated its usefulness as an osteoconductor and for enhancing bone formation, both in vitro and in vivo [11–14], as well as an inducer of apatite and calcium/phosphorus ion deposition, with active biomineralization properties, and its broad potential as a bone regenerator has been demonstrated [15–18]. In vitro and in vivo studies have shown that chitosan stimulates polymorphonuclear and progenitor cell migration, enhancing angiogenesis and extracellular matrix reformation, resulting in accelerated wound healing [19].

Melatonin (Mt, N-acetyl 5-methoxytryptamine), derived from tryptophan, is a hormone synthesized and produced mainly in the pineal gland in a circadian manner [20], with outstanding importance in angiogenesis, bone formation, and remodeling, due to its antioxidant and anti-inflammatory effects and its extraordinary capacity to destroy reactive oxygen species [21,22], the benefits of its application being known as a coating of dental implants to improve their osseointegration [23–25].

In 1972, Godfrey Hounsfield communicated to the scientific community an imaging technique called transverse computed axial tomography. Currently, CT is the only diagnostically justifiable imaging technique that allows approximate conclusions about the structure and density of the maxillary bones and is considered an excellent tool for assessing the distribution of compact and cancellous bone. Bone density (BD) can be assessed using Hounsfield units (HU), which are directly related to tissue attenuation coefficients. The Hounsfield scale is based on density values for air, water, and dense bone, which are arbitrarily assigned values of -1000, 0, and $+1000$, respectively [26].

X-ray microtomography (micro-CT) is a conservative technique used in the evaluation of bone morphometry, and several studies have demonstrated its usefulness in the quantification of bone tissue [27–30]. Micro-CT systems developed in the early 1980s have a high spatial resolution, producing voxels approximately 1,000,000 times smaller in volume than CT voxels [31], making it possible to measure trabecular and cortical bone and provide a spatial representation of bone structure in the peri-implant region while assessing the qualitative and quantitative morphometry of the bone integration of dental implants, having become one of the most widely used anatomical imaging modalities for both research and clinical purposes [32,33].

The purpose of this study was to evaluate and compare, via micro-CT, the BD around Ti dental implants coated with Ch and Mt, with implants with the SLA-type conventional etched surface (Bioetch®, Bioner, Spain), after 12 weeks of immediate post-extraction placement, in the jaws of Beagle dogs.

2. Materials and Methods

2.1. Study Design

Six Beagle breed dogs, aged approximately 5 years and weighing between 15 and 16 kg, were used, following the 3R principle in animal experimentation (replacement, reduction, and refinement). A total of 48 implants were inserted, 4 implants in each hemiarch, and randomly divided into three groups: melatonin test group (MtG), chitosan test group (ChG), and control group (CG). It has been approved by the Ethics Committee of the Catholic University of Murcia (Spain), study protocol, date 24 July 2020, code CE072004. All dogs were in good health prior to the start of the study.

2.2. Implant Surface Preparation

The manufacturer packaged the melatonin test group (MtG) implants immersed in 5% Mt-containing saline (TM-M5250 Sigma-Aldrich®, St. Louis, MO, USA), according to Salomó-Coll et al. [34], and Ch group (ChG) implants immersed in a film-forming solution according to the procedure described by Zhang et al. with slight modifications [35]. Ch (1.6 g) and glycerol (0.4 g) were dispersed in 80 mL of an acetic acid solution (1% w/v), shaking for at least 12 h (4 °C). Similarly to the control group (CG) implants, they were sterilized by gamma irradiation. The control group implants (CG) did not receive any type of surface coating.

2.3. Surgical Protocol

All surgical procedures were performed under general anesthesia via an intravenous catheter in the cephalic vein, infusing Propofol® (Propovet, Abbott Laboratories Ltd., Queensborough, Kent, UK). Maintenance anesthesia was performed with volatile anesthetics. Local anesthesia (Articaine 40 mg, with 1% epinephrine, Ultracain®, Normon, Madrid, Spain) was administered at the surgical sites. All procedures were performed under the supervision of a veterinary surgeon. Extractions of premolars and the mandibular first molar (P2, P3, P4, and M1) were performed in the mandibular hemiarch of each animal. Implant placement was determined by the randomization program (http://www.randomization.com) (29 October 2020), in which the experimental animals were assigned to the three different implant surfaces: 16 implants with Mt (MtG), 16 implants with Ch from the test group (ChG), and 16 uncoated implants from the commercial company Bioner (Bioetch®, Bioner Sistemas Implantológicos, Barcelona, Spain) (CG), randomly distributed in six dogs. Each dog received eight conical screw implants (Bioner®, Barcelona, Spain) (Ø3.5 mm × 8.5 mm in the premolar area and Ø5 mm × 8.5 mm in the molar area), four per hemiarch, randomly and bilaterally in the mandible. After placement, closure screws were placed to allow for a submerged healing protocol (Figure 1A–D). No grafting materials were used in the gaps between the bone cortices and the implants. The flaps were closed with simple nonabsorbable interrupted sutures (Silk 4-0®, Lorca Marín, Lorca, Spain). Sacrifice was performed 12 weeks after implant placement using pentothal natrium (Abbot Laboratories, Madrid, Spain) perfused through the carotid arteries after anesthesia. Sectioned bone blocks were obtained. The animals were maintained on a soft diet from the time of surgery until the end of the study.

2.4. Micro-Computed Tomography Analysis

After euthanasia of animals (after 12 weeks of implants placement), the sections of the block were preserved and fixed in 10% neutral formalin. Image acquisitions were performed using a multimodal SPECT/CT Albira II ARS scanner (Bruker® Corporation, Karksruhe, Germany). The acquisition parameters were 45 kV, 0.2 mA, and 0.05 mm voxels. The acquisition slices were axial, 0.05 mm thick, and 800 to 1000 images were obtained from each piece through a flat panel digital detector with 2400 × 2400 pixels and a FOV (field of view) of 70 mm × 70 mm. The implants were grouped according to the three axes (transverse, coronal, and sagittal). The sagittal section was used for BD measurements, as it provided the best details of the bone structure. In all the images, the same color scale was used (0 min and 3 max) with the same parameters in FOV (%): 90 and zoom: 0.6, with a hardness of 1. BD around the implant was quantified in HU, using seven 10 mm × 10 mm squares or regions of interest (ROI) in the bone implant contact area, two in the crestal area, four in the medial area, and one in the apical area of the implant, using a medical image data examiner (Figure 2A,B).

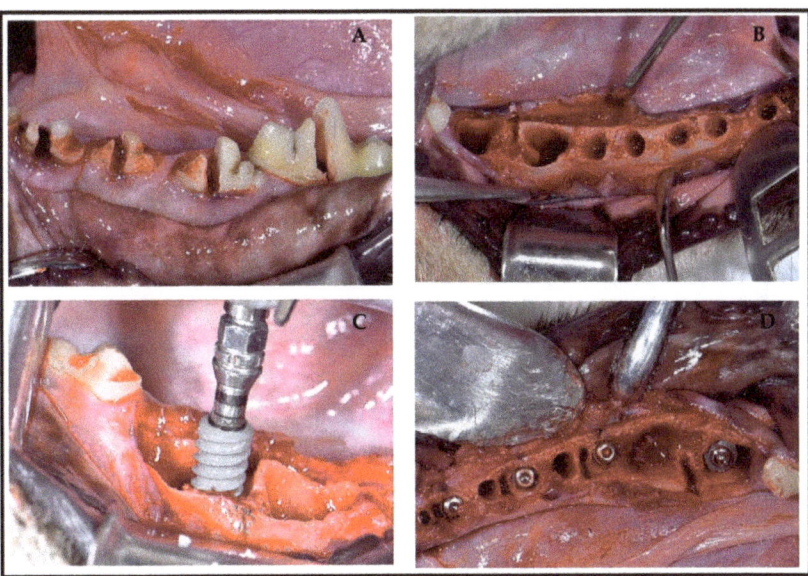

Figure 1. (**A–D**) Dental extractions and implant placement.

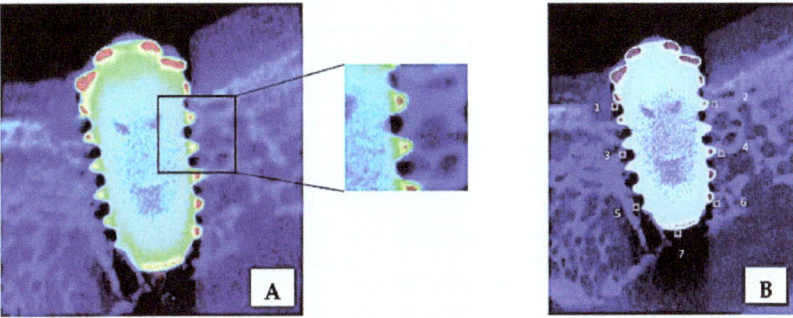

Figure 2. Bone implant contact area (**A**) and regions of interest (ROIs, 1–7) (**B**).

The Norton and Gamble classification [36], modified by Misch [37], was used to assess BD according to Lekholm and Zarb [38]. Once the 7 ROIs (Figure 2B) were positioned, the AMIDE tool allowed us to obtain the data in statistical form, with maxima, minima, and standard deviations; AMIDE is a tool for visualizing, analyzing, and registering volumetric medical image data sets (AMIDE, UCLA University, Los Angeles, CA, USA). It allows one to draw three-dimensional ROIs directly on the images and to generate statistics for these ROIs. In addition, the program supports the following color maps: Black/White, Red/Orange, Blue/Pink, and Green/Yellow, and each color has a given UH range (Figure 3).

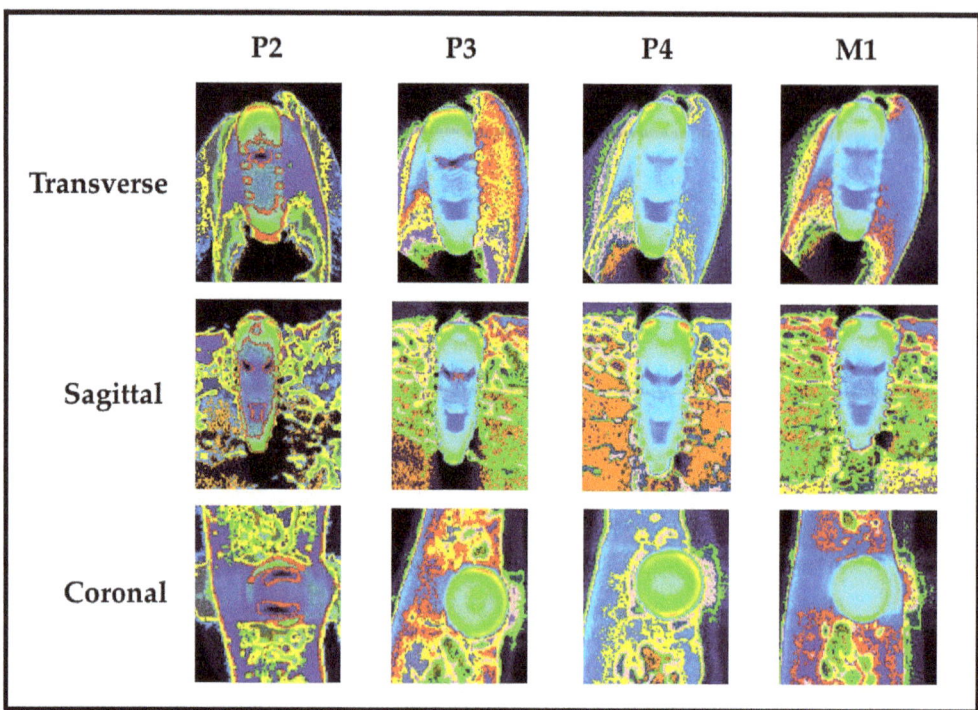

Figure 3. Example of coded BD values from the AMIDE program at 12 weeks after implant placement in transverse, sagittal, and coronal sections of P2, P3, P4, and M1: 250–400 HU (orange color); 400–500 HU (green color); 500–700 HU (pink color); 700–900 HU (yellow color); 900–1200 HU (red color). >850 HU, bone type 1; 500–850 HU, bone type 2/3; 0–500 HU, bone type 4 (according to Norton and Gamble [36]).

2.5. Statistical Analysis

BD variables were analyzed in crestal, mid, and apical areas. Descriptive analysis was performed with SPSS Windows 20.0 and the calculation of *p*-values was performed with SUDAAN 7.0 (RTI, RTP, NC) to account for clustering (multiple sites around implants). We estimated a posteriori, and using Sample Power 2.0 (SPSS, Chicago, IL, USA), the statistical power obtained with those 336 studied locations (=6 dogs × 8 implants/dog × 7 locations/implant), i.e., 112 locations/group. We initially considered from our experience a large design effect (owing to locations being clustered within implants) of 1.33 in estimating the HU measurements. This means that the effective sample size per group would be 84 (=112/1.33). These sample sizes allow, by using the t-test for independent groups and with a power of 80% and 5% alpha error, the detection of an estimated Cohen's d of 0.45 (below a medium effect size according to Cohen's scale [39] when comparing HU measurements between two groups). For crestal sites, the effective sample size per group is 24 (=32/1.33), and this allows the detection of an effect size of 0.8 (large) [39]; for medial sites, the corresponding figure is 48 (=64/1.33) with the capacity to detect an effect size of 0.6, which is between medium (0.5) and large (0.8) [39]; and for apical sites, it is 12 (=16/1.33) and the detectable effect size is 1.2 (very large) (1.2) [40].

3. Results

The total sample consisted of 336 sites (ROIs). A wide range of BD was observed in the different ROIs, depending on their location or level (crestal, medial, and apical) and implant position (P2, P3, P4, and M1). In terms of surface coating, the highest BD (+986 HU) was recorded in the medial of left P2, in CG, with mean values of 0.58 ± 0.20,

0.54 ± 0.13, and 0.59 ± 0.14 for ChG, MtG, and CG, respectively, and the lowest BD was recorded in the apical area (−243 HU) in left P4 in MtG, with mean values of −0.20 ± 0.32, −0.18 ± 0.38, and −0.11 ± 0.33 for ChG, MtG, and CG, respectively. The lower BD in the apical area could be explained by the proximity of the dental nerve canal in this region. Regarding implant position, the highest BD (+995 HU) was recorded in left P3 and the lowest (−330 HU) in left M1; mean values ranged from 0.12 ± 0.35 for P2 with the Mt coating to 0.05 ± 0.23 for M1 with the Ch coating. Mean values and standard deviations are shown in Table 1. Statistical analysis by linear regression showed no statistical significance for surface coatings (ChG, MtG, and CG); however, we found statistical significance in UH for ROIs in the different levels (crestal, medial, and apical) ($p < 0.001$) and implant positions (P2, P3, P4, and M1) ($p = 0.032$) (Table 2).

Table 1. Description and comparison of BD measurements studied [a] in 336 sites [b].

Variable	ChG			MtG			CG		p-Global [c]
	-	Mean ± SD	n		Mean ± SD	n		Mean ± SD	
All	112	0.35 ± 0.32	112		0.33 ± 0.32	112		0.37 ± 0.30	0.631
ROI's (in levels)	-	-	-		-	-		-	-
Crestal [C]	32	0.58 ± 0.20	32		0.54 ± 0.13	32		0.59 ± 0.14	0.438
Medial [M]	64	0.38 ± 0.18	64		0.35 ± 0.22	64		0.38 ± 0.19	0.680
Apical [A]	16	−0.20 ± 0.32	16		−0.18 ± 0.38	16		−0.11 ± 0.33	0.723
p-global [c]	-	<0.001	-		<0.001	-		<0.001	-
paired comparisons [d]	-	C ≠ M ≠ A	-		C ≠ M ≠ A	-		C ≠ M ≠ A	-
Tooth type (position)	-	-	-		-	-		-	-
P2	35	0.11 ± 0.34	21		0.12 ± 0.35	28		0.09 ± 0.31	<0.001
P3	28	0.11 ± 0.34	35		0.08 ± 0.28	21		0.12 ± 0.34	0.207
P4	35	0.11 ± 0.33	35		0.12 ± 0.34	14		0.05 ± 0.22	0.963
M1	14	0.05 ± 0.23	21		0.07 ± 0.27	49		0.08 ± 0.29	0.693
p-global [c]	-	0.003	-		0.004	-		0.582	-
paired comparisons [d]	-	PM2 ≠ M1	-		PM2 ≠ PM3, M1	-		-	-

[a]: The measuring device makes a sweep with multiple measurements. The median of all measurements is taken. [b]: Corresponding to 6 dogs × 8 teeth/dog × 7 sites/tooth (6 × 8 × 7 = 336). [c]: With procedure REGRESS in SUDAAN to account for clustering (multiple sites within teeth). [d]: With procedure DESCRIPT in SUDAAN, where "≠" means $p < 0.05$.

Table 2. Multiple linear regression with BD as the dependent variable, in 336 sites [a].

Variable	β ± se [b]	p-Value [c]
Group	-	
ChG	0.00 ± 0.04	0.653
MtG	−0.04 ± 0.04	
CG	0	
ROIs (in levels)	-	
Crestal	0.73 ± 0.04	<0.001
Medial	0.54 ± 0.04	
Apical (reference)	0	
Tooth type (position)	-	
P2	−0.10 ± 0.04	0.032
P3	−0.04 ± 0.05	
P4	−0.04 ± 0.05	
M1 (reference)	0	

[a]: Corresponding to 6 dogs × 8 teeth/dog × 7 sites/tooth (6 × 8 × 7 = 336). [b]: se = standard error. [c]: With procedure REGRESS in SUDAAN to account for clustering (multiple sites within teeth).

4. Discussion

The aim of this study was to evaluate, via micro-CT, the BD around Ch- and Mt-coated Ti dental implants and to compare it with conventional SLA-type etched surface implants, after 12 weeks of immediate post-extraction placement, in the jaws of Beagle dogs.

Micro-CT has proven to be the most suitable technique for the assessment of bone mass in animal models; it is also a valuable tool for evaluating human biopsies and necropsies [41,42], having been used not only qualitatively, but also quantitatively in different clinical situations [43–46]. It is a noninvasive diagnostic tool that allows the reuse of samples for other types of measurements and is also of great interest in the clinic, where, for obvious reasons, conventional histomorphometry cannot be performed [47]. It is currently used to evaluate morphometric characteristics as a complementary alternative to conventional histological analysis [48]. Particularly in dentistry, it is an extremely useful method for the study of human maxillary bone tissue associated with different conditions and pathologies, and to evaluate the changes when the bone evolves after certain injuries or is subjected to surgical procedures. In addition, it is an accurate and time-saving technique for determining bone morphometry compared to manual methods [49–51].

Ch is considered an excellent material for osteoblast growth, due to its structural characteristics similar to hyaluronic acid; some authors have reported its osteoconductive capacity as a coating for implant materials, so it is widely used for bone regeneration methods, due to its biocompatibility and anti-inflammatory power [52–54]. Khajuria et al. [55] demonstrated in a periodontitis rat model that the local administration of Ch preparations produced significant improvements in periodontal bone support ratios and bone mineral density. In addition, López-Valverde et al. [56] reviewed the literature and concluded that Ch-coated Ti dental implants may have a higher osseointegration capacity and could become a commercial option in the future.

Mt has the capacity to stimulate osteoblastic differentiation and inhibit osteoclast differentiation. Koyama et al. [57] demonstrated in mice that, at pharmacological doses, causes an increase in bone mass by inhibiting bone resorption. Cutando et al. [58] first applied it topically to the surface of dental implants. In vivo studies have shown that local Mt administered at the ostectomy site at the time of implant placement can induce increased contact between the trabecular bone and the implant and increased density of the trabecular area [59]. Similarly, a recent meta-analysis [60] reported that the topical application of Mt to implant sites could induce increased BD around Ti dental implants in the early stages of healing. In this sense, certain studies support the hypothesis that wettability, together with surface micro-texture, would be the determining factors in osteoblast response [61]; therefore, the surface preparation of implants has become a technical challenge.

Different studies have assessed the effectiveness of Ch and Mt as biofunctionalizers of the surface of Ti dental implants, but, to our knowledge, our study was the first to compare both coatings with each other and with a conventional SLA-type coating.

In our investigation, HU measurements ranged from −330 to +995, when all 336 sites were evaluated, 12 weeks after implantation. A total of 112 sites were analyzed in the crestal, medial, and apical levels (ROIs) and at the implant locations (P2, P3, P4, and M1), for the three surfaces studied. In the Norton and Gamble study [36], taken as a reference, a single standard implant of Ø3.5 mm × 11 mm L was used to allow the software to calculate the BD values and, in our study, two implants of different thicknesses (Ø3.5 mm × 8.5 mm and Ø5 mm × 8.5 mm) were used, depending on the premolar or molar area, so there could be a bias in the reporting of the Hounsfield values.

The results of our study provided valuable information on different coatings of dental implants in order to achieve better and faster osseointegration: the surfaces coated with Ch and Mt achieved similar BD values around the implants to the control surface, with conventional SLA etching (Bioetch®), with no significant statistical association observed in the BD measurement values of Mt- and Ch-coated implants and conventional etched surface implants. In this regard, Sultankulov et al. [62] in a recent review concluded that the Ch could introduce valuable properties, such as antimicrobial activity and mucoadhesiveness, recommending further studies on this biopolymer and its osteogenic properties. Similarly, Lu et al. [63] in another recent review highlighted the protective role of melatonin in periodontitis, bone lesions, and osteoporosis, but, because a number of studies have shown adverse effects, they recommended exploring and investigating the optimal conditions of administration.

However, it is possible that these types of surface coatings are eliminated by the action of the forces used during implantation, due to their low mechanical resistance, which would explain the absence of statistical differences between the coated surfaces and the control surfaces.

The most validated strategy to improve the bone-implant interface continues to be the modification of the surface topography by increasing macro-, micro-, and nano-roughness [64].

However, in order to improve the bioactivity of implants, some studies have proposed surface modification by incorporating organic and inorganic ions and molecules, through peptides, proteins, enzymes, and pharmaceuticals, on the Ti oxide layer (TiO_2). All this would lead to an improvement in the biological performance of Ti implants, which would directly influence the local response of the surrounding tissues, improving the apposition of the newly formed bone. In this regard, it is believed that the combination of organic and inorganic components in Ti surface re-coatings would lead to bone-like coatings and, thus, to new generations of surface-modified implants with improved functionality and biological efficacy [65,66].

Another finding of our study was the statistical significance we found for BD in different levels (crestal, medial, and apical) ($p < 0.001$) and positions (P2, P3, P4, and M1) ($p = 0.032$) of the implants. In this regard, our results agreed with Shapurian et al. and Di Stefano et al. [67,68] who, in their respective studies in mandibles, found significant variations in bone density within the mandible, which would underline the importance of identifying specific locations prior to implant placement.

We also found that micro-CT proved to be a very useful diagnostic method in the measurement of peri-implant BD measured in HU. Panoramic radiography provides a two-dimensional view of the anatomical structures of the mandible; however, micro-CT provides much more specific data, such as height, width, or BD in the peri-implant area. This parameter is a key factor to take into account when predicting implant stability and survival. This survival is conditioned by bone quality, i.e., BD, as it has been shown that BD around implants is decisive for their osseointegration [69,70]. In our study, the highest BD was located at the P3 level in the Ch-coated implant group (+995 HU) in the crestal ROI and the lowest (−330 HU) in the apical ROI in M1, probably due to the proximity of the dental canal.

However, the results of our study were biased by a number of limitations that we describe below: first, when defining an ROI in a micro-CT image, one has to take into account that an artefact is always generated when there is a pronounced density gradient.

Due to the nature of the convolution kernels used in the filtered back-projection algorithms, the area adjacent to a high-density object (e.g., the implant) is shown with too low a HU number. This problem could be overcome, in part, if high-resolution kernels are used when reconstructing the images, but this will result in an extremely noisy image and will seriously impair the quantification of the BD in trabecular areas that are not affected by the artefact. In this study, we draw ROIs at a "safe" distance from the implant in cross-sections, but, despite this, an image may be distorted by metallic scatter, and certain studies have highlighted the difficulty in performing an accurate morphometric analysis of the bony areas surrounding an implant [71,72]. Secondly, Rebaudi et al. and Stoppie et al. [73,74] reported that these artefacts created in the areas close to the implant would lead to biases in the measurement of BD in these areas, as it is measured including this artefact. Song et al. [75], in a study with implants in beagle dogs, demonstrated that 45 to 63 μm was a reasonable distance to compensate for artefacts in bone morphometric analysis of an implant containing the tissue sample assessed by micro-CT, and the acquisition distance in our study far exceeded this figure. Thirdly, the micro-CT techniques used to quantify peri-implant BD do not provide specific histological information on the nature of the bone formed around the surfaces tested, despite the color coding of the HU provided by the AMIDE software. Fourth and lastly, regarding clinical applicability, we are aware that with the dog, despite having a similar bone structure to humans, both corticoradicular configuration and mandibular bone remodeling follow different patterns [76].

5. Conclusions

The surface coatings tested/coated with Ch or Mt showed no difference in peri-implant BD compared to the control group with a conventional etched surface, but they did for implant locations and for position. On the other hand, despite the aforementioned limitations, micro-CT, with appropriate complementary software, proved to be a very useful method for the measurement of BD, providing quantitative data of the trabecular bone around the implants.

Author Contributions: Conceptualization, N.L.-V. and A.L.-V.; methodology, N.L.-V.; formal analysis, A.L.-V.; investigation, N.L.-V. and F.M.-M.; writing—original draft preparation A.L.-V.; data curation, J.M.A. and M.C.G.-E.; supervision, J.M.R. and A.L.-V. All authors have read and agreed to the published version of the manuscript.

Funding: This research received no external funding.

Institutional Review Board Statement: This study was approved by the Ethics Committee of the Catholic University of Murcia (Spain). Study protocol, date 24 July 2020, code CE072004.

Informed Consent Statement: Not applicable.

Data Availability Statement: Not applicable.

Acknowledgments: To BIONER, Sistemas Implantológicos, Barcelona, Spain, for their collaboration in this study.

Conflicts of Interest: The authors declare no conflict of interest.

Abbreviations

BD	Bone Density
Ch	Chitosan
CT	Computed Tomography
FOV	Field of View
HU	Hounsfield Unity
Mt	Melatonin
ROI	Region of Interest
SLA	Sandblasted Large grit Acid etched
TiO_2	Titanium Oxide

References

1. Rautray, T.R.; Narayanan, R.; Kwon, T.-Y.; Kim, K.-H. Surface modification of titanium and titanium alloys by ion implantation. *J. Biomed. Mater. Res. Part B Appl. Biomater.* **2010**, *93*, 581–591. [CrossRef]
2. Shah, F.A.; Trobos, M.; Thomsen, P.; Palmquist, A. Commercially pure titanium (cp-Ti) versus titanium alloy (Ti6Al4V) materials as bone anchored implants—Is one truly better than the other? *Mater. Sci. Eng. C* **2016**, *62*, 960–966. [CrossRef]
3. López-Valverde, N.; Flores-Fraile, J.; Ramírez, J.M.; De Sousa, B.M.; Herrero-Hernández, S.; López-Valverde, A. Bioactive Surfaces vs. Conventional Surfaces in Titanium Dental Implants: A Comparative Systematic Review. *J. Clin. Med.* **2020**, *9*, 2047. [CrossRef]
4. Zhang, Y.; Zheng, Y.; Li, Y.; Wang, L.; Bai, Y.; Zhao, Q.; Xiong, X.; Cheng, Y.; Tang, Z.; Deng, Y.; et al. Tantalum Nitride-Decorated Titanium with Enhanced Resistance to Microbiologically Induced Corrosion and Mechanical Property for Dental Application. *PLoS ONE* **2015**, *10*, e0130774. [CrossRef] [PubMed]
5. Elieh-Ali-Komi, D.; Hamblin, M.R. Chitin and Chitosan: Production and Application of Versatile Biomedical Nanomaterials. *Int. J. Adv. Res.* **2016**, *4*, 411–427.
6. Qian, J.; Pan, C.; Liang, C. Antimicrobial activity of Fe-loaded chitosan nanoparticles. *Eng. Life Sci.* **2017**, *17*, 629–634. [CrossRef] [PubMed]

7. Lu, B.; Ye, H.; Shang, S.; Xiong, Q.; Yu, K.; Li, Q.; Xiao, Y.; Dai, F.; Lan, G.; Dai, F. Novel wound dressing with chitosan gold nanoparticles capped with a small molecule for effective treatment of multiantibiotic-resistant bacterial infections. *Nanotechnology* **2018**, *29*, 425603. [CrossRef]
8. Covarrubias, C.; Trepiana, D.; Corral, C. Synthesis of hybrid copper-chitosan nanoparticles with antibacterial activity against cariogenic Streptococcus mutans. *Dent. Mater. J.* **2018**, *37*, 379–384. [CrossRef] [PubMed]
9. Gomes, L.P.; Andrade, C.T.; Del Aguila, E.M.; Alexander, C.; Paschoalin, V.M. Assessing the antimicrobial activity of chitosan nanoparticles by fluorescence-labeling. *Int. J. Biotechnol. Bioeng.* **2018**, *12*, 111–117.
10. Bojar, W.; Kucharska, M.; Ciach, T.; Koperski, Ł.; Jastrzebski, Z.; Szałwiński, M. Bone regeneration potential of the new chitosan-based alloplastic biomaterial. *J. Biomater. Appl.* **2014**, *28*, 1060–1068. [CrossRef]
11. Aguilar, A.; Zein, N.; Harmouch, E.; Hafdi, B.; Bornert, F.; Offner, D.; Clauss, F.; Fioretti, F.; Huck, O.; Benkirane-Jessel, N.; et al. Application of Chitosan in Bone and Dental Engineering. *Molecules* **2019**, *24*, 3009. [CrossRef]
12. Park, J.-S.; Choi, S.-H.; Moon, I.-S.; Cho, K.S.; Chai, J.-K.; Kim, C.-K. Eight-week histological analysis on the effect of chitosan on surgically created one-wall intrabony defects in beagle dogs. *J. Clin. Periodontol.* **2003**, *30*, 443–453. [CrossRef]
13. Abinaya, B.; Prasith, T.P.; Ashwin, B.; Chandran, S.V.; Selvamurugan, N. Chitosan in Surface Modification for Bone Tissue Engineering Applications. *Biotechnol. J.* **2019**, *14*, e1900171. [CrossRef] [PubMed]
14. Soundarya, S.P.; Menon, A.H.; Chandran, S.V.; Selvamurugan, N. Bone tissue engineering: Scaffold preparation using chitosan and other biomaterials with different design and fabrication techniques. *Int. J. Biol. Macromol.* **2018**, *119*, 1228–1239. [CrossRef]
15. He, L.-H.; Yao, L.; Xue, R.; Sun, J.; Song, R. In-situ mineralization of chitosan/calcium phosphate composite and the effect of solvent on the structure. *Front. Mater. Sci.* **2011**, *5*, 282–292. [CrossRef]
16. Leonor, I.; Baran, E.; Kawashita, M.; Reis, R.L.; Kokubo, T.; Nakamura, T. Growth of a bonelike apatite on chitosan microparticles after a calcium silicate treatment. *Acta Biomater.* **2008**, *4*, 1349–1359. [CrossRef] [PubMed]
17. Lu, H.-T.; Lu, T.-W.; Chen, C.-H.; Lu, K.-Y.; Mi, F.-L. Development of nanocomposite scaffolds based on biomineralization of N,O-carboxymethyl chitosan/fucoidan conjugates for bone tissue engineering. *Int. J. Biol. Macromol.* **2018**, *120*, 2335–2345. [CrossRef]
18. Xie, C.-M.; Lu, X.; Wang, K.-F.; Meng, F.-Z.; Jiang, O.; Zhang, H.-P.; Zhi, W.; Fang, L. Silver Nanoparticles and Growth Factors Incorporated Hydroxyapatite Coatings on Metallic Implant Surfaces for Enhancement of Osteoinductivity and Antibacterial Properties. *ACS Appl. Mater. Interfaces* **2014**, *6*, 8580–8589. [CrossRef]
19. Ishihara, M.; Nakanishi, K.; Ono, K.; Sato, M.; Kikuchi, M.; Saito, Y.; Yura, H.; Matsui, T.; Hattori, H.; Uenoyama, M.; et al. Photocrosslinkable chitosan as a dressing for wound occlusion and accelerator in healing process. *Biomaterials* **2002**, *23*, 833–840. [CrossRef]
20. Tan, D.X.; Xu, B.; Zhou, X.; Reiter, R.J. Pineal Calcification, Melatonin Production, Aging, Associated Health Consequences and Rejuvenation of the Pineal Gland. *Molecules* **2018**, *23*, 301. [CrossRef]
21. Maria, S.; Samsonraj, R.; Munmun, F.; Glas, J.; Silvestros, M.; Kotlarczyk, M.; Rylands, R.; Dudakovic, A.; Van Wijnen, A.J.; Enderby, L.T.; et al. Biological effects of melatonin on osteoblast/osteoclast cocultures, bone, and quality of life: Implications of a role for MT2 melatonin receptors, MEK1/2, and MEK5 in melatonin-mediated osteoblastogenesis. *J. Pineal Res.* **2018**, *64*, e12465. [CrossRef]
22. Manchester, L.C.; Coto-Montes, A.; Boga, J.A.; Andersen, L.P.H.; Zhou, Z.; Galano, A.; Vriend, J.; Tan, D.-X.; Reiter, R.J. Melatonin: An ancient molecule that makes oxygen metabolically tolerable. *J. Pineal Res.* **2015**, *59*, 403–419. [CrossRef] [PubMed]
23. Calvo-Guirado, J.L.; Salvatierra, A.A.; Gargallo-Albiol, J.; Delgado-Ruiz, R.A.; Sanchez, J.E.M.; Satorres-Nieto, M. Zirconia with laser-modified microgrooved surface vs. titanium implants covered with melatonin stimulates bone formation. Experimental study in tibia rabbits. *Clin. Oral Implant. Res.* **2014**, *26*, 1421–1429. [CrossRef] [PubMed]
24. Guardia, J.; Gómez-Moreno, G.; Ferrera, M.J.; Cutando, A.; Dds, G.G. Evaluation of Effects of Topic Melatonin on Implant Surface at 5 and 8 Weeks in Beagle Dogs. *Clin. Implant. Dent. Relat. Res.* **2009**, *13*, 262–268. [CrossRef]
25. Calvo-Guirado, J.L.; Gómez-Moreno, G.; López-Marí, L.; Guardia, J.; Marínez-González, J.M.; Barone, A.; Tresguerres, I.F.; Paredes, S.D.; Fuentes-Breto, L. Retracted: Actions of melatonin mixed with collagenized porcine bone versus porcine bone only on osteointegration of dental implants. *J. Pineal Res.* **2010**, *48*, 194–203. [CrossRef]
26. Hounsfield, G.N. Computerized transverse axial scanning (tomography): Description of system. *Br. J. Radiol.* **1973**, *46*, 1016–1022. [CrossRef] [PubMed]
27. Bouxsein, M.L.; Boyd, S.K.; Christiansen, B.A.; Guldberg, R.E.; Jepsen, K.J.; Muller, R. Guidelines for assessment of bone microstructure in rodents using micro-computed tomography. *J. Bone Miner. Res.* **2010**, *25*, 1468–1486. [CrossRef]
28. Irie, M.S.; Rabelo, G.; Spin-Neto, R.; Dechichi, P.; Borges, J.S.; Soares, P.B.F. Use of Micro-Computed Tomography for Bone Evaluation in Dentistry. *Braz. Dent. J.* **2018**, *29*, 227–238. [CrossRef]
29. Peyrin, F. Evaluation of bone scaffolds by micro-CT. *Osteoporos. Int.* **2011**, *22*, 2043–2048. [CrossRef] [PubMed]
30. Shi, G.; Subramanian, S.; Cao, Q.; Demehri, S.; Siewerdsen, J.H.; Zbijewski, W. Application of a novel ultra-high resolution multi-detector CT in quantitative imaging of trabecular microstructure. *Proc. SPIE Int. Soc. Opt. Eng.* **2020**, *11317*, 113171E.
31. Young, S.; Kretlow, J.D.; Nguyen, C.; Bashoura, A.G.; Baggett, L.S.; Jansen, J.A.; Wong, M.; Mikos, A.G. Microcomputed tomography characterization of neovascularization in bone tissue engineering applications. *Tissue Eng. Part B Rev.* **2008**, *14*, 295–306. [CrossRef] [PubMed]
32. Park, Y.-S.; Yi, K.-Y.; Lee, I.-S.; Jung, Y.-C. Correlation between microtomography and histomorphometry for assessment of implant osseointegration. *Clin. Oral Implant. Res.* **2005**, *16*, 156–160. [CrossRef] [PubMed]

33. Swain, M.; Xue, J. State of the art of Micro-CT applications in dental research. *Int. J. Oral Sci.* **2009**, *1*, 177–188. [CrossRef]
34. Salomó-Coll, O.; Maté-Sánchez de Val, J.E.; Ramírez-Fernández, M.P.; Satorres-Nieto, M.; Gargallo-Albiol, J.; Calvo-Guirado, J.L. Osseoinductive elements for promoting osseointegration around immediate implants: A pilot study in the foxhound dog. *Clin. Oral Implant. Res.* **2016**, *27*, e167–e175. [CrossRef]
35. Zhang, C.; Wang, Z.; Li, Y.; Yang, Y.; Ju, X.; He, R. The preparation and physiochemical characterization of rapeseed protein hydrolysate-chitosan composite films. *Food Chem.* **2019**, *272*, 694–701. [CrossRef] [PubMed]
36. Norton, M.R.; Gamble, C. Bone classification: An objective scale of bone density using the computerized tomography scan. *Clin. Oral Implant. Res.* **2001**, *12*, 79–84. [CrossRef] [PubMed]
37. Misch, C.E. Density of bone: Effect on treatment planning, surgical approach, and healing. In *Contemporary Implant Dentistry*; Mosby: St. Louis, MO, USA, 1993; pp. 469–485.
38. Bra-Nemark, P.-I.; Zarb, G.A.; Albrektsson, T.; Rosen, H.M. Tissue-Integrated Prostheses. Osseointegration in Clinical Dentistry. *Plast. Reconstr. Surg.* **1986**, *77*, 496–497. [CrossRef]
39. Cohen, J. *Statistical Power Analysis for the Behavioral Sciences*, 2nd ed.; Lawrence Erlbaum: Hillsdale, MI, USA; Hove, UK, 1988.
40. Sawilowsky, S. New effect size rules of thumb. *J. Mod. App. Stat. Methods* **2009**, *8*, 597–599. [CrossRef]
41. Balbinot, G.S.; Leitune, V.C.B.; Ponzoni, D.; Collares, F.M. Bone healing with niobium-containing bioactive glass composition in rat femur model: A micro-CT study. *Dent Mater.* **2019**, *35*, 1490–1497. [CrossRef]
42. Jiang, Y.; Zhao, J.; Liao, E.Y.; Dai, R.C.; Wu, X.P.; Genant, H.K. Application of micro-CT assessment of 3-D bone micro-structure in preclinical and clinical studies. *J. Bone Miner. Metab.* **2005**, *23*, 122–131. [CrossRef]
43. Sennerby, L.; Wennerberg, A.; Pasop, F. A new microtomo-graphic technique for non-invasive evaluation of the bone structure around implants. *Clin. Oral Implant. Res.* **2001**, *12*, 91–94. [CrossRef]
44. Van Dessel, J.; Nicolielo, L.F.; Huang, Y.; Coudyzer, W.; Salmon, B.; Lambrichts, I.; Jacobs, R. Accuracy and reliability of different cone beam computed tomography (CBCT) devices for structural analysis of alveolar bone in comparison with multislice CT and micro-CT. *Eur. J. Oral Implantol.* **2017**, *10*, 95–105.
45. Rebaudi, A.; Trisi, P.; Cella, R.; Cecchini, G. Preoperative evaluation of bone quality and bone density using a novel CT/microCT-based hard-normal-soft classification system. *Int. J. Oral Maxillofac. Implant.* **2010**, *25*, 75–85.
46. Fanuscu, M.I.; Chang, T.-L. Three-dimensional morphometric analysis of human cadaver bone: Microstructural data from maxilla and mandible. *Clin. Oral Implant. Res.* **2004**, *15*, 213–218. [CrossRef] [PubMed]
47. Cano, J.; Campo, J.; Vaquero, J.J.; González, J.M.M.; Bascones, A. High resolution image in bone biology II. Review of the literature. *Med. Oral Patol. Oral Cir. Bucal* **2008**, *13*, E31–E35. [PubMed]
48. Tjong, W.; Nirody, J.; Burghardt, A.J.; Carballido-Gamio, J.; Kazakia, G.J. Structural analysis of cortical porosity applied to HR-pQCT data. *Med. Phys.* **2014**, *41*, 013701. [CrossRef]
49. Rabelo, G.D.; Coutinho-Camillo, C.; Kowalski, L.P.; Portero-Muzy, N.; Roux, J.-P.; Chavassieux, P.; Alves, F.A. Evaluation of cortical mandibular bone in patients with oral squamous cell carcinoma. *Clin. Oral Investig.* **2017**, *22*, 783–790. [CrossRef]
50. Blok, Y.; Gravesteijn, F.; van Ruijven, L.; Koolstra, J. Micro-architecture and mineralization of the human alveolar bone obtained with microCT. *Arch. Oral Biol.* **2013**, *58*, 621–627. [CrossRef]
51. Romão, M.; Marques, M.; Cortes, A.; Horliana, A.; Moreira, M.; Lascala, C. Micro-computed tomography and histomorphometric analysis of human alveolar bone repair induced by laser phototherapy: A pilot study. *Int. J. Oral Maxillofac. Surg.* **2015**, *44*, 1521–1528. [CrossRef]
52. Chesnutt, B.M.; Yuan, Y.; Buddington, K.; Haggard, W.O.; Bumgardner, J.D. Composite Chitosan/Nano-Hydroxyapatite Scaffolds Induce Osteocalcin Production by Osteoblasts In Vitro and Support Bone Formation In Vivo. *Tissue Eng. Part A* **2009**, *15*, 2571–2579. [CrossRef]
53. Cheung, R.C.F.; Ng, T.B.; Wong, J.H.; Chan, W.Y. Chitosan: An Update on Potential Biomedical and Pharmaceutical Applications. *Mar. Drugs* **2015**, *13*, 5156–5186. [CrossRef] [PubMed]
54. Ezoddini-Ardakani, F.; Navabazam, A.; Fatehi, F.; Danesh-Ardekani, M.; Khadem, S.; Rouhi, G. Histologic evaluation of chitosan as an accelerator of bone regeneration in microdrilled rat tibias. *Dent. Res. J.* **2012**, *9*, 694–699.
55. Khajuria, D.K.; Zahra, S.F.; Razdan, R. Effect of locally administered novel biodegradable chitosan based risedronate/zinc-hydroxyapatite intra-pocket dental film on alveolar bone density in rat model of periodontitis. *J. Biomater. Sci. Polym. Ed.* **2017**, *29*, 74–91. [CrossRef]
56. López-Valverde, N.; López-Valverde, A.; Ramírez, J. Systematic Review of Effectiveness of Chitosan as a Biofunctionalizer of Titanium Implants. *Biology* **2021**, *10*, 102. [CrossRef]
57. Koyama, H.; Nakade, O.; Takada, Y.; Kaku, T.; Lau, K.-H.W. Melatonin at Pharmacologic Doses Increases Bone Mass by Suppressing Resorption Through Down-Regulation of the RANKL-Mediated Osteoclast Formation and Activation. *J. Bone Miner. Res.* **2002**, *17*, 1219–1229. [CrossRef]
58. Cutando, A.; Gómez-Moreno, G.; Arana, C.; Muñoz, F.; Lopez-Peña, M.; Stephenson, J.; Reiter, R.J. Melatonin stimulates osteointegration of dental implants. *J. Pineal Res.* **2008**, *45*, 174–179. [CrossRef]
59. Tresguerres, I.F.; Clemente, C.; Blanco, L.; Khraisat, A.; Tamimi, F.; Tresguerres, J.A. Effects of Local Melatonin Application on Implant Osseointegration. *Clin. Implant. Dent. Relat. Res.* **2010**, *14*, 395–399. [CrossRef] [PubMed]
60. López-Valverde, N.; Pardal-Peláez, B.; López-Valverde, A.; Ramírez, J. Role of Melatonin in Bone Remodeling around Titanium Dental Implants: Meta-Analysis. *Coatings* **2021**, *11*, 271. [CrossRef]

61. Rupp, F.; Liang, L.; Geis-Gerstorfer, J.; Scheideler, L.; Hüttig, F. Surface characteristics of dental implants: A review. *Dent. Mater.* **2018**, *34*, 40–57. [CrossRef]
62. Sultankulov, B.; Berillo, D.; Sultankulova, K.; Tokay, T.; Saparov, A. Progress in the development of chitosan-based biomaterials for tissue engineering and regenerative medicine. *Biomolecules* **2019**, *9*, 470. [CrossRef]
63. Lu, X.; Yu, S.; Chen, G.; Zheng, W.; Peng, J.; Huang, X.; Chen, L. Insight into the roles of melatonin in bone tissue and bone-related diseases (Review). *Int. J. Mol. Med.* **2021**, *47*, 82. [CrossRef]
64. Annunziata, M.; Guida, L. The Effect of Titanium Surface Modifications on Dental Implant Osseointegration. *Craniofacial Sutures* **2015**, *17*, 62–77. [CrossRef]
65. Junker, R.; Dimakis, A.; Thoneick, M.; Jansen, J.A. Effects of implant surface coatings and composition on bone integration: A systematic review. *Clin. Oral Implant. Res.* **2009**, *20*, 185–206. [CrossRef] [PubMed]
66. De Jonge, L.T.; Leeuwenburgh, S.; Wolke, J.G.C.; Jansen, J.A. Organic–Inorganic Surface Modifications for Titanium Implant Surfaces. *Pharm. Res.* **2008**, *25*, 2357–2369. [CrossRef]
67. Shapurian, T.; Damoulis, P.D.; Reiser, G.M.; Griffin, T.J.; Rand, W.M. Quantitative evaluation of bone density using the Hounsfield index. *Int. J. Oral Maxillofac. Implant.* **2006**, *21*, 290–297.
68. Di Stefano, D.A.; Arosio, P.; Pagnutti, S.; Vinci, R.; Gherlone, E. Distribution of Trabecular Bone Density in the Maxilla and Mandible. *Implant Dent.* **2019**, *28*, 340–348. [CrossRef]
69. Molly, L. Bone density and primary stability in implant therapy. *Clin. Oral Implant. Res.* **2006**, *17*, 124–135. [CrossRef]
70. Turkyilmaz, I.; Tozum, T.; Tumer, C. Bone density assessments of oral implant sites using computerized tomography. *J. Oral Rehabil.* **2007**, *34*, 267–272. [CrossRef]
71. De Smet, E.; Jaecques, S.; Wevers, M.; Jansen, J.A.; Jacobs, R.; Sloten, J.V.; Naert, I.E. Effect of controlled early implant loading on bone healing and bone mass in guinea pigs, as assessed by micro-CT and histology. *Eur. J. Oral Sci.* **2006**, *114*, 232–242. [CrossRef]
72. Barrett, J.F.; Keat, N. Artifacts in CT: Recognition and Avoidance. *Radiographics* **2004**, *24*, 1679–1691. [CrossRef]
73. Rebaudi, A.; Koller, B.; Laib, A.; Trisi, P. Microcomputed tomographic analysis of the peri-implant bone. *Int. J. Periodontics Restor. Dent.* **2004**, *24*, 316–325.
74. Stoppie, N.; Van Der Waerden, J.-P.; Jansen, J.A.; Duyck, J.; Wevers, M.; Naert, I.E. Validation of Microfocus Computed Tomography in the Evaluation of Bone Implant Specimens. *Clin. Implant. Dent. Relat. Res.* **2005**, *7*, 87–94. [CrossRef] [PubMed]
75. Song, J.W.; Cha, J.Y.; Bechtold, T.E.; Park, Y.C. Influence of peri-implant artifacts on bone morphometric analysis with micro-computed tomography. *Int. J. Oral Maxillofac. Implant.* **2013**, *28*, 519–525. [CrossRef] [PubMed]
76. Pearce, A.I.; Richards, R.; Milz, S.; Schneider, E.; Pearce, S.G. Animal models for implant biomaterial research in bone: A review. *Eur. Cells Mater.* **2007**, *13*, 1–10. [CrossRef] [PubMed]

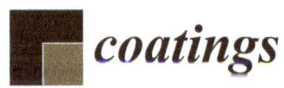

Article

Surface Structure and Properties of Hydroxyapatite Coatings on NiTi Substrates

Ekaterina S. Marchenko [1], Kirill M. Dubovikov [1], Gulsharat A. Baigonakova [1], Ivan I. Gordienko [2] and Alex A. Volinsky [1,3,*]

[1] Laboratory of Superelastic Biointerfaces, National Research Tomsk State University, Tomsk 634045, Russia
[2] Ural State Medical University, Yekaterinburg 620014, Russia
[3] Department of Mechanical Engineering, University of South Florida, Tampa, FL 33620, USA
* Correspondence: volinsky@usf.edu

Abstract: Hydroxyapatite coatings were deposited for 1, 2, and 3 h on NiTi substrates using plasma-assisted radio frequency sputtering. The matrix consisted of NiTi B2 and NiTi B19' phases and Ti_2Ni, Ni_3Ti, and Ni_4Ti_3 intermetallic compounds. The surface coating was monoclinic hydroxyapatite. Increasing the deposition time to 3 h made it possible to form a dense hydroxyapatite layer without visible defects. The phase contrast maps showed that the coating consisted of round grains of different fractions, with the smallest grains in the sample deposited for 3 h. The wettability tests showed that the coating deposited for 3 h had the highest surface energy, reflected in the proliferation density of the MCF-7 cell line.

Keywords: NiTi; sputtering; coating; hydroxyapatite; structure; biocompatibility

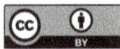

1. Introduction

NiTi-based alloys are widely used for various applications in the medical field such as dentistry, orthopedics, as parts for artificial organs, etc. [1–3]. The main reasons are their shape memory and superelasticity effects, along with high corrosion resistance in the aggressive body environment [4–8]. Large reversible deformation of NiTi alloys up to 10% results in high fatigue strength of implants subjected to high-cycle dynamic loads. The corrosion resistance of NiTi alloys increases the service life of implants due to the presence of a thin electrochemically passive surface titanium oxide layer, which does not provide good corrosion resistance after long usage of an implant in the human body. It causes Ni segregation out of the matrix, which is toxic for the organic tissues [4]. It is necessary to achieve a high level of both bioactivity and bio-inertness and corrosion resistance in implants; therefore, surface modifications and bioactive coatings are used in medical materials science.

One of the most popular candidates as a bioactive coating is hydroxyapatite (HAp), in which the Ca/P molar ratio of 1.67 is considered to be the most stable during healing [9,10]. The advantage of calcium phosphate phases is their structural and compositional similarity to the mineral compounds of human bones and teeth [10], which significantly increases the bioactivity of implants coated with calcium phosphates [9,11–13]. There are various methods of depositing hydroxyapatite on various medical alloys. The most commonly used are plasma spraying, sol-gel, electrochemical and electrophoretic deposition, micro-arc oxidation, plasma electrolytic oxidation, and other methods [9–17] with their corresponding advantages and disadvantages. High variability allows control of coating parameters such as morphology, thickness, density, Ca/P ratio, crystallinity, wettability, solubility, etc. For example, different oxidation methods allow the creation of porous coatings. While this positively affects cell viability, it is not good for the wear resistance of the implants, which may lead to their failure [18]. Other deposition methods can create dense defect-free coatings that may have poor adhesion to a substrate. To solve this problem, substrates with lattice parameters that closely match the deposited film must be chosen, or additional treatments or buffer layers must be implemented [11,15,17]. This negatively affects the cost and labor intensity of the entire process.

Plasma-assisted radio frequency (RF) sputtering is one of the methods used for depositing different coatings on metal surfaces [19]. This method makes it possible to obtain a dense defect-free layer of hydroxyapatite, which has high biocompatibility, and by changing the deposition parameters, it is possible to control the morphology of the coatings [19]. While it is a promising method, there are not many articles devoted to the deposition of calcium phosphate on NiTi substrates. This work aims to study the phase composition, structure, wettability, and cytocompatibility of the Ca-P coatings on NiTi substrates by varying the modes of plasma-assisted RF sputtering.

2. Materials and Methods

Monolithic plates of polycrystalline NiTi were used as substrates. Plasma-assisted RF sputtering with a 200 mm diameter calcium phosphate powder target was used for the deposition of calcium phosphate coatings. The base pressure was 5×10^{-3} Pa. Argon gas was supplied to the sputtering chamber at 0.3 Pa pressure. The plasma generator was turned on, and a negative bias voltage was applied to the substrate to clean and activate the surface with argon plasma for 10 min. After surface treatment, the RF generator connected to the target was turned on to initiate the material sputtering process. The formation of a coating on the surface of the substrate occurred as a result of applying a bias voltage. The optimal deposition parameters were 30 A current and 600 W RF power. The calcium phosphate film deposition rate was 0.5 µm/h. The negative bias on the target was 800–1100 V, which was optimal for sputtering the material, ensuring stable operation of the plasma generator without damage to the RF input insulators and no overheating of the target. For further determination of the optimal phase composition and surface properties, sputtering was carried out for 1, 2, and 3 h at a deposition rate of 0.5 µm/h. The sample number corresponds to the deposition time in hours. These deposition parameters were chosen because Ni can negatively affect cell proliferation during cultivation. The increasing deposition time results in a thicker coating, improving the corrosion resistance and protecting the cells.

The microstructure characterization was carried out using the equipment of Tomsk Regional Core Shared Research Facilities Center of National Research Tomsk State University, sponsored by the grant of the Ministry of Science and Higher Education of the Russian Federation No. 075-15-2021-693 (No. 13.RFC.21.0012). An X-ray diffractometer XRD-7000 (Shimadzu, Kyoto, Japan) was used to analyze the phase composition of the coated samples. The survey was carried out using a Cu anode at a voltage of 30 kV and a current of 30 mA. The scanning speed was 2 degrees/min. Cu Kα radiation was used with the symmetric geometry of the Bragg–Brentano survey in the standard mode. Qualitative analysis was performed using the Profex software and two crystallography databases: Crystallography Open Database and Materials Project.

The surface structure of the samples was examined using scanning electron microscopy (SEM, Axia ChemiSEM, Thermo Fisher Scientific, Waltham, MA, USA) in the secondary electron detection mode. EDS was carried out to determine the elemental composition of the samples' surface. The measurements were conducted using 10–20 kV accelerating voltage, 100 mA beam current, 10 Pa vacuum, and 4.5–6 µm spot size. The surface wetting angle was measured with the sessile drop method using an EasyDrop DSA20E instrument (KRÜSS, Hamburg, Germany). Water and diiodomethane were used as test liquids. The surface free energy was calculated using the Owens, Wendt, Rabel, and Kaelble method. The contact angle was measured at room temperature. Liquids with known surface energy and their polar and dispersive parts were used in the experiment.

$$\sigma_S = \sigma_{SL} + \sigma_L \times \cos\theta \tag{1}$$

$$\sigma_{SL} = \sigma_S + \sigma_L - 2\left(\sqrt{\sigma_S^D \times \sigma_L^D} + \sqrt{\sigma_S^P \times \sigma_L^P}\right) \tag{2}$$

Here, σ_S is the surface free energy, σ_{SL} is the interfacial tension, σ_L is the surface tension of the liquid, θ is the contact angle, σ_S^D and σ_S^P are dispersive and polar parts of the surface energy of the solid, and σ_L^D and σ_L^P are dispersive and polar parts of the surface energy of the liquid.

Atomic force microscopy in the tapping mode (AFM, NT-MDT, Zelenograd, Russia) with a SOLVER HV vacuum chamber was used to study the morphology of the coatings. MCF-7 cells were used to investigate the biocompatibility of the samples. MCF-7 cells were cultured in a medium consisting of DMEM/F12 (Paneco, Tokyo, Japan) supplemented with 10% fetal bovine serum, antibiotics (100 U/mL of penicillin and 100 mg/mL of streptomycin), and 2 mM L-glutamine at 37 °C in a 5% CO_2 and humid atmosphere. Cells were incubated for 72 h in 12-well cell culture plates with a medium in each well. The SEM images were obtained at a low vacuum.

3. Results and Discussion

X-ray diffraction patterns were obtained from three NiTi samples coated with hydroxyapatite in Figure 1. Interpretation of X-ray diffraction patterns made it possible to establish that all samples consisted of the TiNi phase in two crystallographic modifications: cubic B2 austenite (cod_1100132) and monoclinic B19' martensite (cod_9015813). Secondary intermetallic inclusions Ti_2Ni (cod_1527848), Ni_3Ti (cod_1010452), and Ni_4Ti_3 (cod_2100704) were also found, which are the result of the technological process of obtaining monolithic alloys. Monoclinic hydroxyapatite (HAp, mp-721624, a = 9.39 Å, b = 6.87 Å, c = 2a, and γ = 120°) was found on the surfaces of all samples. With an increase in the coating deposition time, the intensity of the HAp diffraction reflections increased, indicating a thicker surface layer. In addition to reflections corresponding to crystalline HAp, X-ray diffraction patterns did not reveal reflections related to other calcium phosphates. In hard tissues such as bones and teeth, the crystal structure of hydroxyapatite is hexagonal with lattice parameters a = b = 9.4 Å, c = 6.86 Å, and γ = 120° (mp-41472). Monoclinic HAp is more thermodynamically stable than hexagonal HAp, even at room temperature. However, the main difference between the forms of HAp lies in the orientation of the hydroxyl groups.

A pronounced splitting of the structural reflection was observed in sample 3 at the 42–42.5° diffraction angle range, which was not present in the other two samples in Figure 1. Probably, with an increase in the deposition time, the Ni_4Ti_3 reflection began to manifest itself more clearly, but it was not possible to establish the reason for this. A slight shift of the high-intensity reflection from the NiTi phase with the B2 austenite structure is worth noting. The shift is associated with a change in the crystal lattice parameters caused by the incorporation of coating atoms into the NiTi bcc structure. Thus, the XRD method shows that, with an increase in the deposition time of the coating, the diffraction reflections from the *hkl* planes of the HAp become more intense, indicating an increase in the deposited coating thickness.

The surface of NiTi alloys coated with HAp was studied using scanning electron microscopy. Samples 1 and 2 had a similar surface morphology in Figures 2 and 3 with small inclusions up to 2 µm in size. Elemental composition analysis showed that the coatings consisted of calcium, phosphorus, and oxygen. Ti and Ni substrate elements were also detected since the spectra registration depth reaches 2 µm. The detected inclusions consisted of the Ti, Ni, and O elements. In terms of size and quantity, these inclusions predominated in sample 1. According to the Ca, P, and O element distribution maps, the coatings were formed unevenly, and a deposition time of 2 h was not enough to obtain a dense HAp layer.

The coating on sample 3 was characterized by a uniform dense surface morphology over the entire area without visible defects, cracks, or chips as seen in Figure 4 in contrast to the coatings on samples 1 and 2.

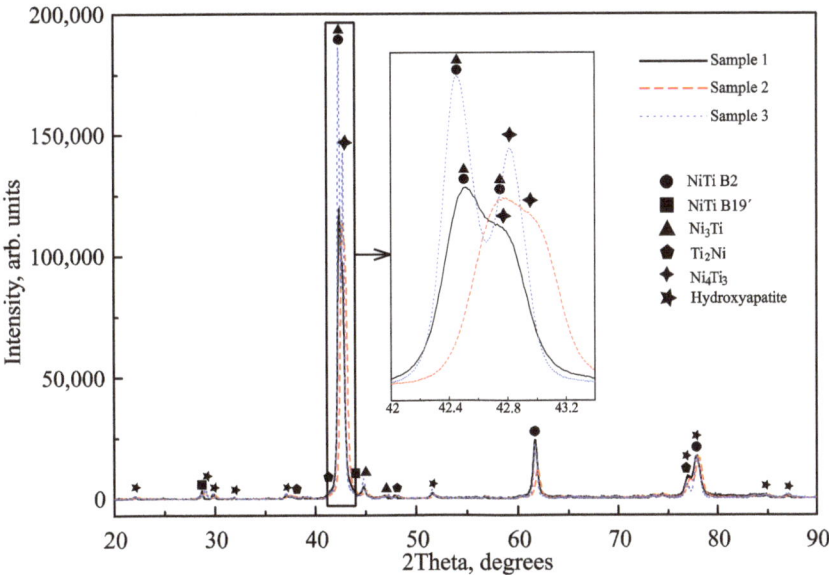

Figure 1. XRD patterns of NiTi samples with hydroxyapatite coatings deposited for 1, 2, and 3 h (samples 1, 2, and 3).

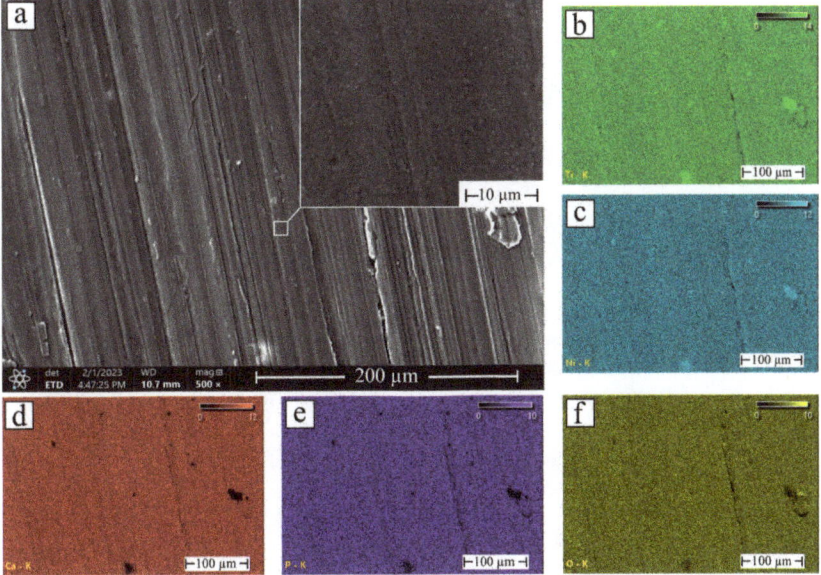

Figure 2. (**a**) SEM image of the NiTi with hydroxyapatite coating deposited for 1 h and elemental maps of: (**b**) Ti; (**c**) Ni; (**d**) Ca; (**e**) P; and (**f**) O.

Quantitative EDS analysis showed a decrease in Ti and Ni content and an increase in Ca, P, and O content with deposition time in Figure 5. These data were consistent with the XRD results, according to which the number and intensity of diffraction reflections increased with deposition time. Quantitative EDS analysis of hydroxyapatite-coated NiTi samples also suggested an increase in the coating thickness.

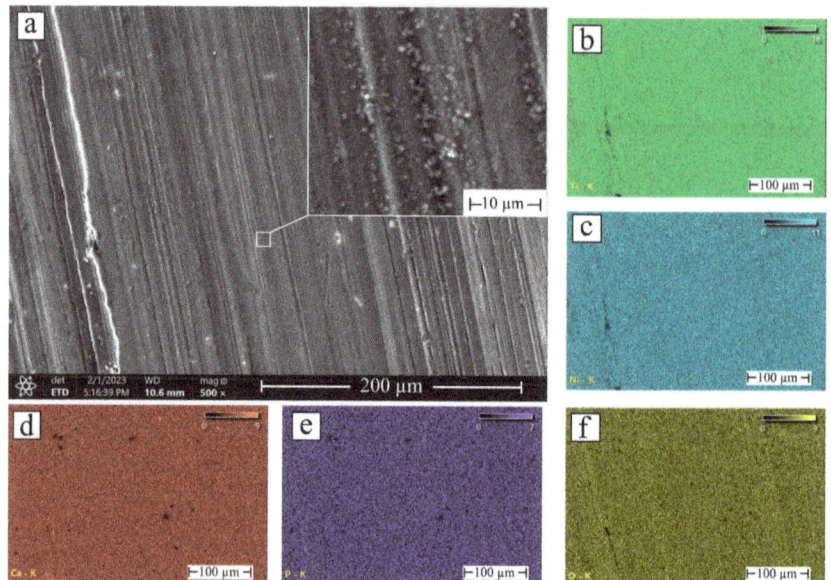

Figure 3. (**a**) SEM image of the NiTi with hydroxyapatite coating deposited for 2 h and elemental maps of: (**b**) Ti; (**c**) Ni; (**d**) Ca; (**e**) P; and (**f**) O.

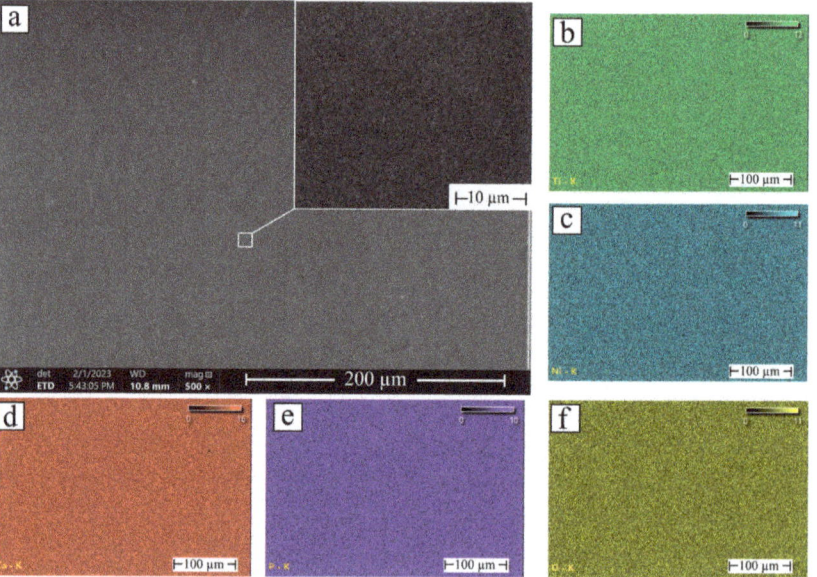

Figure 4. (**a**) SEM image of the NiTi with hydroxyapatite coating deposited for 3 h and elemental maps of: (**b**) Ti; (**c**) Ni; (**d**) Ca; (**e**) P; and (**f**) O.

Phase images 1×1 µm^2 in size were obtained using AFM in Figure 6. Since the survey was carried out in the tapping mode, the tip of the probe touched the surface during oscillations. Because of this, it experienced not only the influence of Coulomb forces, but also adhesive, capillary, and other forces. This caused a phase shift of the oscillations, which made it possible to obtain phase images showing the differences between the areas of the surface. The surface of sample 1 showed large gaps at the grain boundaries, confirming the

SEM data of an uneven coating. With an increase in the deposition time, samples 2 and 3 formed a more uniform coating with many small formations of various shapes ranging in size from 0.1 μm to 0.2 μm.

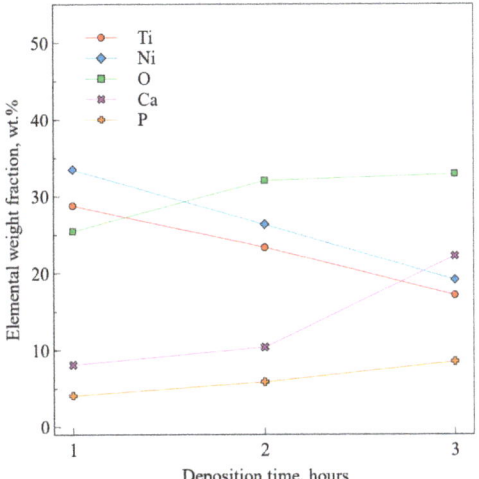

Figure 5. Quantitative elemental EDS analysis of NiTi with hydroxyapatite coatings.

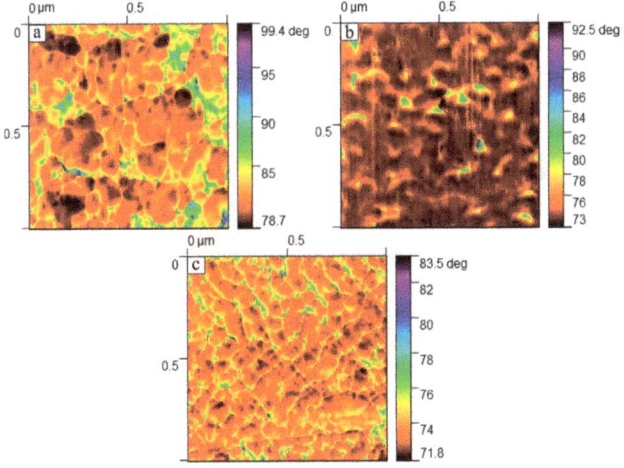

Figure 6. Phase contrast maps obtained using AFM of NiTi with hydroxyapatite coatings deposited for: (**a**) 1 h; (**b**) 2 h; and (**c**) 3 h.

The contact angle was determined using the sessile drop method, and the surface free energy was calculated in Figure 7. Sample 1 exhibited a water contact angle of approximately 56° with a surface free energy of 52 mJ/m^2, which predominantly consisted of a dispersive component. An increase in the deposition time to 2 h contributed to the formation of a more hydrophobic HAp coating for sample 2 with a wetting angle of 86°, while the surface energy decreased to 41.39 mJ/m^2 due to a significant decrease in the polar energy part to 6.12 mJ/m^2. Hydrophobic surfaces are known to exhibit low cell culture attachment efficiency and a long induction period before cells enter the exponential growth phase [20]. Sample 3 was characterized by the most hydrophilic surface of all three coatings with a contact angle of 40.2° and with a maximum surface energy of 57.17 mJ/m^2 due to an increase in the polar part to 17.66 mJ/m^2.

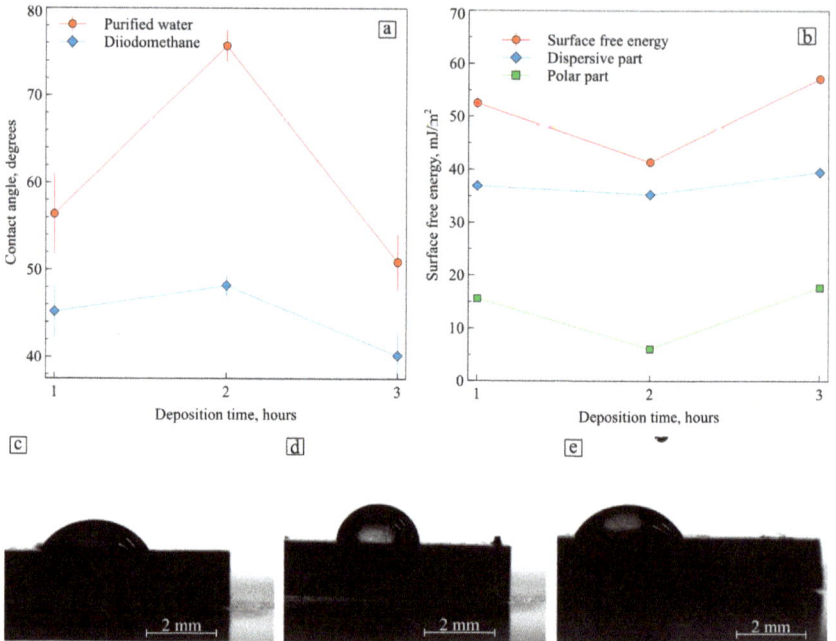

Figure 7. (**a**) Contact angle; (**b**) surface energy values of NiTi with hydroxyapatite coatings; the purified water drops on hydroxyapatite coatings deposited for: (**c**) 1 h; (**d**) 2 h; and (**e**) 3 h.

Considering that the ratio between the dispersive and the polar parts of the surface energy made it possible to predict the adhesion between the two phases, it was concluded that samples 1 and 3 would have the best adhesion during in vitro biocompatibility tests. This is because an increase in surface energy—in particular, an increase in the polar component of the surface energy—has a positive effect on cell adhesion [5]. However, since defects in the coating were found on the surface of sample 1, which could affect the contact angle and surface energy, it made sense to consider only sample 3 for in vitro tests. It should be noted that not only polar groups but also non-polar groups, as well as ligands on the cell surface and protein secretion, are responsible for the behavior of cells on the surface [21], which makes it quite difficult to predict the behavior of cells on artificial materials.

Samples 2 and 3 were chosen for in vitro studies since the coating of sample 1 had pronounced defects. SEM studies after 3-day cultivation of the cells made it possible to establish their normal morphology in Figure 8. The cells spread across the whole surface of sample 2. Some of them formed colonies consisting of several cells, but individual cells can also be seen. After 3 h of deposition, the adhesion of the cells became much better. There were no areas without the cells, so the calcium phosphate coating on sample 3 positively affected cell proliferation.

Despite the in vitro tests, one cannot claim that the increase in deposition time allowed for a boost in the number of viable cells, as some of them could have died. We can only estimate the level of proliferation, which certainly increased after 3 h of deposition. Other researchers have provided the results of in vitro experiments and proved that sputtered hydroxyapatite coatings increase cell viability [22].

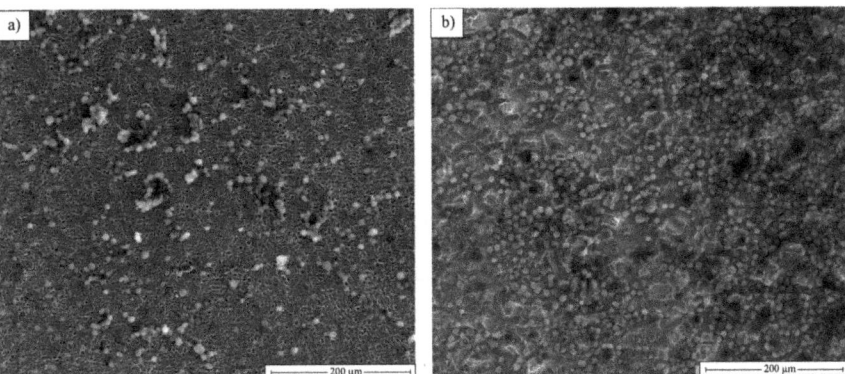

Figure 8. SEM images of hydroxyapatite coatings deposited for (**a**) 2 h and (**b**) 3 h after 72 h culture with MCF-7 cells.

4. Conclusions

Three samples with hydroxyapatite coatings were obtained using plasma-assisted RF sputtering for different deposition times of 1, 2, and 3 h. It was established using XRD that a coating of thermodynamically stable monoclinic HAp was formed on all three samples. The NiTi substrate had a mixed structure. The TiNi phase was in the form of two crystallographic modifications of B2 austenite and B19′ martensite, as well as intermetallic Ti_2Ni, Ni_3Ti, and Ni_4Ti_3 compounds. The structural studies showed that the densest defect-free coating was formed on sample 3 after 3 h of deposition, and according to EDS data, calcium, and phosphorus were evenly distributed over the surface. Sample 3 had the most hydrophilic surface with a contact angle of 40.2° and showed a significantly increased polar surface energy component of 17.66 mJ/m^2 and a high total surface energy of 57.17 mJ/m^2. Tests for cytocompatibility in vitro conditions showed that the surface of sample 2 was filled with cells unevenly, while the coating on sample 3 had a positive effect on adhesion and proliferative activity. Based on the obtained results, it can be concluded that a 3 h deposition time is promising for obtaining biocompatible HAp coatings on NiTi.

Author Contributions: Conceptualization, E.S.M., G.A.B. and K.M.D.; methodology, E.S.M.; validation, E.S.M., G.A.B. and K.M.D.; formal analysis, K.M.D.; investigation, G.A.B. and K.M.D.; resources, K.M.D. and I.I.G.; data curation, I.I.G.; writing—original draft preparation, K.M.D.; writing—review and editing, E.S.M., G.A.B. and A.A.V.; visualization, K.M.D.; supervision, E.S.M.; project administration, G.A.B.; funding acquisition, E.S.M. and A.A.V. All authors have read and agreed to the published version of the manuscript.

Funding: This research was supported by the Russian Science Foundation, No. 19-72-10105, https://rscf.ru/project/19-72-10105/ (accessed on 28 March 2023).

Institutional Review Board Statement: Not applicable.

Informed Consent Statement: Not applicable.

Data Availability Statement: The raw/processed data required to reproduce the above findings cannot be shared at this time as the data also forms part of an ongoing study.

Conflicts of Interest: The authors declare no conflict of interest.

References

1. Nguyen, T.-T.; Hu, C.-C.; Chou, B.-Y.; Chou, C.-Y.; Lin, G.-Y.; Hu, Y.-C.; Chen, Y.-L.; Hsu, W.-T.; Lin, Z.-S.; Lee, Y.-L.; et al. Evaluating hydrogenated nickel-titanium alloy for orthopedic implant. *J. Mater. Res. Technol.* **2022**, *18*, 1115–1123. [CrossRef]
2. Chen, S.; Zhang, B.; Hu, J.; Zheng, X.; Qin, S.; Li, C.; Wang, S.; Mao, J.; Wang, L. Bioinspired NiTi-reinforced polymeric heart valve exhibiting excellent hemodynamics and reduced stress. *Compos. B Eng.* **2023**, *255*, 110615. [CrossRef]
3. Mareci, D.; Earar, K.; Zetu, I.; Bolat, G.; Crimu, C.; Istrate, B.; Munteanu, C.; Matei, M.N. Comparative Electrochemical Behaviour of Uncoated and Coated NiTi for Dental Orthodontic Wires. *Mater. Plast.* **2015**, *52*, 150–153.
4. Wever, D.J.; Veldhuizen, A.G.; Sanders, M.M.; Schakenraad, J.M.; van Horn, J.R. Cytotoxic, allergic and genotoxic activity of a nickel-titanium alloy. *J. Biomater.* **1997**, *18*, 1115–1120. [CrossRef] [PubMed]
5. Hallab, N.J.; Bundy, K.J.; O'Connor, K.; Moses, R.L.; Jacobs, J.J. Evaluation of metallic and polymeric biomaterial surface energy and surface roughness characteristics for directed cell adhesion. *Tissue Eng.* **2001**, *71*, 55–71. [CrossRef]
6. Mehta, K.; Gupta, K. *Fabrication and Processing of Shape Memory Alloys*, 1st ed.; Springer International Publishing: Cham, Switzerland, 2019; p. 84. [CrossRef]
7. Witkowska, J.; Sowińska, A.; Czarnowska, E.; Płociński, T.; Rajchel, B.; Tarnowski, M.; Wierzchoń, T. Structure and properties of composite surface layers produced on TiNi shape memory alloy by a hybrid method. *J. Mater. Sci. Mater. Med.* **2018**, *29*, 110–119. [CrossRef]
8. Marchenko, E.; Baigonakova, G.; Dubovikov, K.; Kokorev, O.; Yasenchuk, Y.; Vorozhtsov, A. In Vitro Bio-Testing Comparative Analysis of NiTi Porous Alloys Modified by Heat Treatment. *Metals* **2022**, *12*, 1006. [CrossRef]
9. Sheykholeslami, S.O.R.; Khalil-Allafi, J.; Fathyunes, L. Preparation, Characterization, and Corrosion Behavior of Calcium Phosphate Coating Electrodeposited on the Modified Nanoporous Surface of NiTi Alloy for Biomedical Applications. *Metall. Mater. Trans. A Phys. Metall. Mater. Sci.* **2018**, *49*, 5878–5887. [CrossRef]
10. Shirdar, M.R.; Sudin, I.; Taheri, M.M.; Keyvanfar, A.; Yusop, M.Z.M.; Kadir, M.R.A. A novel hydroxyapatite composite reinforced with titanium nanotubes coated on Co-Cr-based alloy. *Vacuum* **2015**, *122*, 82–89. [CrossRef]
11. Shanaghi, A.; Mehrjou, B.; Ahmadian, Z.; Souri, A.R.; Chu, P.K. Enhanced corrosion resistance, antibacterial properties, and biocompatibility by hierarchical hydroxyapatite/ciprofloxacin-calcium phosphate coating on nitrided NiTi alloy. *Mater. Sci. Eng. C* **2021**, *118*, 111524. [CrossRef]
12. Etminanfar, M.R.; Khalil-Allafi, J.; Montaseri, A.; Vatankhah-Barenji, R. Endothelialization and the bioactivity of Ca-P coatings of different Ca/P stoichiometry electrodeposited on the Nitinol superelastic alloy. *Mater. Sci. Eng. C* **2016**, *62*, 28–35. [CrossRef]
13. Jue, L.; Chao, L.; Jing, L.; Min, L.; Jian-ming, R. Calcium phosphate deposition on surface of porous and dense TiNi alloys in simulated body fluid. *J. Cent. South Univ.* **2016**, *23*, 1–9. [CrossRef]
14. Horandghadim, N.; Khalil-Allaf, J.; Urgen, M. Influence of tantalum pentoxide secondary phase on surface features and mechanical properties of hydroxyapatite coating on NiTi alloy produced by electrophoretic deposition. *Surf. Coat. Technol.* **2020**, *386*, 125458. [CrossRef]
15. Etminanfar, M.R.; Sheykholeslami, S.O.R.; Khalili, V.; Mahdavi, S. Biocompatibility and drug delivery efficiency of PEG-b-PCL/hydroxyapatite bilayer coatings on Nitinol superelastic alloy. *Ceram. Int.* **2020**, *46*, 12711–12717. [CrossRef]
16. Mehrvarz, A.; Khalil-Allafi, J.; Etminanfar, M.; Mahdavi, S. The study of morphological evolution, biocorrosion resistance, and bioactivity of pulse electrochemically deposited Hydroxyapatite/ZnO composite on NiTi superelastic alloy. *Surf. Coat. Technol.* **2021**, *423*, 127628. [CrossRef]
17. Harun, W.; Asri, R.; Alias, J.; Zulkifli, F.; Kadirgama, K.; Ghani, S.; Shariffuddin, J. A comprehensive review of hydroxyapatite-based coatings adhesion on metallic biomaterials. *Ceram. Int.* **2018**, *44*, 1250–1268. [CrossRef]
18. Schwartz, A.; Kossenko, A.; Zinigrad, M.; Gofer, Y.; Borodianskiy, K.; Sobolev, A. Hydroxyapatite Coating on Ti-6Al-7Nb Alloy by Plasma Electrolytic Oxidation in Salt-Based Electrolyte. *Materials* **2022**, *15*, 7374. [CrossRef] [PubMed]
19. Kima, T.H.; Yeom, G.Y. A Review of Inductively Coupled Plasma-Assisted Magnetron Sputter System. *Appl. Sci. Converg. Technol.* **2019**, *28*, 131–138. [CrossRef]
20. Dowling, D.P.; Miller, I.S.; Ardhaoui, M.; Gallagher, W.M. Effect of Surface Wettability and Topography on the Adhesion of Osteosarcoma Cells on Plasma-modified Polystyrene. *J. Biomater. Appl.* **2011**, *26*, 327–347. [CrossRef] [PubMed]
21. Majhy, B.; Priyadarshini, P.; Sen, A.K. Effect of surface energy and roughness on cell adhesion and growth-facile surface modification for enhanced cell culture. *RSC Adv.* **2021**, *11*, 15467–15476. [CrossRef]
22. Buyuksungur, S.; Huri, P.Y.; Schmidt, J.; Pana, I.; Dinu, M.; Vitelaru, C.; Kiss, A.E.; Tamay, D.G.; Hasirci, V.; Vladescu, A.; et al. In vitro cytotoxicity, corrosion and antibacterial efficiencies of Zn doped hydroxyapatite coated Ti based implant materials. *Ceram. Int.* **2023**, *49*, 12570–12584. [CrossRef]

Disclaimer/Publisher's Note: The statements, opinions and data contained in all publications are solely those of the individual author(s) and contributor(s) and not of MDPI and/or the editor(s). MDPI and/or the editor(s) disclaim responsibility for any injury to people or property resulting from any ideas, methods, instructions or products referred to in the content.

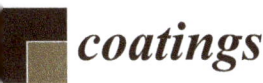

Article

Poly(2-Methoxyethyl Acrylate) (PMEA)-Coated Anti-Platelet Adhesive Surfaces to Mimic Native Blood Vessels through HUVECs Attachment, Migration, and Monolayer Formation

Md Azizul Haque [1,2], Daiki Murakami [1,3,*], Takahisa Anada [1,3] and Masaru Tanaka [1,3,*]

1 Department of Chemistry and Biochemistry, Graduate School of Engineering, Kyushu University, Fukuoka 819-0395, Japan; md.azizul.haque.509@s.kyushu-u.ac.jp (M.A.H.); takahisa_anada@ms.ifoc.kyushu-u.ac.jp (T.A.)
2 Department of Applied Chemistry and Chemical Engineering, Noakhali Science and Technology University, Noakhali 3814, Bangladesh
3 Institute for Materials Chemistry and Engineering, Kyushu University, Fukuoka 819-0395, Japan
* Correspondence: daiki_murakami@ms.ifoc.kyushu-u.ac.jp (D.M.); masaru_tanaka@ms.ifoc.kyushu-u.ac.jp (M.T.); Tel./Fax: +81-92-802-6238 (D.M. & M.T.)

Abstract: Confluent monolayers of human umbilical vein endothelial cells (HUVECs) on a poly(2-methoxyethyl acrylate) (PMEA) antithrombogenic surface play a major role in mimicking the inner surface of native blood vessels. In this study, we extensively investigated the behavior of cell–polymer and cell–cell interactions by measuring adhesion strength using single-cell force spectroscopy. In addition, the attachment and migration of HUVECs on PMEA-analogous substrates were detected, and the migration rate was estimated. Moreover, the bilateral migration of HUVECs between two adjacent surfaces was observed. Furthermore, the outer surface of HUVEC was examined using frequency-modulation atomic force microscopy (FM-AFM). Hydration was found to be an indication of a healthy glycocalyx layer. The results were compared with the hydration states of individual PMEA-analogous polymers to understand the adhesion mechanism between the cells and substrates in the interface region. HUVECs could attach and spread on the PMEA surface with stronger adhesion strength than self-adhesion strength, and migration occurred over the surface of analogue polymers. We confirmed that platelets could not adhere to HUVEC monolayers cultured on the PMEA surface. FM-AFM images revealed a hydration layer on the HUVEC surfaces, indicating the presence of components of the glycocalyx layer in the presence of intermediate water. Our findings show that PMEA can mimic original blood vessels through an antithrombogenic HUVEC monolayer and is thus suitable for the construction of artificial small-diameter blood vessels.

Keywords: poly(2-methoxyethyl acrylate) (PMEA); human umbilical vein endothelial cell (HUVEC); cell-cell interaction; cell adhesion strength; cell migration; frequency-modulation atomic force microscopy (FM-AFM); hydration; artificial small-diameter blood vessel

1. Introduction

According to the World Health Organization (WHO), due to the rapid increase in cardiovascular diseases (CVDs) and the associated number of deaths, the 17.9 million deaths from CVDs in 2019 is estimated to increase to 23.6 million by 2030 [1,2]. Approximately 32% of total deaths worldwide are caused by the diverse categories of CVDs, such as coronary heart disease (CHD) and peripheral artery disease (PAD). Currently, researchers are focusing on obtaining the most suitable treatments for CVDs. To date, angioplasty, atherectomy, stent insertion, and bypass of the injured vessels are the most well-known treatments [3]. Bypass of injured vessels is an effective treatment, and autologous saphenous vessels are generally selected. However, there is a risk of secondary trauma. Therefore, synthetic artificial vascular grafts can be suitable alternatives to autologous saphenous vessels. To date, polyethylene terephthalate (PET) and expanded polytetrafluoroethylene (ePTFE) have been used as synthetic grafts for large-diameter vessels. However, these grafts show poor patency for small-diameter blood vessels due to thrombus formation inside them [4]. PET and ePTFE are unable to promote endothelialization and induce thrombosis and inflammation due to platelet and neutrophil activation [5]. Therefore, vascular graft diameter smaller than 6 mm presents a high risk of thrombus formation. In addition, protein adsorption boosts the platelet adhesion in surface induced clotting [6].

Many methods have been implemented to improve the surface of synthetic grafts through surface modification, new polymer development, and cell–substrate interaction investigation using mechanobiology assessments. Various surface modification techniques have been used to functionalize the substrate interface for cell attachment, growth, migration, rapid endothelization, and long-term anticoagulation [7–9]. Polymer coating is an effective approach to functionalize biomaterial surfaces. Functionalization with poly(ethylene glycol) and zwitterionic polymers, including poly(2-methacryloyloxyethyl phosphorylcholine) (PMPC), suppresses biofilm formation, immune responses to biomaterial surfaces, and adhesion of platelets [10–16]. Moreover, several approaches have been introduced to obtain smart or responsive surfaces. Temperature-responsive grafted polymer brushes based on LCST open opportunities for the fabrication of responsive surfaces [17]. On the other hand, stimuli-responsive macromolecules have significantly impacted new developments in polymeric coatings where the surface shows responsiveness to bacterial attacks, ice or fog formation, anti-fouling properties, autonomous self-cleaning and self-healing, or drug delivery systems [18].

A stable, confluent endothelium lining may act as a completely antithrombogenic surface. However, such an endothelial cell (EC) layer does not form spontaneously at the surface of a vascular implant in humans in vivo. Subsequently, one researcher has proposed pre-seeding ECs or progenitor cells prior to implantation in order to increase the patency of synthetic vascular grafts [19,20]. However, poor cell adhesion ability under flow condition indicates low compatibility [21]. Consequently, polymers with antifouling and antithrombogenic properties with strong endothelial cell attachment abilities are desirable for researchers to develop artificial small-diameter blood vessels (ASDBVs) that can mimic native blood vessels.

In this regard, poly(2-methoxyethyl acrylate) (PMEA), an antithrombogenic synthetic polymer, is a suitable alternative to ePTFE and PET because of its intermediate water (IW, loosely bound water) content, which is a measure of biocompatibility and blood compatibility [22,23]. It was found that IW is present in natural biocompatible polymers, such as DNA (and RNA), heparin, and chondroitin sulfate [24]. PMEA is a US Food and Drug Administration (FDA)-approved biocompatible polymer used in artificial lungs, catheters, and stents as an antithrombogenic coating material. PMEA is water insoluble and hydrophobic in nature. It makes thin film coatings on substrates, such as PET or other surfaces where coating needs to be performed. When the biomaterials contact with the body fluids, the primary interaction happens on the biomaterial–fluid interface in hydrated state. First, proteins are adsorbed and then denatured on the hydrated material surface. Cell adherent protein adsorption depends on the wettability, polymer rich and poor regions, as well as the microphase separation of a homopolymer at an interface. The amount and degree of denaturation of adsorbed proteins affect subsequent cell behavior, including cell adhesion, migration, proliferation, and differentiation. The modification in the chemical structure of PMEA shows distinct morphological and interaction behavior with the blood component [25,26]. A polymer with similar chemical and structural properties to PMEA is named PMEA analogous polymer. Our recent investigation reveals that PMEA analogous polymers suppress platelet adhesion, and the degree of suppression depends on the amount of IW present in each polymer [22,26]. In particular, a polymer with high IW content (e.g., PMPC, IW = 11.11% w) suppresses platelets more effectively than a polymer with low IW content [27]. However, PMPC does not allow the attachment of cells, proteins, or any other blood components on its surface.

A monolayer of ECs can effectively protect surfaces from the adhesion of blood components (platelets, white blood cells, red blood cells, and proteins), thus suppressing platelet coagulation and thrombus formation [28]. Alternatively, PMEA, a blood-compatible polymer, does not activate leukocytes, erythrocytes, or platelets, in vitro [22]. Furthermore, because PMEA and analogous polymers promote the attachment of non-blood cells, they are believed to facilitate endothelization [29]. Therefore, endothelization over the polymer surface may play a major role in surface antithrombogenic properties.

In recent years, the human umbilical vein endothelial cells (HUVEC) model has been used in cardiovascular and clinical research as compared to animal models. In vitro HUVEC models have been convenient to study platelet adhesion to the endothelium, endothelial dysfunctions, the potential effect of atherosclerosis in initial stages and atherosclerosis progression [30,31]. On the other hand, EC activation, migration, and proliferation are responsible for the formation and organization of tubular structures to form new blood vessels through the angiogenesis process [32,33]. Finally, HUVEC as a model to study the endothelium has greatly facilitated the study of cardiovascular disease. In contrast, the glycocalyx is a combination of hydrated sugar-rich molecules (heparin sulfate, chondroitin sulfate, and hyaluronic acid) coating the surface of ECs lining the inside of blood vessels. Our previous study showed that promoting the glycocalyx of HUVECs with transforming growth factor-β1(TGF-β1) decreased platelet adhesion, while degrading the glycocalyx with heparinase I increased platelet adhesion. These results suggested that the glycocalyx of cultured HUVECs modulates platelet compatibility, and the amount of glycocalyx secreted by HUVECs depends on the chemical structure and cross-linker concentration of the scaffolds [34]. Matrix stiffness is also known to affect the expression of the glycocalyx in cultured ECs [35].

In the present study, we aim to find the best polymer from PMEA analogous polymers that can be used to construct an artificial small diameter vascular graft as a coating material. For this purpose, the polymer should fulfil the basic needs, such as antithrombogenic surface, good HUVECs attachment, growth, proliferation, migration, monolayer formation, and strong adhesion strength to the surface. We used HUVECs to measure cell–cell and cell–substrate interactions using single-cell force spectroscopy (SCFS). We found a possible mechanism of HUVECs monolayer formation over a biocompatible polymer surface by comparing the strength of cell–cell and cell–substrate interactions. We then evaluated the migration behavior of HUVECs on the PMEA polymer analogs. In addition, the bilateral migration of HUVECs between two adjacent polymer surfaces was observed, indicating migration of HUVECs from native blood vessels to artificial implants in vitro. Furthermore, a platelet adhesion test was performed on HUVECs monolayers cultured on PMEA and PET. Finally, the upper surface of a single HUVEC was investigated using frequency-modulation atomic force microscopy (FM-AFM) to determine the hydration states of the HUVEC surface to verify the expression of the glycocalyx layer as well as IW states.

2. Materials and Methods

2.1. Chemicals and Materials

Hydrophilized PET sheet (thickness = 120 μm) was purchased from Mitsubishi Plastic Inc. (Tokyo, Japan). PMEA (M_n = 26.9 kg/mol, M_w/M_n = 2.73), poly(3-methoxypropyl acrylate) (PMC3A, M_n = 20.8 kg/mol, M_w/M_n = 3.83), and poly(n-butyl acrylate) (PBA, M_n = 62.8 kg/mol, M_w/M_n = 1.41) were synthesized as previously reported [26]. Poly(n-butyl mathacrylate-co-2-methacryloyloxyethyl phosphorylcholine) (BMA 70 mol%, MPC 30 mol%) (PMPC, Mw = 600 kg/mol) was a gift from the NOF Corporation, Tokyo, Japan. Tissue culture polystyrene (TCPS) was purchased from IWATA, Japan. The chemical structures of the polymers used in the present study are shown in Figure 1. Fibronectin was purchased from Wako Pure Chemical Industries (Osaka, Japan). The platelet adhesion test was performed using human whole blood, which was purchased from Tennessee Blood Services (Memphis, TN, USA). Human whole blood was collected from healthy donors and stored in a vacuum blood collection tube (Venoject II; Terumo Co., Tokyo, Japan) containing 3.2% sodium citrate as an anticoagulant. Blood was used within a week after collection. Blocking reagent was purchased from Nacalai Tesque (Kyoto, Japan). All other reagents and solvents were obtained from Kanto Chemical Co. (Tokyo, Japan).

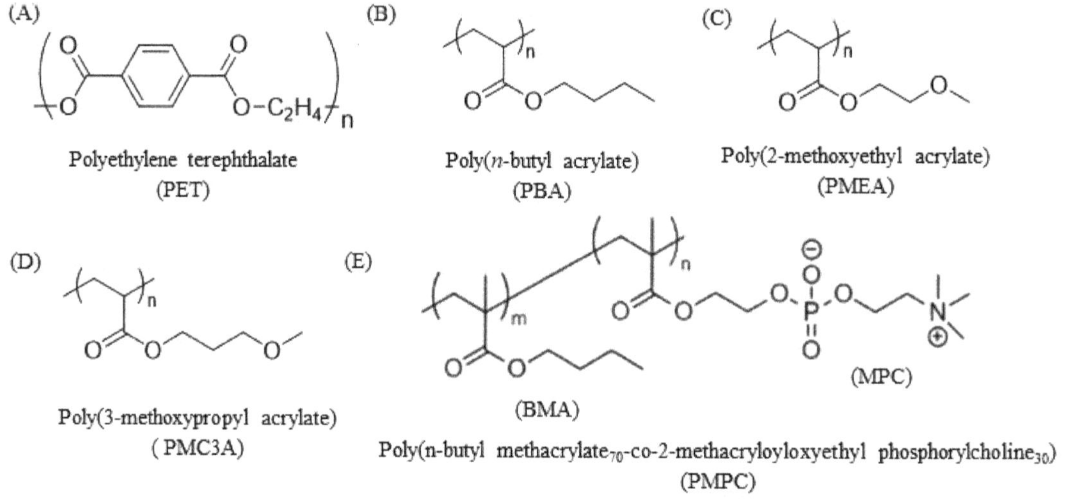

Figure 1. Chemical structure of (**A**) polyethylene terephthalate (PET); (**B**) poly(n-butyl acrylate) (PBA); (**C**) poly(2-methoxyethyl acrylate) (PMEA); (**D**) poly(3-methoxypropyl acrylate) (PMC3A), and (**E**) poly(n-butyl mathacrylate-co-2-methacryloyloxyethyl phosphorylcholine) (BMA 70 mol%, MPC 30 mol%) (PMPC).

2.2. Fabrication of Polymer-Coated Substrates

PET was used as a substrate for the polymer coating. Initially, the PET sheet was cut into a circular shape with a diameter of 14 mm using a hand press cutter and cleaned by washing with toluene. PMEA, PMC3A, and PBA were dissolved in toluene (0.5% w/v) to obtain the polymer solution. PMPC was dissolved in methanol at the same concentration. The PMEA analogous polymer solutions of 40 µL were charged on the PET substrates for spin-coating using a Spin Coater (Mikasa MS-A100) at a constant speed of 3000 rpm for 40 s, ramped down for 4 s, and then dried for at least for 24 h in a vacuum dryer at 25 °C. Bare PET was used as the positive control and TCPS was used as the cell culture dish. The morphologies of the polymer-coated surfaces were observed by atomic force microscopy (AFM) and the thickness was estimated at around 100 nm using transmission electron microscopy [25,36]. The surface roughness of all polymer coatings was almost the same within 10–20 nm. However, AFM observation showed that the interfacial structures of the PMEA and PMC3A were highly ordered, homogeneous, and compactly dispersed in nanometer scale, although the low blood-compatible polymer PBA interface had an irregular structure [25].

2.3. Contact Angle

Contact angle measurements were conducted using milli Q water. Two methods (sessile drop and air bubble) were used to measure the contact angle values of PMEA analogous surfaces at 25 °C using a DropMaster DMo-501SA (Kyowa Interface Science Co., Tokyo, Japan (shown in Table 1). Following the sessile drop method, 2 µL of water droplet was dropped on the polymer surface for 60 s, and the contact angles were calculated from the photograph. In the captive bubble method, PMEA analogous substrates were immersed in Milli-Q water for 24 h. Then, a 2 µL air bubble was injected beneath the substrate surfaces located in water, and the contact angles were also measured using photographic images. Finally, the contact angle at 30 s was counted as the contact angle of that substrate.

Table 1. Contact angle and water content of studied polymers.

Polymers	Contact Angle * [deg]			IW
	Sessile Water Drops	Captive Air Bubble		
	(30 s)	(30 s)	24 h	(wt.%)
PET	73.3 (±0.9)	125.5 (±2.2)	125.4 (±0.5)	0
PBA	83.8 (±1.9)	126.7 (±2.8)	125.0 (±1.7)	0.31
PMEA	44.3 (±2.1)	134.0 (±0.9)	132.9 (±1.8)	3.7
PMC3A	52.1 (±0.5)	126.9 (±1.0)	127.8 (±0.7)	2.8
PMPC	108.9 (±0.5)	152.4 (±2.9)	150.0 (±3.8)	11.11

* 2 µL water droplet in air (sessile drop) and 2 µL air bubble in water (Captive bubble). The data represent the means ± SD (n = 5).

2.4. HUVECs Culture

ECs were solely used for all experiments described in this article. Commercially available HUVECs (Lonza, Cologne, Germany) were cultured under static cell culture conditions (37 °C, 5% CO_2) in polystyrene-based cell culture flasks. Cells were used for 4–6 passages and cultured in endothelial basal medium (EBM-2) supplemented with endothelial growth medium (EGM-2) Single Quots® kit and 2% fetal calf serum (FCS; Lonza). Before starting the experiments, cells were detached using 0.25% trypsin/EDTA solution (Thermo Fisher Scientific, Rockford, IL, USA) from the culture dish. Then, HUVECs solution was centrifugated for 3 min at 1200 rpm to isolate HUVECs from the medium. Initial cell counting was performed using a hemocytometer to adjust the cell density.

2.5. Cell Attachment, Proliferation, and Immunocytochemical Analysis

Cell attachment and proliferation assays were performed using a 24-well plate (IWATA). The 24-well plate was first coated with PMPC (0.5% w/v) and allowed to dry. The pre-coated polymer substrates were then fixed onto the 24-well plate using glue on the back side of each substrate and cured under UV light for 30 min. Phosphate-buffered saline (PBS) was then added to the wells and incubated for 1 h at 37 °C. Afterwards, culture media were added and incubated for another hour at 37 °C. HUVECs were seeded on the substrates at 1×10^4 cells/cm^2 in serum-containing media and allowed to adhere and proliferate on the surface of the substrates for 1 h, 1 day, or 3 days. After cultivation at these specific time intervals, the cells were analyzed using ImageJ software (version 1.53C; National Institutes of Health, Bethesda, MD, USA).

In addition, before starting the immunocytochemical analysis, the prepared substrates were preconditioned, as in the cell attachment and proliferation assays. HUVECs were seeded (5×10^3 cells/cm^2) on polymer-coated PET substrates and incubated for 1, 24, or 72 h. After culturing for specific times, the cells were fixed using preheated (37 °C) 4% (w/v) paraformaldehyde (Fujifilm Wako Pure Chemical Co., Ltd., Osaka, Japan) and stored outside for 10 min. Thereafter, 1% (v/v) Triton X-100 (Fujifilm Wako Pure Chemicals Co., Ltd.) in PBS (−) was added to increase plasma membrane permeability. After washing, the sections were blocked for 30 min. Then, the substrates were stained with mouse monoclonal anti-human vinculin antibody (VIN-11-5; Sigma-Aldrich, St. Louis, MO, USA) (1:200) diluted in PBS (−) for 90 min at room temperature (RT), and subsequently stained with Alexa Fluor 568-conjugated anti-mouse immunoglobulin G (IgG) (H + L) antibody (1:1000 dilution), Alexa Fluor 488-conjugated phalloidin (1:1000 diluted), and 4,6-diamidino-2-phenylindole (DAPI, 1:1000 dilution) (all from Thermo Fisher Scientific, Waltham, MA, USA), all diluted in 10% blocking solution in PBS, treated for 1 h at RT. After performing these steps, stained cells were fixed on glass slides. Fluorescence photographs were taken using a confocal laser-scanning microscope (CLSM) (FV-3000; Olympus, Tokyo, Japan). The HUVEC morphology was quantitatively assessed using ImageJ.

2.6. HUVECs Migration Analysis

HUVECs migration analyses were executed in six-well plates. Initially, one half of the PET substrate (φ = 30 mm) was coated with a PMEA-analogous polymer and the other half was exposed to bare PET. First, HUVECs were cultured on all studied substrates, placed into six-well plates with a seeding density 1×10^4 cells/cm^2 and incubated at 37 °C until full confluency. After confluency, the cell monolayer surface was scratched using a 4 mm wide rubber cell scraper in the PET–polymer interface region and kept in incubator for migration. Finally, cell migration towards the scratched area was observed at 0, 24, and 48 h of scratching, and time-lapse images were taken using a phase-contrast microscope (Figure 2). The migrated area was quantified using ImageJ software and denoted as $A_0 - A_t$, where A_0 is the initial area before migration and A_t is the area at the certain time t (i.e., 0, 24, or 48 h). The migration rate was then plotted against the types of substrates where migration happened.

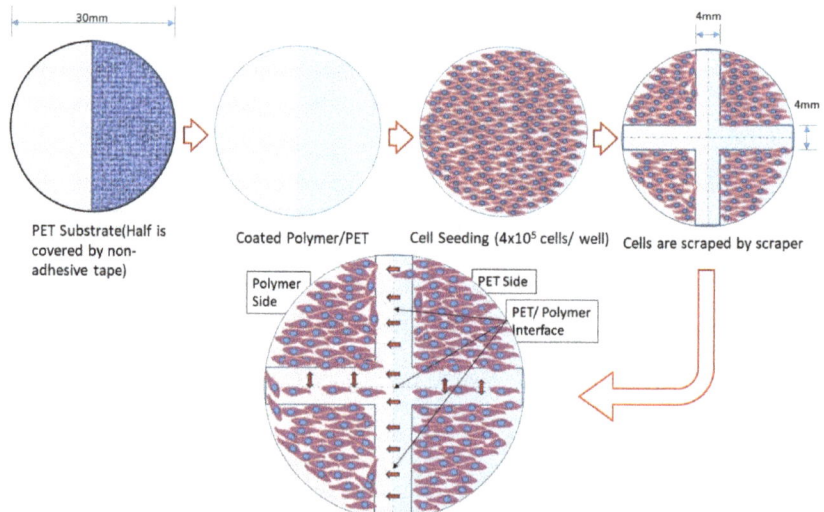

Figure 2. Schematic representation of the HUVECs migration rate measurements and observation of HUVECs migration through the coated polymer-PET interface.

2.7. HUVEC-PMEA and HUVEC-HUVEC Interaction Determined by SCFS

Prior to the HUVEC–PMEA interaction measurement, the PMEA-coated substrates were placed under UV light for 30 min before the PBS was poured and placed in incubator for 1 h at 37 °C. Subsequently, EGM-2 medium was added to the substrate and freshly detached cells (five to six passages) were injected into it. In addition, the tipless cantilever named TL-CONT (spring constant k = 0.2 N/m; Bruker, Billerica, MA, USA) was coated with fibronectin solution (1 mg/mL) and kept for around 20 min to dry. Then, a single HUVEC was captured with a tipless cantilever for 10 min with set point: 2 nN. The force–distance curves between the cells and the substrates were measured using an AFM (CellHesion JPK; Bruker, Billerica, MA, USA) equipped with a tipless cantilever (set point: 2 nN, approaching rate: 5.0 µm/s, holding time: 120 s, retraction rate: 15 µm/s). The value of set point for the measurement of HUVEC adhesion strength was used from our previous report, where the relationship between the set points and the cell adhesion strength of HeLa cells were evaluated [37]. In this investigation, the maximum force for cell detachment from the substrate is denoted as adhesion force, which is indicated at the lowest point of the retraction curve. Adhesion work was estimated as the amount of work required to detach the cell from the substrate, corresponding to the area enclosed by the baseline and retraction curve [38]. The same experimental conditions were used to determine HUVEC–HUVEC interactions. The only exception was that HUVECs were cultured on both the

PMEA-coated PET substrate and TCPS. HUVEC adhesion strength was measured on the attached HUVECs using the same procedure as described earlier in this section.

2.8. Platelet Adhesion Test on Cultured HUVECs Monolayer

The platelet adhesion test was performed under static conditions as previously described [22,34,39]. In brief, fresh blood was centrifuged at $400 \times g$ for 5 min to obtain platelet-rich plasma (PRP), and the remaining blood was centrifuged at $2500 \times g$ for 10 min to obtain platelet-poor plasma (PPP). The platelet concentration was determined using a hemocytometer. Cell density (4×10^7 cells/cm^2) was adjusted by mixing PPP and PRP. Prior to this experiment, HUVECs were cultured on the PMEA-coated and bare PET substrates. Before loading the platelet suspension, the cultured HUVECs layer was washed with PBS (−). Then, 450 µL of platelet suspension was loaded onto HUVECs proliferated on the confluent layer and incubated for 1 h at 37 °C. After 1 h of incubation, the weakly adhered platelets were rinsed three times with PBS. Adhered platelets were then fixed using 1% glutaraldehyde for 2 h at 37 °C. After this period, samples were rinsed with PBS, 50% PBS, and Milli-Q water. Finally, the samples were dried at RT for 1–2 days before being subjected to sputter gold coating for scanning electron microscopy (SEM) observation. Then, the number of adhered platelets was counted from SEM images using ImageJ software (n = 15 of each substrate).

2.9. FM-AFM of Single HUVEC Surface

FM-AFM was conducted using an SPM-8100FM (Shimadzu Co., Kyoto, Japan) in water at 23 °C. A PPP-NCHAuD cantilever (typical spring constant, k = 42 N/m, NanoWorld AG, Neuchâtel, Switzerland) was used. The resonance frequency in water was approximately 140 kHz, and the scan in the z-direction was performed with a force limit of 2.5 V, which corresponds to a frequency shift of approximately 500 Hz. The amplitude of the cantilever oscillation was maintained constant at approximately 2 nm.

2.10. Statistical Analyses

Data from at least three independent trials were used in calculation of mean ± standard deviation (SD). Significant differences were assessed using one-way analysis of variance (ANOVA) (Tukey–Kramer multiple comparison test) with Origin Pro (version 2019b; OriginLab Co., Northampton, MA, USA). $p < 0.05$ was set to evaluate statistical significance.

3. Results and Discussion

3.1. HUVECs Cultured on PMEA-Analogous Polymers

The formation of confluent EC monolayers on implanted materials has been identified as a method to avoid thrombus formation [28,40]. PMEA polymer analogs (PMEA, PMC3A, and PBA) and PMPC were coated on PET substrates to culture HUVECs and investigate HUVECs adhesion ability. The physical properties of the studied polymer are shown in Table 1. HUVECs attachment ability depends on the surface type, morphology, and biomechanical interaction in the interface. In our previous study, we mentioned the surface morphology of our polymer studied by AFM observation [25]. Figure 3 shows the phase-contrast micrographs of the sub-confluent to confluent layer of HUVECs attached to the PMEA polymers at 120 h. Bare PET and PMPC were used as the positive and negative controls, respectively. It was found that HUVECs can attach to PMEA polymer analogs and form a confluent monolayer. This confirms our previous findings that ECs can attach, proliferate, and form a layer on PMEA-coated surfaces compared with other analogous polymers. The proliferation of HUVECs on the various substrates decreased in the following order: TCPS > PET ≈ PMEA > PMC3A ≈ PBA > PMPC. No considerable number of HUVECs was found on PMPC at 120 h. HUVECs could not survive on PMPC because of their strong antithrombogenic properties. These results agree with those of our previous study in which HUVECs and aorta smooth muscle cells (AoSMCs) were cultured on PET, PMEA, and PMPC [41].

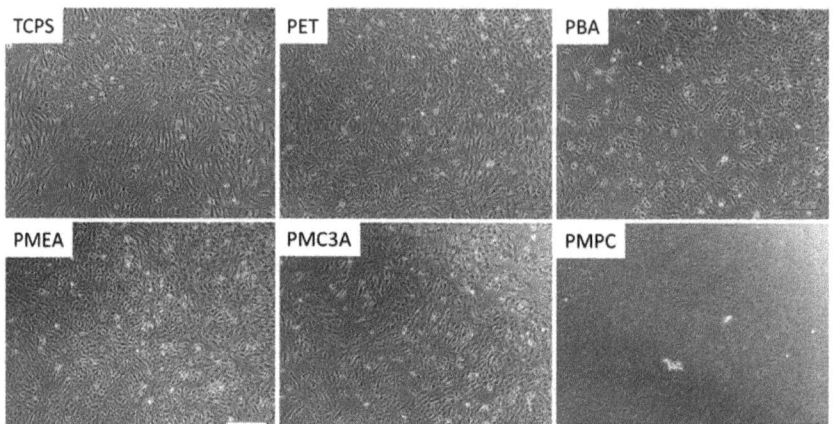

Figure 3. Phase-contrast micrographs of the HUVECs cultured for 120 h on PMEA-analogous polymers and on TCPS, PET, and PMPC as controls (scale bar = 200 μm).

The different attachment behaviors of HUVECs on PMEA-analogous polymers depend on the hydration state, surface morphology, and stiffness of each polymer [35,40,42]. Generally, cells adhere to a polymeric surface via cell-binding proteins, such as fibronectin or fibrinogen, through integrin [43]. HUVECs are more likely to adhere to fibronectin than fibrinogen through the RGD sequence, which is a universal binding site [44]. It has been proven that cells can attach to PMEA in an integrin-dependent and -independent manner through direct interaction between the cell membrane and the polymer interface [45]. In this study, we found a more confluent HUVECs monolayer on PMEA-coated substrates than on other analogous polymers. This can be attributed to the selective protein adsorption and integrin-independent and -dependent adhesion mechanism of PMEA, which is regulated by the IW content [41].

3.2. Possible Mechanism of HUVECs Monolayer Formation on PMEA (Cell-Cell Interaction)

The initial interactions between individual HUVECs cultured on the PMEA surface were measured using the SCFS. Figure 4 shows the HUVEC adhesion strength in nN, measured at three different places of the attached HUVEC on PMEA. We found that the adhesion strength was highest in the external cellular matrix (ECM) of the attached single HUVEC, lower on arbitrary positions of the monolayer, and lowest on the top of the cell where the nucleus is present. Therefore, variation in interaction strength can occur because of the concentration of adhesion proteins in the serum medium. Previous studies have shown that cell adhesion on PMEA in serum-free medium is similar to that on serum-containing medium [45]. In contrast, the adhesion energy differed among the various interaction locations of the attached HUVEC, which may be due to the dissimilar surface interaction area and number of focal adhesion points.

In contrast, intercellular adhesion plays a major role in tissue development and homeostasis [46]. Sancho et al. measured the cell adhesion forces of HUVECs on substrates in well-attached individual cells and monolayers. In the present study, we measured and compared the initial HUVEC adhesion strength between HUVEC–PMEA and HUVEC–HUVEC, where the HUVECs were cultured on both TCPS and PMEA surfaces, as shown in Figure 5. The average HUVEC–HUVEC interaction strength was calculated, as shown in Figure 4, and results revealed that there is no effect of culture substrates on cell–cell interaction strength. However, the HUVEC–PMEA adhesion strength was much higher than the cell–cell interaction. Therefore, initially, HUVECs seem to be more involved in attachment to the substrates than individual cells, even though a few portions of seeded cells were in a tri-dimensional (3D) aggregated form. After seeding, the cells spread and formed a two-dimensional (2D) layer. Therefore, the initial cell adhesion strength is a measure of monolayer formation. This result shows that the measurement of cell adhesion strength is vital for the development of endothelial monolayers for the construction of ASDBV. In addition, ECs forming the inner wall of every blood vessel are constantly exposed to the mechanical forces generated by blood flow [47]. If the cell–substrate interaction is not sufficient to resist the force exerted by blood flow, then no cell can be attached or migrate to form a confluent layer of cells. Therefore, EC responses to these hemodynamic forces and interaction strength play a critical role in the homeostasis of the circulatory system in the development of ASDBV.

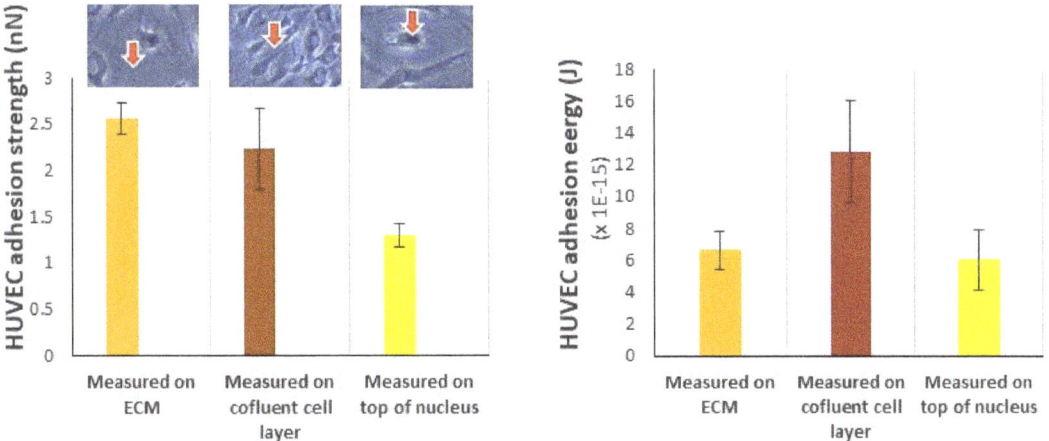

Figure 4. Cell-cell interaction strength measured in three positions (ECM, arbitrary point of confluent layer, top of nucleus) of confluent HUVECs monolayer. The data represent the mean ± SD (n = 4). Red arrows represent the typical positions at which the force measurements were done.

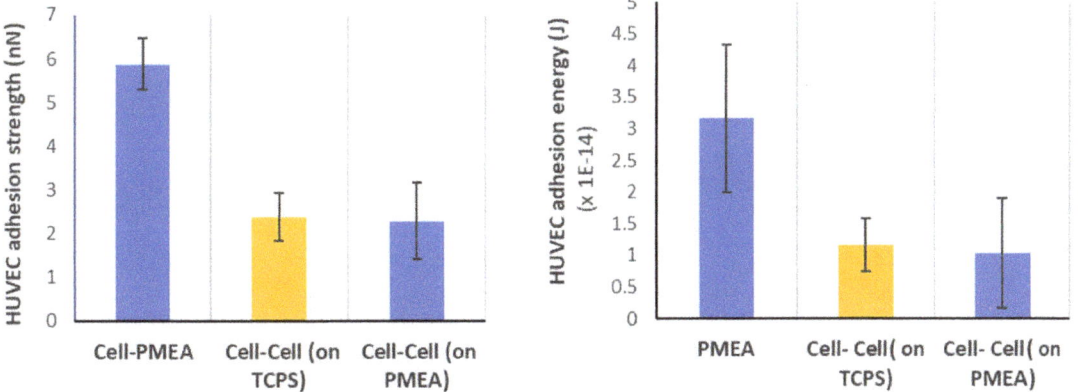

Figure 5. Comparison of HUVEC adhesion strength between cell-PMEA, cell-cell cultured on TCPS, and cell-cell cultured on PMEA. The data represent the mean ± SD (n > 4).

3.3. HUVECs Migration Analysis

HUVECs migration analysis was performed to evaluate the migration ability of HUVECs on the different polymeric surfaces. Figure 6 shows the HUVECs migration analysis on the PMEA, PMC3A, PBA, and PET. The left side of each substrate was coated on the polymer side, and the right side was always bare PET. The white dotted line in each image indicates the interface between the PMEA-analogous and bare PET. The migration time was recorded from 0 to 48 h using a time-lapse microscope. The red dotted line indicates the area occupied by HUVECs before and after migration at the various time intervals. In Figure 2, we demonstrate the HUVECs migration procedure, in which the layer of HUVECs was scratched in both the vertical and horizontal directions. After migration, five locations were selected for each substrate to calculate the migration rate. From Figure 6, we can see that those cultured monolayers of HUVECs were scratched using a rubber scraper to set the initial area of cultured HUVECs on PMEA-analogous polymer and PET surfaces. Then, images were taken every hour for 48 h.

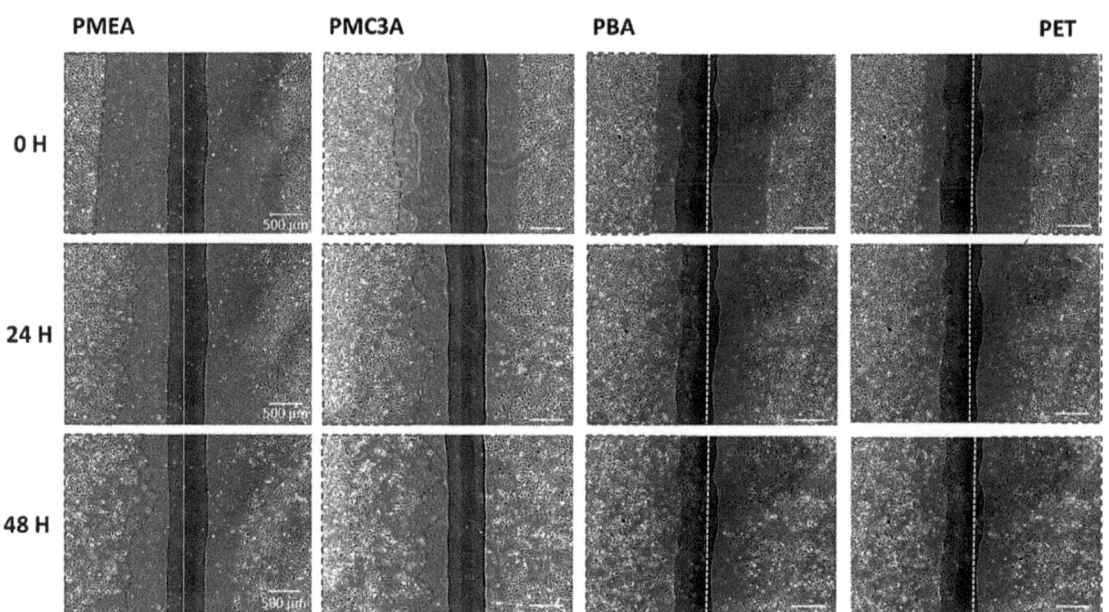

Figure 6. HUVECs migration analysis on PMEA, PMC3A, PBA, and PET (scale bar = 500 μm). The white dotted line indicates the interface between PMEA-analogous polymers and bare PET. Migration was recorded from 0 to 48 h. The red dotted line indicates the HUVECs occupied area before and after migration.

3.4. Observation of Cell Migration between Surfaces

In addition, we observed HUVECs migration between the surfaces through the interface. Focusing on the interface (white dotted line) of each polymer, we identified the migration of HUVECs from the bare PET side to the PMEA side through the interface. The migration is marked by a red rectangle in Figure 7, and it increased with time. Furthermore, we calculated the HUVECS migration rate for all the substrates from the newly covered area after migration. We found that the migration rates were slightly different, although the differences were not statistically significant (Figure 8). However, PMEA showed the highest average migration rate among all samples.

The most vital task of ECs is to protect the vascular system through the formation of an antithrombogenic monolayer that is periodically renewed to maintain proper endothelial functions [48,49]. To treat CVDs, after the implementation of cardiovascular devices or artificial blood vessels, the capacity to migrate ECs toward injured or foreign surfaces is crucial. Endothelization and migration of HUVECs are influenced by many factors, including the physical and chemical properties of polymers, surface characteristics, and adhesion of binding proteins on specific polymeric substrates. In the present study, PMEA analogs showed similar migration behavior, although PMEA-analogous polymers have dissimilar wet abilities, surface characteristics, and binding protein adsorption abilities, as already known from our previous study. These effects did not affect the migration rate of HUVECs. In addition, migration from the bare PET to the PMEA side confirmed the mimetic behavior of native blood vessels.

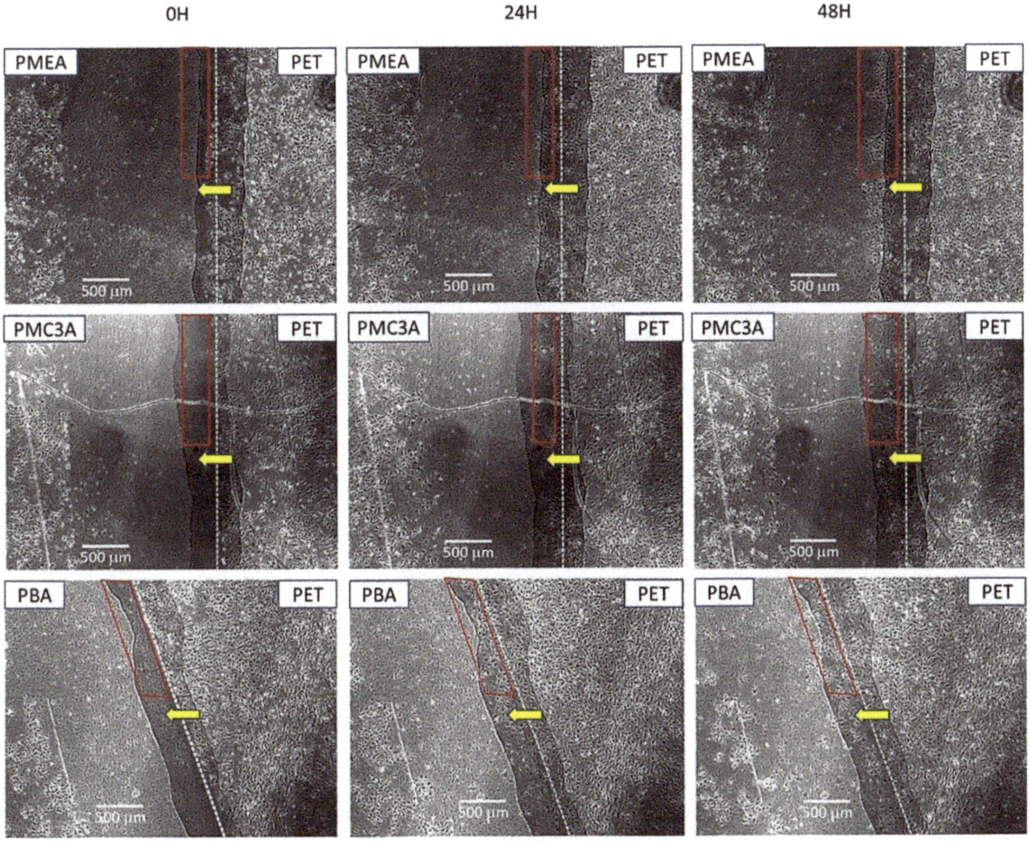

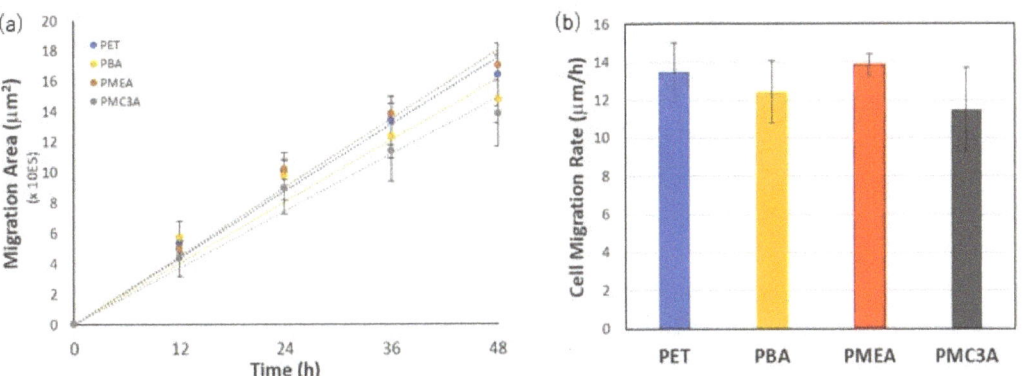

Figure 7. Observation of HUVECs migration between the substrate surfaces (scale bar = 500 μm). Time laps imaging confirmed the HUVECs migration from PET to polymers through the interface of PMEA-PET, PMC3A-PET, and PBA-PET. Migration was recorded from 0 to 48 h. The migration processes are marked with red rectangles and yellow arrows.

Figure 8. (a) Migration area (b) migration rate on PMEA-analogous polymers and bare PET. The data represent the mean ± SD (n = 5). $p < 0.05$ was used to define statistical significance.

3.5. Platelet Adhesion on HUVECs Monolayer Cultured on Polymers Film

The biocompatibility and antithrombogenic behavior of PMEA-analogous polymers have already been studied based on different factors, such as contact angle, protein adsorption, surface roughness, polymer chain length, platelet adhesion behavior, and IW content of each polymer. In the present study, we limited our investigation to only PMEA and PET because of the results of previous platelet adhesion tests under static conditions. PMEA showed an antithrombogenic surface compared with PET, where more platelets were adhered. In contrast, there is no significant study on platelet adhesion on a HUVECs monolayer that acts as an internal antithrombogenic surface of real blood vessels.

Figure 9 shows confocal images from the immunocytochemical analysis of HUVECs cultured on PMEA and PET. These CLSM images reveal that a similar type of HUVECs monolayer was formed on PET and PMEA. In addition, the shape of adhered HUVECs was comparable in both substrates. In our previous study, we found that cell adhesion depends on the integrin-mediated binding protein adhesion to the specific surface, known as integrin-dependent adhesion [45]. However, cells can adhere to PMEA through direct physicochemical contact (integrin-independent contact) and via integrin-dependent adhesion. Furthermore, the HUVEC adhesion strength on PMEA was similar to that on PET. If the PET-based artificial vascular graft needs to be replaced because of thrombus formation after implementation, PMEA seems to offer the best alternative due to its proven antithrombogenicity. We observed that the number of platelets was much higher on bare PET (Figure 10a) than bare PMEA (Figure 10e), which agrees with our previous studies [23,41,50]. In contrast, few adhered platelets were found on the HUVECs monolayer on PET (Figure 10b–d), and this was lower than in the bare PET. However, no significant number of platelets was found on the surfaces of HUVECs cultured on PMEA (Figure 10f–h). Therefore, PMEA seems to keep its antithrombogenic activity before and after HUVECs monolayer formation on PMEA. A summary of the platelet adhesion test is shown in Figure 10i. This antithrombogenic property of HUVECs monolayer on PMEA is essential to the construction of ASDBVs. Further investigations are still needed regarding blood flow conditions, including in vivo experiments, for additional confirmation of this antithrombogenic property of PMEA.

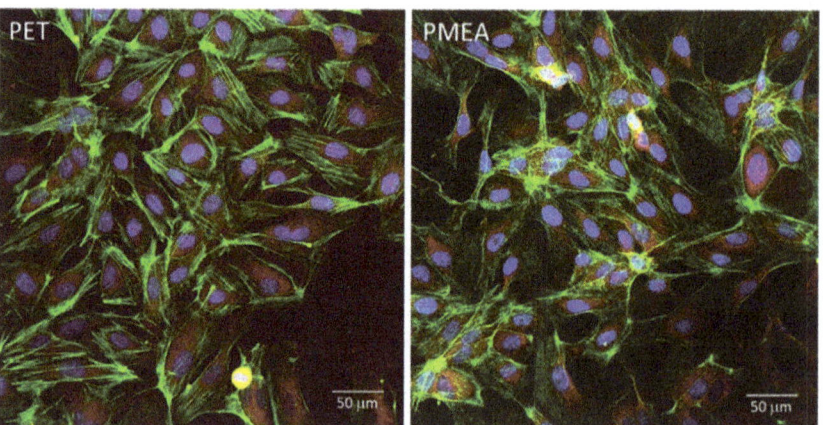

Figure 9. CLSM images of HUVECs cultured on PET and PMEA-coated surface. Blue: Cell nuclei; green: vinculin; red: actin fiber.

3.6. FM-AFM of HUVECs Surface

To investigate the antithrombogenic activity of the HUVEC monolayer on PMEA from the hydration state perspective, FM-AFM was performed. Figure 11 shows the results of the FM-AFM (z–x scan) on the HUVEC–PBS interface. The repulsive layer observed is marked in blue and white, demonstrating the degree of frequency shift. This repulsive layer may be attributed to the glycocalyx, which is composed of a hydrated sugar-rich layer. Our previous work demonstrated that such a hydrated polymer layer could contribute to the antithrombogenicity of the surfaces [51]. The repulsive layer on HUVEC was thicker than 10 nm. This is thicker than that observed on the PMEA spin-coated surface (approximately 5 nm) and thinner than that on the PMPC spin-coated surface (approximately 20 nm) on PET (see Figure S1 in Supplementary Material). Thus, the FM-AFM results corroborated the high antithrombogenic activity of the HUVEC monolayer on PMEA, as well as the platelet adhesion test results.

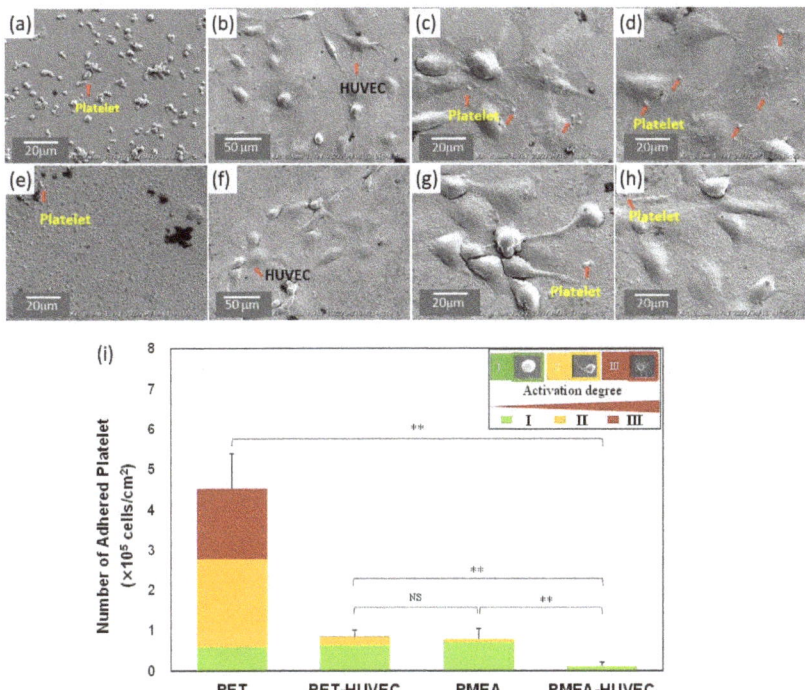

Figure 10. SEM image of (**a**) bare PET; (**b**) HUVEC monolayer on PET (scale bar = 50 μm); (**c,d**) HUVEC monolayer on PET (scale bar = 20 μm); (**e**) bare PMEA; (**f**) HUVEC monolayer on PMEA (scale bar = 50 μm); and (**g**) and (**h**) HUVEC monolayer on PMEA (scale bar = 20 μm). Red arrows indicate the typical positions of observed cells. (**i**) Number of adhered platelets counted from SEM images. The data represent the means ± SD, n = 15, ** $p < 0.05$; NS means not significant deference).

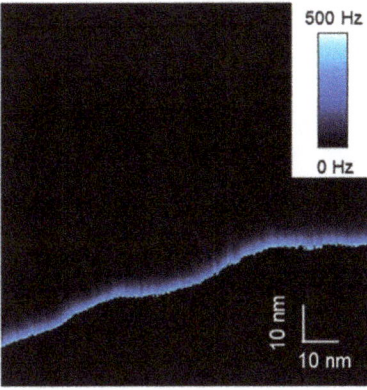

Figure 11. FM-AFM z-scan image on the HUVEC/PBS interface.

4. Conclusions

In conclusion, the comparison study of HUVEC–substrate and HUVEC–HUVEC adhesion strength revealed the mechanism of HUVECs monolayer formation on PMEA-coated substrates. HUVECs attachment, proliferation, and migration indicated the blood compatibility of PMEA as a coating material. HUVECs migration from bare PET to the PMEA-coated side is a sign of cell migration from the native blood vessel to the artificial graft. In addition, the HUVECs monolayers effectively suppressed platelet adhesion. Finally, the FM-AFM observation of the hydration layer of HUVECs may be attributed to the presence of the glycocalyx layer. A healthy glycocalyx contributes to the antithrombogenic property of the PMEA-coated surface. Based on our results, a confluent monolayer of HUVECs can prevent platelet adsorption. Therefore, the PMEA coating can mimic the native blood vessel and can be used as a construction material for the development of ASDBVs for the antithrombogenic and confluent monolayer formation of ECs.

Supplementary Materials: The following supporting information can be downloaded at: https://www.mdpi.com/article/10.3390/coatings12060869/s1. Figure S1: Images of FM-AFM z—x scan on (left) PMEA/PBS and (right) PMPC/PBS interface.

Author Contributions: Conceptualization: D.M. and M.T.; methodology: M.A.H., D.M., T.A. and M.T.; formal analysis: M.A.H.; investigation: M.A.H. and D.M.; data curation: M.A.H.; writing—original draft preparation: M.A.H.; writing—review and editing: D.M., T.A. and M.T.; supervision: D.M., T.A. and M.T.; project administration: M.T.; funding acquisition: M.T. All authors have read and agreed to the published version of the manuscript.

Funding: This study was funded by the Japan Society for the Promotion of Science (JSPS) (19H05720) from the Ministry of Education, Culture, Sports, Science and Technology of Japan.

Institutional Review Board Statement: Not applicable.

Informed Consent Statement: Not applicable.

Data Availability Statement: The authors confirm that the data supporting the findings of this study are available within the article.

Acknowledgments: We thank the Government of Japan (MEXT) for providing a scholarship for conducting this study and research at Kyushu University.

Conflicts of Interest: The authors declare no conflict of interest.

References

1. WHO. Cardiovasculaer Diseases (CVDs)—World Health Organization. 2017. Available online: www.who.int/News-Room/Fact-Sheets/Detail/Cardiovascular-Diseases-(Cvds) (accessed on 1 May 2022).
2. Smith, S.C.; Collins, A.; Ferrari, R.; Holmes, D.R.; Logstrup, S.; McGhie, D.V.; Ralston, J.; Sacco, R.L.; Stam, H.; Taubert, K.; et al. Our time: A call to save preventable death from cardiovascular disease (heart disease and stroke). *Glob. Heart* **2012**, *7*, 297–305. [CrossRef] [PubMed]
3. Mallis, P.; Kostakis, A.; Stavropoulos-Giokas, C.; Michalopoulos, E. Future perspectives in small-diameter vascular graft engineering. *Bioengineering* **2020**, *7*, 160. [CrossRef] [PubMed]
4. Xue, L.; Greisler, H.P. Biomaterials in the development and future of vascular grafts. *J. Vasc. Surg.* **2003**, *37*, 472–480. [CrossRef]
5. Eckmann, D.M.; Tsai, I.Y.; Tomczyk, N.; Weisel, J.W.; Composto, R.J. Hyaluronan and dextran modified tubes resist cellular activation with blood contact. *Colloids Surf. B Biointerfaces* **2013**, *108*, 44–51. [CrossRef]
6. PThalla, K.; Fadlallah, H.; Liberelle, B.; Lequoy, P.; de Crescenzo, G.; Merhi, Y.; Lerouge, S. Chondroitin sulfate coatings display low platelet but high endothelial cell adhesive properties favorable for vascular implants. *Biomacromolecules* **2014**, *15*, 2512–2520. [CrossRef] [PubMed]
7. Gao, A.; Hang, R.; Li, W.; Zhang, W.; Li, P.; Wang, G.; Bai, L.; Yu, X.F.; Wang, H.; Tong, L.; et al. Linker-free covalent immobilization of heparin, SDF-1α, and CD47 on PTFE surface for antithrombogenicity, endothelialization and anti-inflammation. *Biomaterials* **2017**, *140*, 201–211. [CrossRef] [PubMed]
8. Weidenbacher, L.; Müller, E.; Guex, A.G.; Zündel, M.; Schweizer, P.; Marina, V.; Adlhart, C.; Vejsadová, L.; Pauer, R.; Spiecker, E.; et al. In Vitro Endothelialization of Surface-Integrated Nanofiber Networks for Stretchable Blood Interfaces. *ACS Appl. Mater. Interfaces* **2019**, *11*, 5740–5751. [CrossRef]
9. Radke, D.; Jia, W.; Sharma, D.; Fena, K.; Wang, G.; Goldman, J.; Zhao, F. Tissue Engineering at the Blood-Contacting Surface: A Review of Challenges and Strategies in Vascular Graft Development. *Adv. Healthc. Mater.* **2018**, *7*, 1701461. [CrossRef]

10. Noy, J.-M.; Chen, F.; Akhter, D.T.; Houston, Z.H.; Fletcher, N.L.; Thurecht, K.J.; Stenzel, M.H. Direct Comparison of Poly(ethylene glycol) and Phosphorylcholine Drug-Loaded Nanoparticles In Vitro and In Vivo. *Biomacromolecules* **2020**, *21*, 2320–2333. [CrossRef]
11. Furuzono, T.; Ishihara, K.; Nakabayashi, N.; Tamada, Y. Chemical modifcation of silk fibroin with 2-methacryloyloxyethyl phosphorylcholine. II. Graft-polymerization onto fabric through 2-methacryloyloxyethyl isocyanate and interaction between fabric and platelets. *Biomaterials* **2000**, *21*, 327–333. [CrossRef]
12. Park, H.H.; Sun, K.; Seong, M.; Kang, M.; Park, S.; Hong, S.; Jung, H.; Jang, J.; Kim, J.; Jeong, H.E. Lipid-Hydrogel-Nanostructure Hybrids as Robust Biofilm-Resistant Polymeric Materials. *ACS Macro Lett.* **2019**, *8*, 64–69. [CrossRef] [PubMed]
13. Hoffmann, J.; Groll, J.; Heuts, J.; Rong, H.; Klee, D.; Ziemer, G.; Moeller, M.; Wendel, H.P. Blood cell and plasma protein repellent properties of Star-PEG-modified surfaces. *J. Biomater. Sci. Polym. Ed.* **2006**, *17*, 985–996. [CrossRef] [PubMed]
14. Zhang, M.; Desai, T.; Ferrari, M. Proteins and cells on PEG immobilized silicon surfaces. *Biomaterials* **1998**, *19*, 953–960. [CrossRef]
15. Ratner Buddy, D.J. Blood compatibility—A perspective. *J. Biomater. Sci. Polym. Ed.* **2000**, *11*, 1107–1119. [CrossRef]
16. Kidane, A.; Lantz, G.C.; Jo, S.; Park, K. Surface modification with PEO-containing triblock copolymer for improved biocompatibility: In vitro and ex vivo studies. *J. Biomater. Sci. Polym. Ed.* **1999**, *10*, 1089–1105. [CrossRef]
17. Stetsyshyn, Y.; Raczkowska, J.; Harhay, K.; Gajos, K.; Melnyk, Y.; Dąbczyński, P.; Shevtsova, T.; Budkowski, A. Temperature-responsive and multi-responsive grafted polymer brushes with transitions based on critical solution temperature: Synthesis, properties, and applications. *Colloid Polym. Sci.* **2021**, *299*, 363–383. [CrossRef]
18. Liu, Q.; Urban, M.W. Stimulus-Responsive Macromolecules in Polymeric Coatings. *Polym. Rev.* 2022, in press. [CrossRef]
19. Bordenave, L.; Fernandez, P.; Rémy-Zolghadri, M.; Villars, S.; Daculsi, R.; Midy, D. In vitro endothelialized ePTFE prostheses: Clinical update 20 years after the first realization. *Clin. Hemorheol. Microcirc.* **2005**, *33*, 227–234.
20. Deutsch, M.; Meinhart, J.; Fischlein, T.; Preiss, P.; Zilla, P. Clinical autologous in vitro endothelialization of infrainguinal ePTFE grafts in 100 patients: A 9-year experience. *Surgery* **1999**, *126*, 847–855. [CrossRef]
21. Feugier, P.; Black, R.A.; Hunt, J.A.; How, T.V. Attachment, morphology and adherence of human endothelial cells to vascular prosthesis materials under the action of shear stress. *Biomaterials* **2005**, *26*, 1457–1466. [CrossRef]
22. Tanaka, M.; Motomura, T.; Kawada, M.; Anzai, T.; Kasori, Y.; Shiroya, T.; Shimura, K.; Onishi, M.; Mochizuki, A. Blood compatible aspects of poly(2-methoxyethylacrylate) (PMEA)-relationship between protein adsorption and platelet adhesion on PMEA surface. *Biomaterials* **2000**, *21*, 1471–1481. [CrossRef]
23. Tanaka, M.; Mochizuki, A.; Ishii, N.; Motomura, T.; Hatakeyama, T. Study of blood compatibility with poly(2-methoxyethyl acrylate). Relationship between water structure and platelet compatibility in poly(2-methoxyethylacrylate-co-2-hydroxyethylmethacrylate). *Biomacromolecules* **2002**, *3*, 36–41. [CrossRef] [PubMed]
24. Hatakeyama, T.; Tanaka, M.; Hatakeyama, H. Thermal properties of freezing bound water restrained by polysaccharides. *J. Biomater. Sci. Polym. Ed.* **2010**, *21*, 1865–1875. [CrossRef] [PubMed]
25. Murakami, D.; Kobayashi, S.; Tanaka, M. Interfacial Structures and Fibrinogen Adsorption at Blood-Compatible Polymer/Water Interfaces. *ACS Biomater. Sci. Eng.* **2016**, *2*, 2122–2126. [CrossRef]
26. Kobayashi, S.; Wakui, M.; Iwata, Y.; Tanaka, M. Poly(ω-methoxyalkyl acrylate)s: Nonthrombogenic Polymer Family with Tunable Protein Adsorption. *Biomacromolecules* **2017**, *18*, 4214–4223. [CrossRef]
27. Hatakeyama, T.; Tanaka, M.; Hatakeyama, H. Studies on bound water restrained by poly(2-methacryloyloxyethyl phosphorylcholine): Comparison with polysaccharide-water systems. *Acta Biomater.* **2010**, *6*, 2077–2082. [CrossRef]
28. McGuigan, A.P.; Sefton, M.V. The influence of biomaterials on endothelial cell thrombogenicity. *Biomaterials* **2007**, *28*, 2547–2571. [CrossRef]
29. Kitakami, E.; Aoki, M.; Sato, C.; Ishihata, H.; Tanaka, M. Adhesion and proliferation of human periodontal ligament cells on poly(2-methoxyethyl acrylate). *BioMed Res. Int.* **2014**, *2014*, 102648. [CrossRef]
30. Fearon, I.M.; Gaça, M.D.; Nordskog, B.K. In vitro models for assessing the potential cardiovascular disease risk associated with cigarette smoking. *Toxicol In Vitro* **2013**, *27*, 513–522. [CrossRef]
31. Medina-Leyte, D.J.; Domínguez-Pérez, M.; Mercado, I.; Villarreal-Molina, M.T.; Jacobo-Albavera, L. Use of human umbilical vein endothelial cells (HUVEC) as a model to study cardiovascular disease: A review. *Appl. Sci.* **2020**, *10*, 938. [CrossRef]
32. Carmeliet, P.; Jain, R.K. Molecular mechanisms and clinical applications of angiogenesis. *Nature* **2011**, *473*, 298–307. [CrossRef] [PubMed]
33. Zhao, Z.; Sun, W.; Guo, Z.; Zhang, J.; Yu, H.; Liu, B. Mechanisms of lncRNA/microRNA interactions in angiogenesis. *Life Sci.* **2020**, *254*, 116900. [CrossRef] [PubMed]
34. Chen, Y.M.; Tanaka, M.; Gong, J.P.; Yasuda, K.; Yamamoto, S.; Shimomura, M.; Osada, Y. Platelet adhesion to human umbilical vein endothelial cells cultured on anionic hydrogel scaffolds. *Biomaterials* **2007**, *28*, 1752–1760. [CrossRef] [PubMed]
35. Mahmoud, M.; Cancel, L.; Tarbell, J.M. Matrix Stiffness Affects Glycocalyx Expression in Cultured Endothelial Cells. *Front. Cell Dev. Biol.* **2021**, *9*, 731666. [CrossRef] [PubMed]
36. Hoshiba, T.; Orui, T.; Endo, C.; Sato, K.; Yoshihiro, A.; Minagawa, Y.; Tanaka, M. Adhesion-based simple capture and recovery of circulating tumor cells using a blood-compatible and thermo-responsive polymer-coated substrate. *RSC Adv.* **2016**, *6*, 89103–89112. [CrossRef]
37. Nishida, K.; Anada, T.; Kobayashi, S.; Ueda, T.; Tanaka, M. Effect of bound water content on cell adhesion strength to water-insoluble polymers. *Acta Biomater.* **2021**, *134*, 313–324. [CrossRef]

38. Friedrichs, J.; Legate, K.R.; Schubert, R.; Bharadwaj, M.; Werner, C.; Müller, D.J.; Benoit, M. A practical guide to quantify cell adhesion using single-cell force spectroscopy. *Methods* **2013**, *60*, 169–178. [CrossRef]
39. Tanaka, M.; Motomura, T.; Kawada, M.; Anzai, T.; Kasori, Y.; Shimura, K.; Onishi, M.; Mochizuki, A.; Okahata, Y. A New Blood-Compatible Surface Prepared by Poly (2-methoxyethylacrylate) (PMEA) Coating-Protein Adsorption on PMEA Surface. *Jpn. J. Artif. Organs* **2000**, *29*, 209–216. [CrossRef]
40. Krüger-Genge, A.; Hauser, S.; Neffe, A.T.; Liu, Y.; Lendlein, A.; Pietzsch, J.; Jung, F. Response of Endothelial Cells to Gelatin-Based Hydrogels. *ACS Biomater. Sci. Eng.* **2021**, *7*, 527–540. [CrossRef]
41. Sato, C.; Aoki, M.; Tanaka, M. Blood-compatible poly(2-methoxyethyl acrylate) for the adhesion and proliferation of endothelial and smooth muscle cells. *Colloids Surf. B Biointerfaces* **2016**, *145*, 586–596. [CrossRef]
42. Kono, K.; Hiruma, H.; Kobayashi, S.; Sato, Y.; Tanaka, M.; Sawada, R.; Niimi, S. In vitro endothelialization test of biomaterials using immortalized endothelial cells. *PLoS ONE* **2016**, *11*, e0158289. [CrossRef] [PubMed]
43. Hozumi, K.; Otagiri, D.; Yamada, Y.; Sasaki, A.; Fujimori, C.; Wakai, Y.; Uchida, T.; Katagiri, F.; Kikkawa, Y.; Nomizu, M. Cell surface receptor-specific scaffold requirements for adhesion to laminin-derived peptide-chitosan membranes. *Biomaterials* **2010**, *31*, 3237–3243. [CrossRef] [PubMed]
44. Hersel, U.; Dahmen, C.; Kessler, H. RGD modified polymers: Biomaterials for stimulated cell adhesion and beyond. *Biomaterials* **2003**, *24*, 4385–4415. [CrossRef]
45. Hoshiba, T.; Yoshihiro, A.; Tanaka, M. Evaluation of initial cell adhesion on poly (2-methoxyethyl acrylate) (PMEA) analogous polymers. *J. Biomater. Sci. Polym. Ed.* **2017**, *28*, 986–999. [CrossRef] [PubMed]
46. Sancho, A.; Vandersmissen, I.; Craps, S.; Luttun, A.; Groll, J. A new strategy to measure intercellular adhesion forces in mature cell-cell contacts. *Sci. Rep.* **2017**, *7*, 46152. [CrossRef] [PubMed]
47. Zeng, Y.; Zhang, X.F.; Fu, B.M.; Tarbell, J.M. The role of endothelial surface glycocalyx in mechanosensing and transduction. In *Advances in Experimental Medicine and Biology*; Springer: New York, NY, USA, 2018; pp. 1–27. [CrossRef]
48. Félétou, M. The Endothelium, Part I: Multiple Functions of the Endothelial Cells—Focus on Endothelium-Derived Vasoactive Mediators. In *Colloquium Series on Integrated Systems Physiology: From Molecule to Function*; Morgan & Claypool Life Sciences: San Rafael, CA, USA, 2011; Volume 3, pp. 1–306. [CrossRef]
49. Gori, T.; von Henning, U.; Muxel, S.; Schaefer, S.; Fasola, F.; Vosseler, M.; Schnorbus, B.; Binder, H.; Parker, J.D.; Münzel, T. Both flow-mediated dilation and constriction are associated with changes in blood flow and shear stress: Two complementary perspectives on endothelial function. *Clin. Hemorheol. Microcirc.* **2016**, *64*, 255–266. [CrossRef]
50. Murakami, D.; Kitahara, Y.; Kobayashi, S.; Tanaka, M. Thermosensitive Polymer Biocompatibility Based on Interfacial Structure at Biointerface. *ACS Biomater. Sci. Eng.* **2018**, *4*, 1591–1597. [CrossRef]
51. Murakami, D.; Nishimura, S.; Tanaka, Y.; Tanaka, M. Observing the repulsion layers on blood-compatible polymer-grafted interfaces by frequency modulation atomic force microscopy. *Mater. Sci. Eng C* **2022**, *133*, 112596. [CrossRef]

Article

Novel Technology for Enamel Remineralization in Artificially Induced White Spot Lesions: In Vitro Study

Lavinia Luminita Voina Cosma [1], Marioara Moldovan [2], Alexandrina Muntean [1], Cristian Doru Olteanu [3], Radu Chifor [4,*] and Mindra Eugenia Badea [4]

1 Department Pedodontics, University of Medicine and Pharmacy "Iuliu Hatieganu", 400083 Cluj-Napoca, Romania
2 "Raluca Ripan" Institute for Research in Chemistry, University "Babes-Bolyai", 400294 Cluj-Napoca, Romania
3 Department Orthodontics, University of Medicine and Pharmacy "Iuliu Hatieganu", 400083 Cluj-Napoca, Romania
4 Department Prevention in Dentistry, University of Medicine and Pharmacy "Iuliu Hatieganu", 400083 Cluj-Napoca, Romania
* Correspondence: chifor.radu@umfcluj.ro; Tel.: +40-742195229

Abstract: The enamel white spot lesion is a common complication of orthodontic treatment with a high prevalence. This research aims to create an artificially induced white spot lesion, evaluate three different commercial products in terms of visual appeal, mineral reestablishment, and roughness, and determine which material can recover the initial structure. We created an artificially induced white spot lesion in extracted teeth. The materials used in the study were peptide p11-4 (CurodontTM Repair, Credentis AG), bioactive glass toothpaste (Biomin F, BioMin Technologies Limited), and local fluoridation (Tiefenfluorid, Humanchemie) in conjunction with low-level laser therapy (LLLT). To objectively assess the surface, the roughness, mineral content, and esthetic were measured. The roughness increased with a median difference of −0.233 μm in the bioactive glass group; the color parameter delta L decreased dramatically with a median difference of 5.9–6.7; and the cervical third increased the Ca-P mineral content above the starting stage. Each material contributed significantly to enamel consolidation, with peptide therapy providing the most encouraging results.

Keywords: bioactive glass; fluoride; laser; peptide; remineralization; white spot lesion

1. Introduction

The literature defines a white spot lesion (wsl) as an initial, non-cavitated, and active caries in the tooth's enamel. This surface is recognized and macroscopically altered in a white/opaque formation with an uninterrupted external layer [1,2]. Enamel initial demineralization is the most frequent complication during orthodontic treatment [3,4]. The plaque accumulation of bacteria around the bracket is the etiology of this condition, which encourages an acidic attack on the tooth's outer shell, disintegrating the enamel minerals [4–7]. According to Chapman et al., the ratio of this disease in the upper teeth divides as follows: 34% for the lateral incisor, 31% for the canine, 28% for the first premolars, and only 17% for the central incisors [4,5]. This lesion's consistency appears on the buccal maxillary surface, the middle third of the tooth around the bracket, and the cervical third [8]. The accuracy of white spot lesions for patients undergoing fixed orthodontic treatment ranges between 2–97 percent, and it has been highlighted four weeks after the application [2,7,9]. We chose this theme because treating this pathology remains challenging due to the complexity of the enamel structure and individual customs. Numerous attempts in the literature to find a remedy have resulted in two distinct paths: remineralization or camouflage [4,7,9]. The camouflage technique employs resin infiltration, whereas the second method, which is the most debated and is currently being researched, refers to mineral structure recapturing. The remineralization approach offers a variety of options, ranging from the commonly used fluoride and casein phosphopeptide-amorphous calcium phosphate products in various forms to the newly added substances in adhesion, pastes, or solutions, such as bioactive glass, nanohydroxyapatite, peptide p11-4, and cold plasma [10–15]. The evolution of research in dental prophylaxis is ongoing to identify the best product for caries prevention and the remineralization of the white spot lesion. Fluoride is an essential agent in caries prevention because it inhibits tooth demineralization; therefore, many different types of fluoride with different concentrations, releasing systems, and enrichments with other substances have been developed.

Tiefenfluorid is a material that provides deep-penetration fluoridation by precipitating calcium fluoride in the funnels of the loosened enamel (approx. 7 m) of hard tooth tissue. It generates spontaneously in a precipitation reaction, in addition to magnesium fluoride and silica gel, after applying the solutions [16,17]. In the literature, few articles have tested this novel therapeutic approach. Laser irradiation has been used for a while in studies for caries prevention. It has been demonstrated that it produces a significant decrease in dissolution at the surface of the enamel, as well as fusion and recrystallization of hydroxyapatite crystals that are more resistant to acidic solutions [18,19]. The combination of fluoride with low-level laser therapy has been less studied. BioMin F technology, which contains fluoro calcium phosphosilicate bioactive glass, was recently introduced. Any substance that can form a hydroxyl-carbonated apatite layer within a biological system is considered a bioactive material. The bioactive glass material interacts with cells and tissues and starts a layer inside the saliva. The general similarity in the chemical constituents of enamel and bone material has increased interest in dentistry [11,20–22]. Another material recently gaining popularity is the peptide p11-4, a class of peptides that goes through a hierarchical order and a predetermined process of scaffold assembly and formation. Curodont Repair is a guided enamel regeneration product that uses the p11-4-based Curolox technology. By binding phosphate and calcium ions from saliva, this regeneration process restores the original composition of the enamel by inducing de novo hydroxyapatite crystal growth [14,23].

The advancement and development of technologies and materials are currently putting a strain on society. Testing the products is required to assess the materials and their impact and to narrow the knowledge gap. Experiments are classified into three types: in vitro, in vivo, and in silico, each playing an essential role in research. In vitro research involves studying tissues, human cells, animal cells, or bacteria outside a living organism. The investigations are well controlled, making them suitable for studies requiring a particular target; however, they can only partially replicate natural functioning; it is difficult to predict what would happen within an organism, and the results obtained may differ from time to time. In vivo studies are carried out within a living organism, including animal testing and clinical trials on human applicants. The advantage of these studies is that they can measure the effects of mixtures and are standardized. In contrast, animal experiments require significant resources, and only a few species represent a large ecosystem. An in silico experiment is conducted using computer software or a computer simulation. It is the most recent of the three research methods and has significantly contributed to biomedicine research and clinical trials. They do not require synthesis or preparation; toxicity can be determined before the materials enter production. As a disadvantage, it is critical to check the data quality because it can distort the results; they do not prove an experimental result and require validation to demonstrate predictability [24,25]. We chose to conduct the study in vitro because it gave us greater control over the environment in which we worked. We wanted to verify the biomechanical efficiency of these materials through roughness and the restoration of the composition of the dental hard tissue through X-ray, neither of which can be performed in vivo or in silico.

The novelty of this work originated from the testing of fluoride with low-level laser therapy, as well as the comparison of these three products in terms of esthetics, the remineralization effect by mineral content regain, mechanical testing by roughness, and the plaque accumulation susceptibility.

The objectives of this paper are to create an artificially induced white spot lesion, to treat this lesion with three novel technology materials, and to compare it in relation to esthetics and physical and remineralization terms and to determine which material provides the best outcome for recovering the original structure.

2. Materials and Methods

The study was conducted at the "Raluca Ripan" Institute for Research in Chemistry at the University "Babes-Bolyai" in Cluj-Napoca, Romania, and the Department of Prevention in Dentistry at the University of Medicine and Pharmacy "Iuliu Hatieganu" in Cluj-Napoca, Romania. Fifty-four randomly selected teeth (19 incisors, 6 canines, 4 premolars, and 25 molars) from periodontal disease patients were used in the study. The inclusion criteria for the tooth selections were no macroscopical cracks, hypoplasia, or caries lesions on the tooth's buccal surface. The exclusion criteria were visible cracks, fractures, or decay on the enamel. The probes were scaled and polished before being placed in a silicon cup filled with acrylic resin (Duracryl Plus Spofa Dental) until the buccal outer layer of the teeth was sectioned with a microtome machine, yielding slices of enamel ranging in thickness from 1–3 mm. The buccal outer layer of the enamel, which was kept intact after vertical sectioning, was the tested surface of the tooth and had a size of approximately 8 mm × 10 mm. We wanted to replicate the conditions found in the oral cavity using artificial saliva; the template was Na_2HPO_4 0.426 g, $NaHCO_3$ 1.68 g, $CaCl_2$ 0.147 g, H_2O 800 mL, and HCl-1 M 2.5 mL, and the pieces were kept at room temperature (25 °C) throughout the experiment. The research strategy, divided into three stages, is summarized in Scheme 1, as are the chemical compositions of the materials used and the manufacturer information. The primary step coincided with the teeth preparation. The second step met the intermediate phase, where a 37 percent (H_3PO_4) acid etching solution was prepared to assess white spot lesions, immersing the teeth for 4 min. In the last step, the teeth were divided into three groups to test different therapeutic approaches. The teeth were split into groups using the random.org website. The first option was to combine local fluoridation (Tiefenfluorid Humanchemie) with low-level laser therapy (group F+LLLT). The teeth were dried with a cotton roll before applying Tiefenfluorid Tochierlosung with an applicator. After the solution was assimilated, Tiefenfluorid Nachtouchierlosung was used and irradiated with the laser Sirolaser Blue Sirona at a distance of 4 mm, with a wavelength of 660 nm, a power of 100 mW, and a time of irradiation of 60 s. Biomin F, a toothpaste enriched with a bioactive glass (BAG), was the second treatment option (group BAG). A cotton roll was used to dry the teeth, and a 1 cm toothpaste was applied twice daily for 2 min until the fourth day. Peptide p11-4 (CurodontTM Repair) was used in the final alternative therapy (group p11-4). The teeth were dried with cotton rolls, disinfected with sodium hypochlorite 2% (Chloraxid 2% Cerkamed) for 20 s, etched with acid orthophosphoric 35% for 20 s, washed, and dried. Finally, Curodont repair was utilized and allowed to diffuse for 5 min.

The surface measurements were made in all stages (initial—before creating wsl, intermediate—after completing the wsl, and final—after the treatment application), evaluating the teeth's surface roughness, color, and enamel mineral stability. The roughness was measured optically on the Alicona Infinite Focus microscope (Alicona Imaging GmbH, Graz, Austria), which provides 3D surface quantification by integrating the absolute value of roughness (Ra). This machine precisely measures tools for tolerances in the µm and sub-µm ranges. The surface was scanned over a 4 mm² area in the middle third of the tooth. A 2 mm line was drawn in the area with no scanning gaps, and a cut-off (λ c) of 250,000 µm was used to process the measurement in accordance with DIN EN ISO 4288. A high Ra value influences plaque accumulation, which could favor dental caries over time.

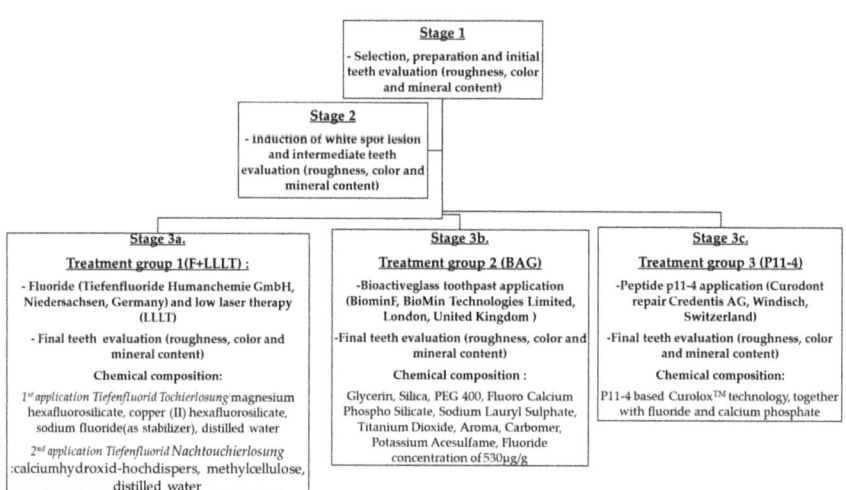

Scheme 1. The research's strategy.

The color parameter was measured using the Vita Easy Shade spectrophotometer (Vita Zahnfabrik, Bad Säckingen, Germany). This digital device was designed to identify the shade of natural teeth and ceramic restorations precisely, quickly, and reliably. The accuracy is very high, 93.75%, and the measurement's reliability is based on LED technology, which is unlikely to be affected by environmental conditions. The spectrophotometer calculates the CIELAB (Commission Internationale de L'Eclairage L*a*b) color notation system. Before each evaluation, the probe tip was calibrated on the calibration port built into the machine. The teeth were measured by holding the device tip 90 degrees to the surface in the middle third of the teeth. All samples were analyzed using measurement methods of lightness (parameter L) and color (parameters a for red/green and b for yellow/blue). The measurements were formalized using the same background, operator, and lighting conditions. The Fischerscope X-ray fluorescence analysis (Helmut Fischer GmbH, Sindelfingen, Germany) was used to determine the enamel's mineral content. The software converts the data from the measured X-ray spectra into parameters for layer thickness measurement and material analysis. The technique is based on the fact that when atoms are excited by primary X-rays, they discharge power in the form of element-specific fluorescence radiation. The spectrum of the energy radiated reveals information about the sample's composition. The detector has a high energy resolution and, therefore, can provide precise, measured data in a short amount of time. For each treatment group, we examined the report between the elements Ca (Calcium) and P (Phosphorus) and Ca/F (Fluoride) in four regions: the middle third of the incisal, cervical, mesial, and distal zone. The results are interpreted by analyzing whether the initial report is re-established. All the data from the study were analyzed using IBM SPSS Statistics 25 and illustrated using Microsoft Office Excel/Word 2013. Quantitative variables were tested for normal distribution using the Shapiro–Wilk test and were written as averages with standard deviations or medians with interquartile ranges. Quantitative independent variables with non-parametric distribution were tested using the Mann–Whitney U/Kruskal–Wallis H tests. Quantitative independent variables with normal distribution were tested using the Student/One-Way ANOVA/Welch ANOVA tests. Post-hoc analysis was made using the Tukey HSD/Games–Howell/Dunn–Bonferroni tests. Quantitative variables with repeated measures and non-parametric distribution were tested using related samples Wilcoxon signed-rank tests. Quantitative variables with repeated measures and normal distribution were tested using paired-samples t-tests. In each treatment group, the comparison was made according to the distribution of the measured intervals.

3. Results

3.1. Surface Roughness Measurement Ra Parameter in Each Treatment Group

The evolution of the Ra parameter in each treatment group is shown in Figure 1. According to the Wilcoxon tests, the Ra parameter did not change significantly in evolution in the F+LLLT and p11-4 peptide groups (median difference of −0.038 and 0.031 μm), and the observed difference in Ra was not statistically significant. The Ra parameter in the BAG group increased significantly in evolution ($p = 0.039$), with a significant difference (median = −0.233 μm, IQR = −0.473–0.140 μm).

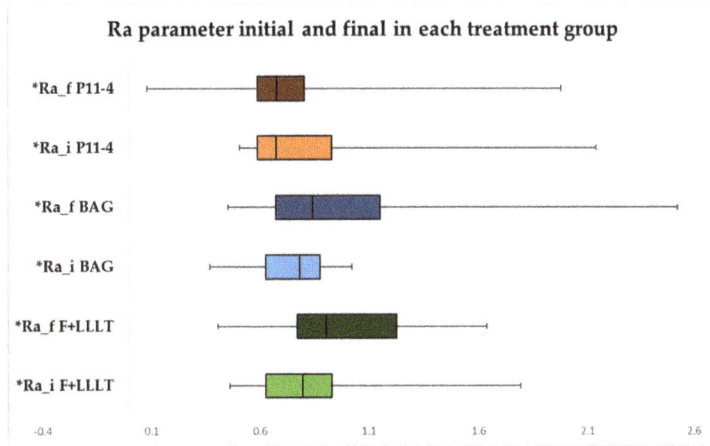

Figure 1. Boxplot representation of Ra parameter initial and final in each treatment group. * Ra_i—parameter Ra initial; Ra_f—parameter Ra final.

3.2. Color Measurement of "L" Parameter in Each Treatment Group

The progression of the L parameter is represented in Figure 2, and according to the paired-samples t-tests/Wilcoxon tests, the F+LLLT and BAG groups reduced dramatically in advancement, with a significant difference in comparison to the p11-4 peptide group, where there was no change in evolution and statistical significance.

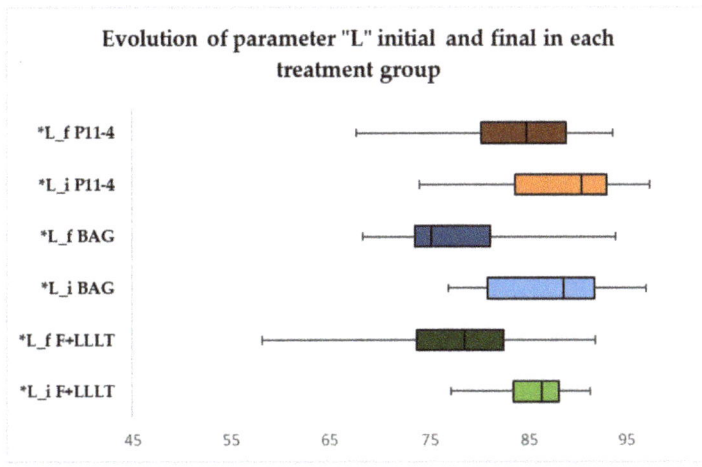

Figure 2. Boxplot representation of the evolution of "L" parameter initial and final in each treatment group. * L_i—color parameter "L" initial; L_f—color parameter "L" final.

3.3. Colour Measurement of "a" Parameter in Each Treatment Group

The evolution of the a parameter is shown in Figure 3; it rose exponentially in progression ($p < 0.001$) in all three treatments, with a significant difference.

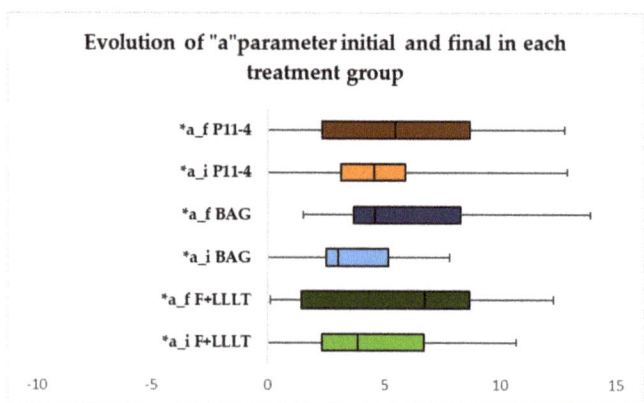

Figure 3. Boxplot representation of the evolution of "a" parameter initial and final in each treatment group. * a_i—color parameter "a" initial; a_f—color parameter "a" final.

3.4. Colour Measurement of "b" Parameter in Each Treatment Group

The boxplot from Figure 4 exposes the evolution of the b parameter in each treatment group. The paired-samples t-tests show that the parameter changed radically in all treatment groups, with a significant difference.

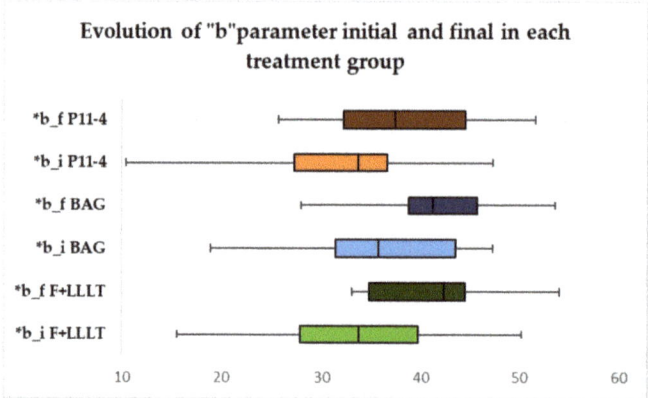

Figure 4. Boxplot representation of the evolution of "b" parameter initial and final in each treatment group. * b_i—color parameter "b" initial; b_f—color parameter "b" final.

3.5. Evolution of the Incisal Third Ca/P and Ca/F Ratio in Each Treatment Group

The data from Figure 5 show the evolution of the incisal third Ca/P ratio in each treatment group. With regard to the Wilcoxon tests, the results show that in all the groups the Ca/P ratio did not change significantly in evolution. The observed difference was not statistically significant. The incisal third Ca/F ratio variation is represented in Figure 6, and according to the Wilcoxon tests, the treatment groups were not altered in progression. The observed difference was not statistically significant.

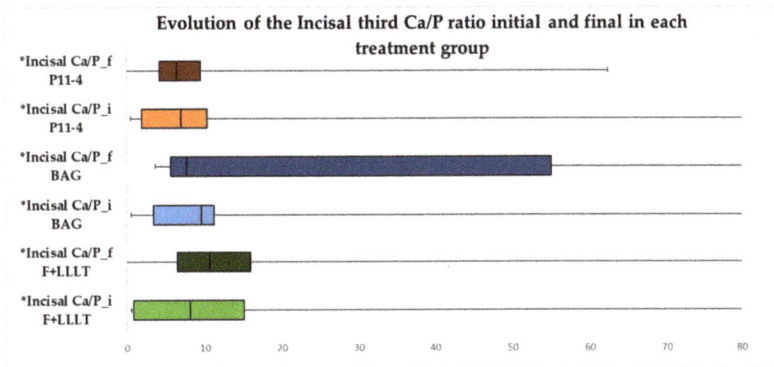

Figure 5. Boxplot representation of the evolution of the incisal third Ca/P ratio initial and final in each treatment group. * Incisal Ca/P_i—incisal third Ca/P ratio initial; incisal Ca/P_f—incisal third Ca/P ratio final.

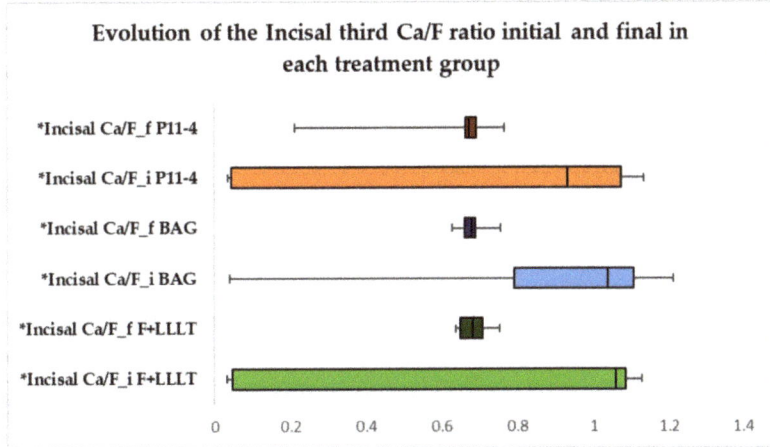

Figure 6. Boxplot representation of the evolution of the incisal third Ca/F ratio initial and final in each treatment group. * Incisal Ca/F_i—incisal third Ca/F ratio initial; incisal Ca/F_f—incisal third Ca/F ratio final.

3.6. Evolution of Cervical Ca/P and Ca/F Ratio in Each Treatment Group

Figure 7 records show the effects of the cervical Ca/P proportion in each treatment. According to the Wilcoxon tests, the Ca/P ratio in the p11-4 peptide group increased significantly in evolution ($p = 0.022$), with a significant difference (median = -2.912, IQR = -4.157–1.250) in reference to the other groups where the ratio did not change significantly in evolution, and the observed difference was not statistically significant. The development of the cervical Ca/F ratio for each treated group can be seen in Figure 8. According to the Wilcoxon tests in all the groups, the Ca/F balance did not significantly change in evolution and the observed difference was not statistically significant.

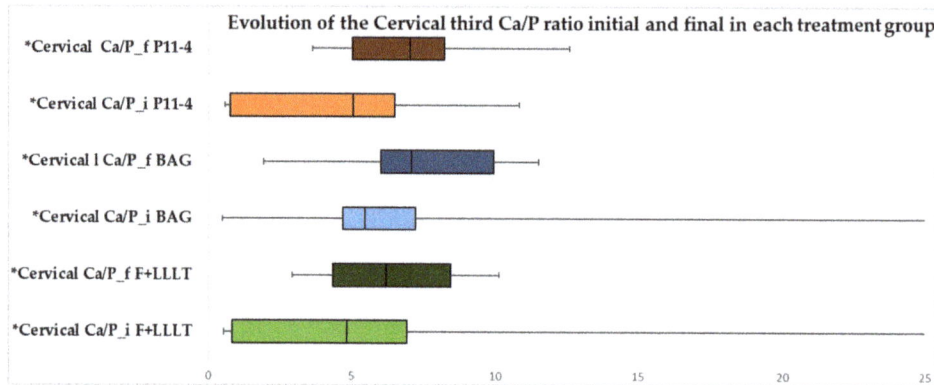

Figure 7. Boxplot representation of the evolution of Ca/P ratio in the cervical third initial and final in each treatment group. * Cervical Ca/P_i—cervical third Ca/P ratio initial; cervical Ca/P_f—cervical third Ca/P ratio final.

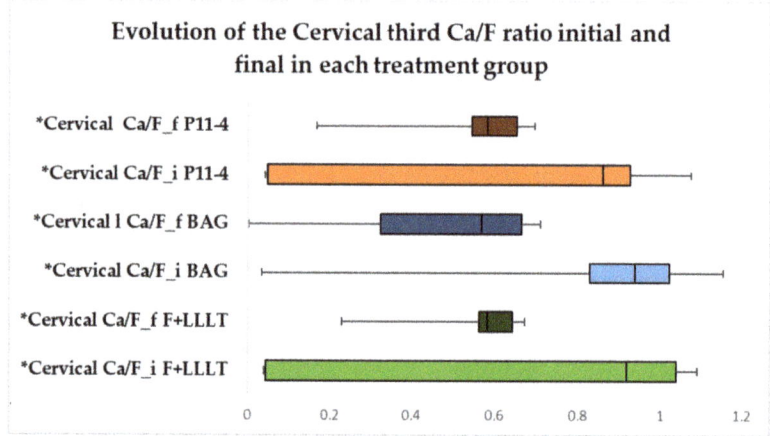

Figure 8. Boxplot representation of the evolution of Ca/F ratio in the cervical third initial and final in each treatment group. * Cervical Ca/F_i—cervical third Ca/F ratio initial; cervical Ca/F_f—cervical third Ca/F ratio final.

3.7. Evolution of Mesial Ca/P and Ca/F Ratio in Each Treatment Group

The data in Figure 9 show the variation of the mesial Ca/P balance in each treatment group. The results indicate that the Ca/P ratio did not change considerably in all the groups over time, and the identified difference is insignificant. The data from Figure 10 show the existence of the mesial Ca/F ratio in each treatment group. The findings suggest that the mesial Ca/F ratio in the BAG group dropped dramatically in evolution ($p = 0.016$), with a significant difference (median = 0.422, IQR = 0.19–0.497) compared to the other groups, where the ratio did not change significantly in advancement, and the observed difference is not statistically significant.

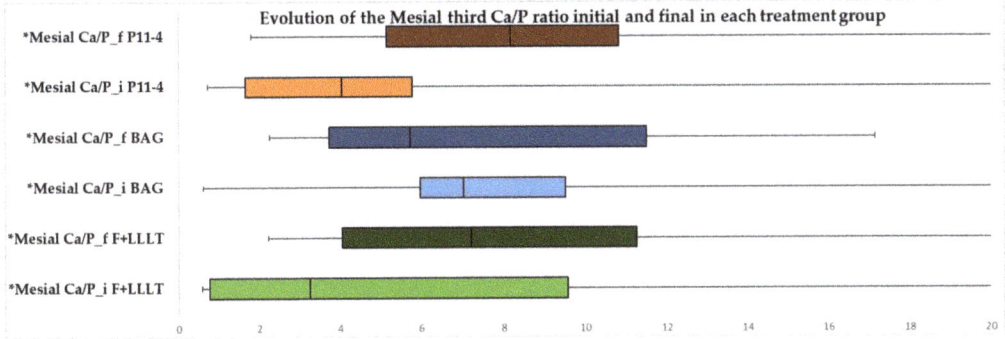

Figure 9. Boxplot representation of the evolution of Ca/P ratio in the mesial third initial and final in each treatment group. * Mesial Ca/P_i—mesial third Ca/P ratio initial; mesial Ca/P_f—mesial third Ca/P ratio final.

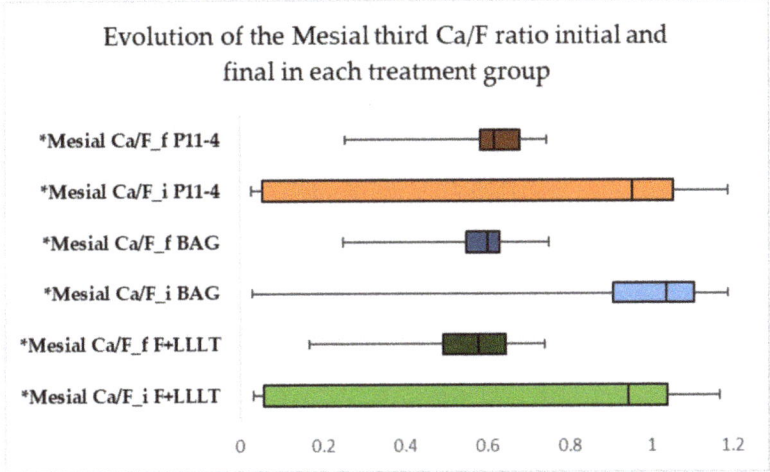

Figure 10. Boxplot representation of the evolution of Ca/F ratio in the mesial third initial and final in each treatment group. * Mesial Ca/F_i—mesial third Ca/F ratio initial; mesial Ca/F_f—mesial third Ca/F ratio final.

3.8. Evolution of Distal Ca/P and Ca/F Ratio in Each Treatment Group

The data in Figure 11 show the evolution of the distal Ca/P ratio in each treatment group. According to the Wilcoxon tests, the distal Ca/P ratio in all three treatments did not alter in evolution, and the reported difference was not statistically significant. The data from Figure 12 show the development of the distal Ca/F ratio in each treatment group; the distal Ca/F ratio in the BAG group decreased significantly in evolution ($p = 0.048$), with a significant difference (median = 0.374, IQR = 0.053–0.515). The ratio did not change significantly over time compared to the other groups, and the reported difference was not statistically considerable.

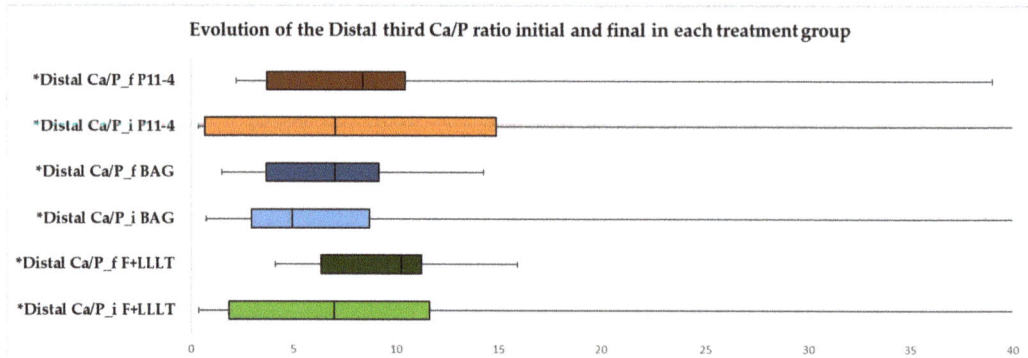

Figure 11. Boxplot representation of the evolution of Ca/P ratio in the distal third initial and final in each treatment group. * Distal Ca/P_i—distal third Ca/P ratio initial; distal Ca/P_f—distal third Ca/P ratio final.

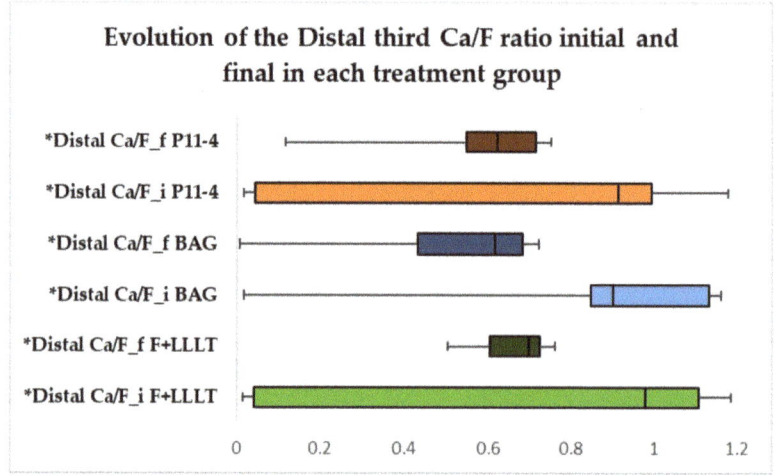

Figure 12. Boxplot representation of the evolution of Ca/F ratio in the distal third initial and final in each treatment group. * Distal Ca/F_i—distal third Ca/F ratio initial; distal Ca/F_f—distal third Ca/F ratio final.

4. Discussion

An imbalance of the demineralization and remineralization process provokes the mechanism involved in the white spot lesion. The alteration depends on the variations of the oral environment with regard to their duration and intensity. Demineralization is reversible as long as the conditions necessary for remineralization are met and the organic matrix is intact. The process's dynamic is based on the phenomenon of the dissolution of the apatite crystal and precipitation of salts in the fluid of the bacterial biofilm [26–28]. Remineralization does not reconstruct the initial enamel prism architecture, but it does form a thick layer of calcium phosphate and fluoride. This dense layer becomes more durable to further demineralization than regular enamel [29].

The study's objectives were met, and each treatment significantly contributed, more or less, to restoring the teeth's surface. The novelty of this research was the comparison of the efficacy of three different commercial products, the use of fluoride combined with low laser therapy, and the comparison of treatment achievements not only esthetically but also structurally. The microstructure of the enamel is fully accountable for its natural roughness. Enamel etching and material use may make restoring the enamel's original condition challenging. Dental materials can potentially roughen the teeth's outer layer, influencing plaque accumulation and discoloration [30]. Our findings showed no difference between the group with the fluoride and low-level laser therapy and the peptide p11-4 before and at the end of the treatment. This discovery could imply that the initial roughness of the enamel was maintained, which is consistent with the findings of Sindhura et al. and Magalhaes et al., who demonstrated the recovery of the tooth's exterior layer in just seven days after treatment [31,32]. The bioactive glass group showed increased roughness after treatment, indicating a greater preference for enhancing bacterial deposition and raising the risk of demineralization. The last statement contradicts the study of Farooq et al., in which commercial fluorided bioactive glass toothpaste reduced roughness values, with the maximum decrease obtained using a combination of theobromine and fluoride bioactive glass toothpaste [33]. Other published studies also confirmed roughness reduction after using bioactive glass [34,35].

The color of a natural tooth is defined by the projection of incident light [36]. This feature has been utilized to develop diagnostic techniques for caries lesions relying on enamel fluorescence. Color analyses on enamel decay are rarely performed, even though they appear in the initial phases as increased whiteness that raises concerns and may need restorative approaches [37,38]. A spectrophotometer was used to properly assess the modification in color parameter (L*a*b) for the conventional quantitative assessment of coloration. The reliability and validity of the measurements have contributed to its popularity [38,39]. The L parameter represents the color's lightness [40]. Many studies have shown that creating the wsl raises the whiteness of the tooth by affecting the absorbing light in that region, implying the treatments' influence on the teeth's brightness [41]. In comparison to the peptide group, our findings show that the groups F-LLLT and BAG had a significant reduction in tooth color. Clinically, this affirmation shows that the color for the last two groups darkened in contrast to the baseline color. This result was similar to the findings of Mohamed et al. but contrary to the research results of Yetkiner et al. They investigated the color stability for fluoride treatments and accomplished a color improvement near the baseline level. Iwami et al. demonstrated that the L and components are related to caries activity; therefore, a low value may indicate a high bacterial activity that leads to enamel decay. This observation may imply that the enamel remineralization in groups F-LLT and BAG was incomplete due to a lack of deep material infiltration in the created white spot lesion and the persistence of discoloration [42–44]. The red-green chromaticity increased in all groups, indicating a transition to the red component, which is consistent with the findings of Mohamed et al. The yellow-blue chromaticity also rose in all groups except the peptide group, resulting in a much more yellow component, which contradicts the outcomes of Mohamed et al.; Polo et al. explored natural tooth color prediction in Caucasians from Spain [45]. The study's conclusion revealed that teeth appear darker, yellow, and reddish with age. This is similar to our observations because we used extracted teeth from Caucasians in Romania with periodontal disease. Consequently, this remark may indicate that all treatment groups display asymmetrical coloristic improvement.

The presence of a white spot lesion induces enamel mineral loss, implying degradation of the dental tissue, which leads to a change in the structure, sensitivity, and esthetics [46]. The mineral constituent of the tooth's outer layer is substituted calcium hydroxyapatite (HAP). Numerous element substitutions can replace the concentration of ions missing from HAP, such as calcium replacing magnesium, carbonate replacing phosphate, and hydroxyl replacing fluoride [47–49]. These changes can affect HAP's actions, particularly its dissolution rate at low pH. Calcium deficiency and carbonate-rich areas are likely exposed to acid demineralization but replacing hydroxide with fluoride increases protection against demineralization [50]. When the caries threat is prevented, it is acknowledged that white spot lesion seems to regress with the appearance of remineralizing agents [51–53]. The remineralization process is not mineral precipitation onto the tooth structure but rather a crystal restoration in the lesion's subsurface [54]. We evaluated three different remineralization therapies in different regions of the buccal surface of the tooth in this study (middle incisal, cervical, mesial, and distal third). Compared to the other regions, the mineral gain of Ca and F in the BAG group decreased significantly in the mesial and distal middle thirds. These results have many possible interpretations. The mineral loss and regain may vary between thirds, the fluoride intake from the BAG group may diffuse slowly in comparison with the other buccal areas, and the use of the commercial products Tiefenfluorid and Curodont repair may have a better intake of the minerals. Calcium is the favored element for dissolution during the first four hours of demineralization [55]. When there is a calcium deficiency, there is selective absorption of calcium and a tendency to return to a Ca/P apatite, as demonstrated by the precipitation of calcium phosphates on hydroxyapatite crystals [56,57]. In our study, all the groups experienced a significant recovery in Ca/P, but only the peptide group gained a higher value after the treatment application in the cervical third. This fact is important because the cervical third of the tooth is known to be the least mineralized zone, with increased porosity and a higher risk of caries [58,59]. The Biomin F treatment was the least effective in returning the tooth to its original state; we encountered roughness, color, and mineral uptake issues. Tiefenfluorid and low-level laser therapy was the second effective remedy; the difficulties were noticed only with the esthetics of the enamel reformation. Finally, the peptide p11-4 Curodont repair commercial product delivered the best performance, improving all measurements and ensuring the recovery of the lost surface.

The limitations of these studies include the small number of teeth used, the lack of oral cavity conditions, the demineralization process being more aggressive than a typical acid attack in the oral cavity, and the need for additional analyses to confirm crystal reintegration. Another limitation of our study was the experiment type, in vitro, because it replicates only a portion of the natural functioning of an organism, in our case the oral cavity, and the results obtained may differ from those obtained in vivo or in silico.

5. Conclusions

P11-4 peptide Curodont Curolox technology had the best outcome in terms of improving white spot lesions compared to the other tested materials. However, more research is needed to confirm the research approach. We believe that developing new technologies and materials will help us understand the remineralization process of the enamel white spot lesion and that this lesion will be history in the future.

Author Contributions: Conceptualization, L.L.V.C. and M.E.B.; methodology, L.L.V.C., M.E.B., M.M. and R.C.; software, C.D.O.; validation, M.E.B., M.M., C.D.O. and A.M.; formal analysis, C.D.O. and A.M.; investigation, L.L.V.C. and R.C.; resources, C.D.O. and A.M.; data curation, A.M.; writing—original draft preparation, L.L.V.C.; writing—review and editing, R.C. and M.E.B.; visualization, M.M., C.D.O. and A.M.; supervision, M.E.B. and M.M. All authors have read and agreed to the published version of the manuscript.

Funding: This research received no external funding.

Institutional Review Board Statement: The study was conducted in accordance with the Declaration of Helsinki and approved by the Ethics Committee of the University of Medicine and Pharmacy "Iuliu Hatieganu" Cluj-Napoca, Romania (protocol code 228 and date of approval 25 July 2022).

Informed Consent Statement: Not applicable.

Data Availability Statement: Not applicable.

Acknowledgments: This research takes a part from the Ph.D. thesis entitled "Prevention and management of white spot lesion during or after orthodontic treatment", from the University of Medicine and Pharmacy "Iuliu Hatieganu" Cluj-Napoca, Romania.

Conflicts of Interest: The authors declare no conflict of interest.

References

1. Nanci, A. *Ten Cate's Oral Histology*; Elsevier: Montreal, QC, Canada, 2017; pp. 289–307.
2. Heidemann, D.; Hellwig, E.; Hickel, R.; Hugo, B.; Klaiber, B.; Klimek, J. *Kariologie und Fullungstherapie*; Urban und Schwarzenberg: Munchen, Germany, 1999; pp. 31–33.
3. Chanachai, S.; Chaichana, W.; Insee, K.; Benjakul, S.; Aupaphong, V.; Panpisut, P. Physical/Mechanical and Antibacterial Properties of Orthodontic Adhesives Containing Calcium Phosphate and Nisin. *J. Funct. Biomater.* **2021**, *12*, 73. [CrossRef]
4. Cosma, L.L.; Suhani, R.D.; Mesaros, A.; Badea, M.E. Current Treatment Modalities of Orthodontically Induced White Spot Lesions and Their Outcome. *Med. Pharm. Rep.* **2019**, *92*, 25–30. [CrossRef] [PubMed]
5. Featherstone, J. The Continuum of Dental Caries–Evidence for a Dynamic Disease Process. *J. Dent. Res.* **2004**, *83*, 39–42. [CrossRef] [PubMed]
6. Chapman, J.A.; Roberts, E.W.; Eckert, G.J.; Kula, K.S.; Gonzalez-Cabezas, C. Risk Factors for Incidence and Severity of White Spot Lesions during Treatment with Fixed Orthodontic Appliances. *Am. J. Orthod. Dentofacial. Orthop.* **2010**, *138*, 88–94. [CrossRef]
7. Khoroushi, M.; Kachuie, M. Prevention and Treatment of White Spot Lesions in Orthodontic Patients. *Contemp. Clin. Dent.* **2017**, *8*, 11–19.
8. Gorelick, L.; Geiger, A.; Gwinnett, A. Incidence of White Spot Formation after Bonding and Banding. *Am. J. Orthod.* **1982**, *81*, 93–98. [CrossRef]
9. Ritter, A.; Eidson, R.; Donovan, T. *Sturdevant's Art and Science of Operative Dentistry*; Elsevier: Saint Louis, MO, USA, 2018; pp. 40–94.
10. Karabekiroglu, S.; Unlu, N.; Kucukyilmaze, E.; Sener, S.; Botsali, M.; Malkoc, S. Treatment of Post-Orthodontic White Spot Lesions with CPP-ACP Paste: A Three Year Follow up Study. *Dent. Mater. J.* **2017**, *36*, 791–797. [CrossRef] [PubMed]
11. Abbassy, M.; Bakry, A.; Almoabady, E.; Almusally, S.; Hassan, A. Characterization of a Novel Enamel Sealer for Bioactive Remineralization of White Spot Lesions. *J. Dent.* **2021**, *109*, 103663. [CrossRef] [PubMed]
12. Brown, M.; Davis, H.; Tufekci, E.; Crowe, J.; Covell, D.; Mitchell, J. Ion Release from a Novel Orthodontic Resin Bonding Agent for the Reduction and/or Prevention of White Spot Lesions. *Angle Orthod.* **2011**, *81*, 1014–1020. [CrossRef] [PubMed]
13. Krishnan, V.; Bhatia, A.; Varma, H. Development, Characterization and Comparison of Two Strontium Doped Nano Hydroxyapatite Molecules for Enamel Repair/Regeneration. *Dent. Mater. J.* **2016**, *32*, 646–659. [CrossRef]
14. Jablonski-Momeni, A.; Heinzel-Gutenbrunner, M. Efficacy of the Self-Assembling Peptide P11-4 in Constructing a Remineralization Scaffold on Artificially-Induced Enamel Lesions on Smooth Surfaces. *J. Orofac. Orthop.* **2014**, *75*, 175–190. [CrossRef] [PubMed]
15. El-Wassefy, N. Remineralizing Effect of Cold Plasma and/or Bioglass on Demineralized Enamel. *Dent. Mater. J.* **2017**, *36*, 157–167. [CrossRef] [PubMed]
16. Coordes, S.; Brinkmann, P.; Prager, T.; Bartzela, T.; Visel, D.; Jacker, T.; Hartwich, R. A Comparison of Different Sealants Preventing Demineralization around Brackets. *J. Orofac. Orthop.* **2018**, *79*, 49–56. [CrossRef] [PubMed]
17. Meto, A.; Meto, A.; Tragaj, E.; Lipo, M.; Bauermann, C. The Use of Tiefenfluorid for Desensitization of Dentinal Hyperesthesia*. *Balk. J. Dent. Med.* **2014**, *18*, 85–88. [CrossRef]
18. Ahrari, F.; Poosti, M.; Motahari, P. Enamel Resistance to Demineralization Following Er:YAG Laser Etching for Bonding Orthodontic Brackets. *Dent. Res. J.* **2012**, *9*, 472–477.
19. Bishara, S.; Abadi, E. The Effect on the Bonding Strength of Orthodontic Brackets of Fluoride Application after Etching. *Am. J. Orthod. Dentofacial. Orthop.* **1989**, *95*, 259–260. [CrossRef]
20. Ferraris, S.; Yamaguchi, S.; Barbani, N.; Cazzola, M.; Cristallini, C.; Miola, M.; Verne, E.; Spriano, S. Bioactive Materials: In Vitro Investigation of Different Mechanisms of Hydroxyapatite Precipitation. *Acta Biomater.* **2020**, *102*, 468–480. [CrossRef]
21. Earl, J.; Leary, R.; Muller, K.; Langford, R.; Greenspan, D. Physical and Chemical Characterization of Dentin Surface Following Treatment with NovaMin Technology. *J. Clin. Dent.* **2011**, *22*, 62–67.
22. Dai, L.; Mei, M.; Chu, C.; Lo, E. Mechanisms of Bioactive Glass on Caries Management: A Review. *Materials* **2019**, *12*, 4183. [CrossRef]
23. Maude, S.; Tai, L.; Davies, R. Peptide Synthesis Andself-Assembly. *Top. Curr. Chem.* **2011**, *310*, 27–69.
24. Benfenati, E.; Gini, G.; Luttik, R.; Hoffmann, S. Comparing In Vivo, In Vitro and In Silico Methods and Integrated Strategies for Chemical Assessment: Problems and Prospects. *Altern. Lab. Anim.* **2010**, *38*, 153–166. [CrossRef] [PubMed]
25. Jamari, I.; Ammarullah, M.; Santoso, G.; Sugiharto, S.; Supriyono, T.; van der Heide, E. In Silico Contact Pressure of Metal-on-Metal Total Hip Implant with Different Materials Subjected to Gait Loading. *Metals* **2022**, *12*, 1241. [CrossRef]
26. Staley, R. Effect of Fluoride Varnish on Demineralization Around Orthodontic Brackets. *Semin. Orthod.* **2008**, *14*, 194–199. [CrossRef]
27. Greene, L.; Bearn, D. Reducing White Spot Lesion Incidence during Fixed Appliance Therapy. *Dent. Update* **2013**, *40*, 487–490. [CrossRef]
28. Iovan, G. *Caria Dentară: Repere Etiologice Și Patogenice*; GR. T. Popa: Iasi, Romania, 2011; pp. 176–182.
29. Featherstone, J. Dental Caries: A Dynamic Disease Process. *Aust. Dent. J.* **2008**, *53*, 286–291. [CrossRef]
30. Caixeta, R.; Berger, S.; Lopes, M.; Paloco, E.; Faria, E.; Contreras, E. Evaluation of Enamel Roughness after the Removal of Brackets Bonded with Different Materials: In Vivo Study. *Braz. Dent. J.* **2021**, *32*, 34–40. [CrossRef]

31. Sindhura, V.; Uloopi, K.; Vinay, C.; Chandrasekhar, R. Evaluation of Enamel Remineralizing Potential of Self-Assembling Peptide P11-4 on Artificially Induced Enamel Lesions in Vitro. *J. Indian Soc. Pedod. Prev. Dent.* **2018**, *36*, 352–356. [CrossRef]
32. Magalhaes, G.; Fraga, M.; Araujo, I.; Pachero, R.; Correr, A.; Puppin-Rontani, R. Effect of a Self-Assembly Peptide on Surface Roughness and Hardness of Bleached Enamel. *J. Funct. Biomater.* **2022**, *13*, 79. [CrossRef]
33. Farooq, I.; Khan, A.; Moheet, I.; Alshwaimi, E. Preparation of a Toothpaste Containing Theobromine and Fluoridated Bioactive Glass and Its Effect on Surface Micro-Hardness and Roughness of Enamel. *Dent. Mater. J.* **2021**, *40*, 393–398. [CrossRef]
34. Pribadi, N.; Citra, A.; Rukmo, M. The Difference in Enamel Surface Hardness after Immersion Process with Cocoa Rind Extract (*Theobroma cacao*) and Fluoride. *J. Int. Oral Health* **2019**, *11*, 100–103. [CrossRef]
35. Taha, A.; Fleming, P.; Hill, R.; Patel, M. Enamel Remineralization with Novel Bioactive Glass Air Abrasion. *J. Int. Oral Health* **2018**, *97*, 1438–1444. [CrossRef] [PubMed]
36. Tranaeus, S.; Al-Khateeb, S.; Bjorkman, S.; Twetman, S.; Angmar-Mansson, B. Application of Quantitative Light-Induced Fluorescence to Monitor Incipient Lesions in Caries-Active Children. A Comparative Study of Remineralisation by Fluoride Varnish and Professional Cleaning. *Eur. J. Oral Sci* **2001**, *109*, 71–75. [CrossRef] [PubMed]
37. Joiner, A.; Hopkinson, I.; Deng, Y.; Westland, S. A Review of Tooth Colour and Whiteness. *J. Dent.* **2008**, *36*, 2–7. [CrossRef] [PubMed]
38. Kim, Y.; Son, H.; Yi, K.; Kim, H.; Ahn, J.; Chang, J. The Color Change in Artificial White Spot Lesions Measured Using a Spectroradiometer. *Clin. Oral Investig.* **2013**, *17*, 139–146. [CrossRef]
39. Torres, C.; Borges, A.; Torres, L.; Gomes, I.; de Oliveira, R.S. Effect of Caries Infiltration Technique and Fluoride Therapy on the Colour Masking of White Spot Lesions. *J. Dent.* **2011**, *39*, 202–207. [CrossRef] [PubMed]
40. Yetkiner, E.; Wegehaupt, F.; Wiegand, A.; Attin, R.; Attin, T. Colour Improvement and Stability of White Spot Lesions Following Infiltration, Micro-Abrasion, or Fluoride Treatments in Vitro. *Eur. J. Orthod.* **2014**, *36*, 595–602. [CrossRef]
41. Mohamed, A.; Wong, K.; Lee, W.; Marizan Nor, M.; Mohd Hussaini, H.; Rosli, T. In Vitro Study of White Spot Lesion: Maxilla and Mandibular Teeth. *Saudi Dent. J.* **2018**, *30*, 142–150. [CrossRef] [PubMed]
42. Iwami, Y.; Hayashi, N.; Takeshige, F.; Ebisu, S. Relationship between the Color of Carious Dentin with Varying Lesion Activity, and Bacterial Detection. *J. Dent.* **2008**, *36*, 143–151. [CrossRef]
43. Chin, M.Y.; Sandham, A.; Rumachik, E.; Ruben, J.; Huysmans, M.C. Fluoride Release and Cariostatic Potential of Orthodontic Adhesives with and without Daily Fluoride Rinsing. *Am. J. Orthod. Dentofacial. Orthop.* **2009**, *136*, 547–553. [CrossRef]
44. Paris, S.; Schwendicke, F.; Keltsch, J.; Dorfer, C.; Meyer-Lueckel, H. Masking of White Spot Lesions by Resin Infiltration In Vitro. *J. Dent.* **2013**, *41*, 28–34. [CrossRef]
45. Gomez-Polo, C.; Montero, J.; Gomez-Polo, M.; de Parga, J.; Celemin-Vinuels, A. Natural Tooth Color Estimation Based on Age and Gender. *J. Prosthodont.* **2017**, *26*, 107–114. [CrossRef] [PubMed]
46. West, N.; Joiner, A. Enamel Mineral Loss. *J. Dent.* **2014**, *42*, 2–11. [CrossRef]
47. Robinson, C.; Shore, R.; Brookes, S.; Strafford, S.; Wood, S.; Kirkham, J. The Chemistry of Enamel Caries. *Crit. Rev. Oral Biol. Med.* **2000**, *11*, 481–495. [CrossRef] [PubMed]
48. Featherstone, J. Prevention and Reversal of Dental Caries: Role of Low Level Fluoride. *Community Dent. Oral Epidemiol.* **1999**, *27*, 31–40. [CrossRef]
49. Robinson, C. Fluoride and the Caries Lesion: Interactions and Mechanism of Action. *Eur. Arch. Paediatr. Dent.* **2009**, *10*, 136–140. [CrossRef] [PubMed]
50. Featherstone, J.; Goodman, P.; Mclean, J. Electron Microscope Study of Defect Zones in Dental Enamel. *J. Ultrastruct. Res.* **1979**, *67*, 117–123. [CrossRef]
51. Beerens, M.; Van Der Veen, M.; Van Beek, H.; Ten Cate, J. Effects of Casein Phosphopeptide Amorphous Calcium Fluoride Phosphate Paste on White Spot Lesions and Dental Plaque after Orthodontic Treatment: A 3-Month Follow-Up. *Eur. J. Oral Sci.* **2010**, *118*, 610–617. [CrossRef]
52. Marinho, V.; Higgins, J.; Logan, S.; Sheiham, A. Topical Fluoride (Toothpastes, Mouthrinses, Gels or Varnishes) for Preventing Dental Caries in Children and Adolescents. *Cochrane Database Syst. Rev.* **2003**, *4*, CD002782. [CrossRef]
53. Derks, A.; Katsaros, C.; Frencken, J.; Van't Hof, M.; Kuijpers-Jagtman, A. Caries-Inhibiting Effect of Preventive Measures during Orthodontic Treatment with Fixed Appliances: A Systematic Review. *Caries Res.* **2004**, *38*, 413–420. [CrossRef]
54. Cochrane, N.; Cai, F.; Huq, N.; Burrow, M.; Reynolds, E. New Approaches to Enhanced Remineralization of Tooth Enamel. *J. Dent. Res.* **2010**, *89*, 1187–1197. [CrossRef]
55. Arends, J.; Davidson, C. HPO2-4 Content in Enamel and Artificial Carious Lesions. *Calcif Tissue Res.* **1975**, *18*, 65–79. [CrossRef] [PubMed]
56. Ingram, G.; Nash, P. A Mechanism for the Anticaries Action of Fluoride. *Caries Res.* **1980**, *14*, 298–303. [CrossRef] [PubMed]
57. Tomazic, B.; Tomson, M.; Nancollas, G. Growth of Calcium Phosphates on Hydroxyapatite Crystals: The Effect of Magnesium. *Arch. Oral Biol.* **1975**, *20*, 803–808. [CrossRef]
58. Akkus, A.; Akkus, O.; Roperto, R.; Lang, L. Investigation of Intra- and Inter-Individual Variations of Mineralisation in Healthy Permanent Human Enamel by Raman Spectroscopy. *Oral Health Prev. Dent.* **2016**, *14*, 321–327.
59. Yeni, Y.; Yerramshetty, J.; Akkus, O.; Pechey, C.; Les, C. Effect of Fixation and Embedding on Raman Spectroscopic Analysis of Bone Tissue. *Calcif Tissue Res.* **2006**, *78*, 363–371. [CrossRef]

MDPI
St. Alban-Anlage 66
4052 Basel
Switzerland
www.mdpi.com

Coatings Editorial Office
E-mail: coatings@mdpi.com
www.mdpi.com/journal/coatings

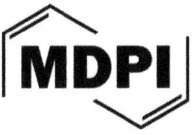

Disclaimer/Publisher's Note: The statements, opinions and data contained in all publications are solely those of the individual author(s) and contributor(s) and not of MDPI and/or the editor(s). MDPI and/or the editor(s) disclaim responsibility for any injury to people or property resulting from any ideas, methods, instructions or products referred to in the content.

www.ingramcontent.com/pod-product-compliance
Lightning Source LLC
LaVergne TN
LVHW070610100526
838202LV00012B/614